NOTES ON FELINE INTERNAL MEDICINE

Second Edition

T0258565

Notes On

"Notes on" is an exciting series specifically designed, through an accessible note-based style, to ensure veterinarians and students have quick and easy access to the most up-to-date clinical and diagnostic information.

Other titles in the series:

Canine Internal Medicine, third edition
Edward J. Hall, Kate Murphy and Peter G. Darke
9780632053711

Rabbit Internal Medicine
Richard Saunders and Ron Rees Davies
9781405115148

Small Animal Dermatology
Judith Joyce
9781405134972

Cardiorespiratory Diseases of the Dog and Cat, second edition
Mike Martin and Brendan Corcoran
9781405122641

NOTES ON FELINE INTERNAL MEDICINE

Second Edition

Kit Sturgess

WILEY Blackwell

This edition first published 2013 © 2003, 2013 by John Wiley & Sons, Ltd

Registered office: John Wiley & Sons, Ltd, The Atrium, Southern Gate, Chichester, West Sussex, PO19 8SQ, UK

Editorial offices: 9600 Garsington Road, Oxford, OX4 2DQ, UK
The Atrium, Southern Gate, Chichester, West Sussex, PO19 8SQ, UK
1606 Golden Aspen Drive, Suites 103 and 104, Ames, Iowa 50010, USA

For details of our global editorial offices, for customer services and for information about how to apply for permission to reuse the copyright material in this book please see our website at www.wiley.com/wiley-blackwell

Library of Congress Cataloging-in-Publication Data
Sturgess, Kit.
  Notes on feline internal medicine / Kit Sturgess. – 2nd ed.
    p.; cm.
  Includes bibliographical references and index.
  ISBN 978-0-470-67117-7 (pbk.) – ISBN 978-1-118-59769-9 (Mobi) –
ISBN 978-1-118-59771-2 (ePDF) – ISBN 978-1-118-59772-9 (ePub) –
ISBN 978-1-118-64516-1 – ISBN 978-1-118-64536-9
  I. Title.
  [DNLM: 1. Cat Diseases–diagnosis–Handbooks.   2. Cat Diseases–therapy–Handbooks. SF 985]
  SF985
  636.8089–dc23
                                                                              2013013320

A catalogue record for this book is available from the British Library.

Wiley also publishes its books in a variety of electronic formats. Some content that appears in print may not be available in electronic books.

Cover image (left): Photo by Kit Sturgess; (middle) iStock stock-photo-15408185-cats-x-ray; (right) stock-photo-18813080-veterinarian

Cover design by Sandra Heath

Set in Sabon LT Std 9/11pt by Aptara® Inc., New Delhi, India

1 2013

CONTENTS

ABBREVIATIONS

$\Rightarrow$	implies	ASA	American society of
%	percent		anesthesiologists
/	per	ASD	atrial septal defect
@	at	AST	aspartate aminotransferase
<	less than	ATIII	antithrombin III
>	greater than	AV	arteriovenous;
±	with or without		atrioventricular
2D	two dimensional	AZT	azidothymidine
AAFP	American association of	B_{12}	vitamin B_{12}
	feline practitioners	BA	bile acids
AcCh	acetylcholine	BCS	body condition score
ACE	angiotensin-converting	BE	base excess
	enzyme	BIPS	barium impregnated
ACEi	angiotensin-converting		polyspheres
	enzyme inhibitor	BMR	basal metabolic rate
ACP	acepromazine	BNP	brain natriuretic peptide
ACT	activated clotting time	BP	blood pressure
ACTH	adrenocorticotropic	bpm	beats per minute
	hormone	BSA	body surface area
ADE	antibody-dependent	BSH	British shorthair
	enhancement	C	cervical vertebra (followed
ADH	antidiuretic hormone		by number)
	(vasopressin)	C.	*Clostridium*
ad lib	free access	Ca^{2+}	calcium ion
AF	atrial fibrillation	cAMP	cyclic adenosine
A:G	albumin to globulin (ratio)		monophosphate
AIDS	acquired immunodeficiency	C(P)K	creatine (phospho)kinase
	syndrome	CD	cluster of differentiation
AKI	acute kidney injury		(followed by number)
ALI	acute lung injury	CDI	central diabetes insipidus
AL(K)P	alkaline phosphatase	cf.	compare with
ALT	alanine aminotransferase	CHF	congestive heart failure
ANA	antinuclear antibody	CKD	chronic kidney disease
Ao	aorta	Cl^-	chloride ion
APC	atrial premature	CN	cranial nerve
	contraction	CNS	central nervous system
APTT	activated partial	CO	cardiac output
	thromboplastin time	CO_2	carbon dioxide
APUDomas	amine precursor and	COAP	cyclophosphamide, Oncovin
	uptake decarboxylation		(vincristine), L-asparaginase
	omas		prednisolone
ARDS	acute respiratory distress	COP	cyclophosphamide,
	syndrome		Oncovin (vincristine),

	prednisolone; colloidal	FCV	feline calicivirus
	osmotic pressure	FDP	fibrin(ogen) degradation
COX	cyclooxygenase		product
CPCR	cardiopulmonary cerebral	FE	fractional excretion
	resuscitation	FeLV	feline leukaemia virus
CPV (2)	canine parvovirus (2)	FeSFV	feline syncytium-forming
CRI	continuous rate infusion		virus
CSF	cerebrospinal fluid	FG	French gauge
CT	computed tomography	FHV-1	feline herpesvirus 1
cTnI	cardiac troponin I	FIA	feline infectious anaemia
CVA	cerebrovascular accident	FIC	feline idiopathic cystitis
CVP	central venous pressure	FIP	feline infectious peritonitis
D	right (isomer)	FIV	feline immunodeficiency
DCM	dilated cardiomyopathy		virus
DDAVP	desmopressin	fl	femtolitre
DEET		FLK	fentanyl, lidocaine and
DI	diabetes insipidus		ketamine
DIC	disseminated intravascular	FLUTD	feline lower urinary tract
	coagulation		disease
DKA	diabetic ketoacidosis	FNA	fine needle aspirate
dl	decilitre	FOCMA	feline oncornavirus cell-
DLH	domestic long hair		membrane-associated
DM	diabetes mellitus		antigen
DMSO	dimethylsulfoxide	FORL	feline odontoclastic
DNA	deoxyribonucleic acid		resorptive lesion
DSH	domestic short hair	FPV	feline parvovirus
DV	dorsoventral	fPLi	feline pancreatic-specific
e.g.	for example		lipase
ECG	electrocardiogram	Fr	French
EDTA	ethylenediaminetetraacetic	FS	fractional shortening
	acid	FSE	feline spongiform
EFA	essential fatty acid		encephalopathy
ELISA	enzyme-linked	fTLI	feline trypsin-like
	immunosorbent assay		immunoreactivity
EM	electron microscopy	fTSH	feline TSH
EMG	electromyelogram	g	gram; gauge
ENT	ear, nose, throat	GA	general anaesthesia
EPI	exocrine pancreatic	GAG	glycosaminoglycans
	insufficiency	GFR	glomerular filtration rate
EPO	erythropoietin	GI	gastrointestinal
ET	endotracheal	GIT	gastrointestinal tract
ETCO$_2$	end-tidal carbon dioxide	GME	granulomatous
F	female; factor		meningoencephalitis
FAIDS	feline AIDS	gp	glycoprotein followed
FB	foreign body		by number (= molecular
FCoV	feline coronavirus		weight × 1000 in daltons)

GT	glutamyl transferase	kcal	kilocalories
h	hour	KCl	potassium chloride
H^+	hydrogen ions	kg	kilogram
H_2	type 2 histamine receptor	l	litre
HAC	hyperadrenocorticism	L	lumbar vertebra (followed
Hb	haemoglobin		by number)
HCM	hypertrophic	L	lumbar vertebra (followed
	cardiomyopathy		by number); left
HCO_3^-	bicarbonate ions	LA	left atrium
HCT	haematocrit	LAFB	left anterior fascicular
Hg	mercury		block
HGAL	high grade alimentary	LAP	left atrial pressure
	lymphoma	LBBB	left bundle branch block
HIV	human immunodeficiency	LDH	lactate dehydrogenase
	virus	LGAL	low grade alimentary
hpf	high power field		lymphoma
I	ionised	LMN	lower motor neuron
i.e.	that is	LUTD	lower urinary tract disease
I^{131}	radioactive iodine	LV	left ventricular
IBD	inflammatory bowel	LVOT	left ventricular outflow
	disease		tract
IC	immunochromatography	m	metres
iCa^{2+}	ionised calcium	M	male
ICP	intracranial pressure	M.	*Mycoplasma;*
IF	immunofluorescence		*Mycobacterium*
IFA	immunofluorescent	MCH	mean cell haemoglobin
	antibody	MCHC	mean cell haemoglobin
iFLUTD	idiopathic feline lower		concentration
	urinary tract disease	MCV	mean cell volume
Ig	immunoglobulin	MDA	maternally derived
IgA	immunoglobulin A		antibody
IGF-1	insulin-like growth factor 1	ME	metabolisable energy
IgG	immunoglobulin G	MEA	mean electrical axis
IgM	immunoglobulin M	MEN	multiple endocrine
iBD	idiopathic IBD		neoplasia
IM	intramuscular	mEq	milliequivalent
IMHA	immune-mediated	MER	maintenance energy
	haemolytic anaemia		requirement
IRIS	International renal interest	mg	milligram
	society	Mg^{2+}	magnesium ion
iU	international units	MHz	mega hertz
IV (i/v)	intravenous	min	minute
IVFT	intravenous fluid therapy	ml	millilitre
IVS	interventricular septum	MLK	morphine, lidocaine and
JGA	juxtaglomerular apparatus		ketamine
K^+	potassium ion	mmol	millimoles

MODS	multiple organ dysfunction syndrome	pH	acid-base balance of a substance
MRI	magnetic resonance imaging	PHA	primary hyperaldosteronism
MV	mitral valve	PIVKAs	proteins induced by vitamin K antagonists
MVO_2	myocardial oxygen consumption	PKD	polycystic kidney disease
MVO_2	myocardial oxygen demand	PLE	protein losing enteropathy
MW	molecular weight	PLR	pupillary light response
n	number (in sequence of carbon atoms)	PM	post mortem
		PMEA	phosphonomethoxyethyl adenine
Na^+	sodium ion	PMI	point of maximum intensity
NA (N/A)	not assessed		
NaCl	salt (sodium chloride)	pmol	picomoles
NB	*nota bene*	PNS	peripheral nervous system
NDI	nephrogenic diabetes insipidus	PO	per os
		pO_2	partial pressure of oxygen
ng	nanograms	POM-V	prescription only medicine – veterinary
NH_4Cl	ammonium chloride		
NMDA	N-methyl-D-asparate	PPDH	pericardioperitoneal diaphragmatic hernia
nmol	nanomoles		
NSAIDs	non-steroidal anti-inflammatory drugs	proBNP	pro brain natriuretic peptide
NT-proBNP	N-terminal pro brain natriuretic peptide	PSS	portosystemic shunt
		PT	prothrombin
°C	degrees Celsius	PTH	parathyroid hormone
°F	degrees Fahrenheit	PTH-rP	parathyroid hormone-related peptide
OP	organophosphate		
OSPT	one stage prothrombin time	PU	polyuria
		PU/PD	polyuria/polydipsia
p	protein followed by number (= molecular weight × 1000 in daltons)	PUFA	polyunsaturated fatty acid
		PUO	pyrexia of unknown origin
		PVC	polyvinyl chloride
PA	pulmonary artery	q	every
pCO2	partial pressure of carbon dioxide	qPCR	real time PCR
		RA	right atrium
PCR	polymerase chain reaction	RAAS	renin–angiotensin–aldosterone system
PCV	packed cell volume		
PD	polydipsia	RBBB	right bundle branch block
PDA	persistent ductus arteriosus	RBCC	red blood cell count
PE	Pericardial effusion	RBC	red blood cell
PEG	percutaneous endoscopic gastrostomy	RCM	restricted cardiomyopathy
		RER	resting energy requirement
PETS	pet travel scheme	RIM	rapid immunodiffusion
pg	picograms	R→L	right to left

RNA	ribonucleic acid	TV	tricuspid valve
RR	respiratory rate	U	international units
R-R	time interval between successive R waves on an ECG	U	units
		UCCR	urine cortisol:creatinine ratio
RTA	road traffic accident	UGA	under general anaesthesia
S	heart sound (followed by number); sacral vertebra (followed by number)	UK	United Kingdom
		UMN	upper motor neuron
SA	sinoatrial	UPC (R)	urine protein:creatinine ratio
SAMe	s-adenosyl methionine		
SAM	systolic anterior motion	URT	upper respiratory tract
SAP	serum alkaline phosphatase	URTD	upper respiratory tract disease
SC	subcutaneous	USA	United States of America
SCC	squamous cell carcinoma	USG	urine specific gravity
SG	specific gravity	USMI	urethral sphincter mechanism incompetence
SIRS	systemic inflammatory response syndrome	UTI	urinary tract infection
SLE	systemic lupus erythematosus	UV	ultraviolet
		VCTM	viral chlamydia transport medium
sp(p).	species		
SpO_2	oxygen saturation measured by pulse oximetry	VD	ventrodorsal
		VI	virus isolation
		VPC	ventricular premature contraction
T	thoracic vertebra (followed by number); total	VSD	ventricular septal defect
T_3	triiodothyronine	vs.	versus
T_4	thyroxin; fourth thoracic vertebra	VWF	von Willebrand factor
		WBC	white blood cell
TCO_2	total carbon dioxide	WBCC	white blood cell count
TLI	trypsin-like immunoreactivity	WHO	world health organisation
TMJ	temporomandibular joint	WSAVA	World small animal veterinary association
TOC	treatment of choice		
TP	total protein	XO	female with single X chromosome
TPR	temperature, pulse and respiration		
		μmol	micromoles
TRH	thyroid stimulating releasing hormone	γ-GT; GGT	gamma glutamyl transferase
TSH	thyroid stimulating hormone	μg	microgram
		μl	microlitre

Since the first edition of this book in 2003, feline medicine has continued to expand rapidly. It is estimated that there are between 9.3 and 11.3 million pet cats and a similar number of pet dogs in the United Kingdom. The increase in pet cat numbers seems to be a worldwide trend. Many practices, particularly those in towns and cities, see more cats than dogs for consultations. Ninety two percent of the pet cats in the United Kingdom are domestic short hairs (moggies) compared to the dog population that is 75% pedigree. Cats are more likely to be kept as pets for companionship than dogs because they are perceived as being easier to look after and as fitting better with current lifestyles; this may explain the increases that are being seen in the pet cat population.

Throughout this book, focus will be placed on evidence-based medicine. Where this is unavailable, current best practice will be presented. Additional sections have been provided on sedation and anaesthesia, health screening, oncology and emergency and critical care. The number of diagrams has been increased and sources of further information highlighted.

Fewer drugs are licensed for use in cats than dogs, so the dose rates of many compounds used off-label are based on clinical experience and may require modification as appropriate. When deciding upon which drug to use, it is important to remember that the cascade system (in the United Kingdom) applies to the choices made.

The text is divided into five sections:
• Section 1 gives an overview of other key areas of feline medicine including health screening, paediatric and geriatric medicine, analgesia, fluid therapy,

anaesthesia and algorithms for emergency and critical care.
• Section 2 focuses on the approach to common presenting signs.
• Section 3 covers the differential diagnosis of commonly used haematologic and biochemical parameters.
• Section 4 presents an organ-system-based approach.
• Section 5 covers feline infectious diseases.

Distinct differences exist between cats and dogs not only in their physiology and metabolism but also in the way disease tends to present. Sick cats tend to mask the nature and extent of their disease, becoming withdrawn and quiet; as a consequence, presentation to a veterinarian is often later in the course of the disease. Cats also seem to be more 'secretive' about their clinical signs, and are less likely to have organ-specific presentations, tending to show lethargy and inappetence instead. Owners are also changing, becoming more informed and demanding of a diagnosis, making problem-based medicine central to the approach to a sick cat.

This text is intended to be a short 'pocket guide' to feline internal medicine, aimed at assisting in the formulation of a diagnostic plan and therapeutic strategy. References will not be given in the text, but a selection of useful texts and websites will be included at the end.

Physical examination

A calm approach, and in the majority of cases minimal restraint, usually allows thorough clinical evaluation (see http://catvets.com/professionals/guidelines/publications/index.aspx?Id=468 for the

Notes on Feline Internal Medicine, Second Edition. Edited by Kit Sturgess. ©2013 John Wiley & Sons, Ltd.
Published 2013 by Blackwell Publishing Ltd.

American Association of Feline Practitioners and International Society of Feline Medicine guide on cat handling 2011). Some cats, however, require chemical restraint in order for a thorough physical examination to be performed – see section 1.6. A systematic examination is mandatory to ensure that no major problems are overlooked. As inappetence is a major presentation in cats, oral examination should always be performed. In cats over 6 years of age, palpation of the ventral neck for a goitre should also become part of the regime. Enlarged thyroid glands can be best palpated with the cat standing and the chin raised; the trachea is located between the thumb and first finger and the neck is palpated craniocaudally. If no gland is felt, and the cat is amenable, the cat can be gently tipped head downwards, allowing a thyroid nodule that is lying just within the thoracic inlet to be palpated.

Auscultation of the cardiorespiratory system can be optimised by using a paediatric, infant or electronic stethoscope that will allow better localisation of any abnormality. The upper and lower respiratory tracts, including the trachea, should be included to determine whether increased parenchymal lung sounds are, in fact, referred from the upper airway. Cardiac murmurs are frequently loudest parasternally and relatively cranially in cats, making them easy to miss if auscultation is carried out only at the left apex. Purring can prevent adequate thoracic auscultation and is difficult to stop. Sometimes turning on a tap, gentle compression of the larynx, covering the nares or blowing on the nostrils will work, but these are not always practical or effective solutions. Thoracic examination should include percussion as well as palpation of the cranial thorax for compressibility. Cats' chests tend to sound relatively resonant even when fluid is present; it is therefore important to percuss all cats so the subtle lowering of pitch and slight loss of resonance that accompany a pleural effusion can be appreciated.

Abdominal palpation is rewarding in most cats. Both kidneys, the small and large intestines and the bladder can be appreciated in non-obese, normal cats. The stomach, liver and spleen are not usually palpated unless abnormal. Lifting the cat's forelimbs can sometimes aid renal palpation.

Assessing the locomotor system is difficult, as many cats are reluctant to walk in the consulting room. In cases where such an evaluation is important, owner history is crucial and video evidence can also be helpful.

Clinical pathology

Haematology

Many automated machines struggle to produce accurate results due to the relatively spherical nature of feline red cells and the tendency for platelets to clump. Whilst the automated result can provide valuable information, examination of a smear is essential if more than a packed cell volume is required. A smear should always be included when blood is sent to an external laboratory for evaluation.

Interpretation

See Section 3 (Laboratory Abnormalities).

Biochemistry

In the text, routine biochemistry refers to:
- Total protein, albumin and globulin
- Alanine aminotransferase (ALT) and alkaline phosphatase (ALP)
- Urea and creatinine
- Cholesterol
- Calcium and phosphorus
- Electrolytes (sodium, potassium ± chloride)
- Creatine kinase (CPK)

The value of estimating lipase and amylase is limited in cats and does not form part of a routine biochemical evaluation.

Radiology and Ultrasound

Cats make good subjects for radiography, as they are small and of relatively even body thickness. The use of a grid in cats is unnecessary. Detail can be improved by using a suitable film–screen combination. Sedation or anaesthesia is required in all but the sickest of cats.

Ultrasound can be very rewarding in cats, relatively high frequency probes are required. A 7.5mHz microconvex or 10mHz linear probe are ideal producing high quality images and allowing the internal structure of the abdominal organs to be examined.

Sedation

Sedation is frequently necessary during the investigation of a sick cat. A variety of drug combinations have been recommended (see Section 1.6).

INTRODUCTION

SECTION 1

KEY TOPICS IN FELINE MEDICINE

Notes on Feline Internal Medicine, Second Edition. Edited by Kit Sturgess. ©2013 John Wiley & Sons, Ltd.
Published 2013 by Blackwell Publishing Ltd.

1.1 HEALTH SCREENING

1.1.1 Introduction
- Performed to minimise anaesthetic risk and to maximise long-term health.
- Benefit of screening programmes is less clear.
- Clear planning and practice policy relating to which patients to screen, what to screen for and what to do with abnormal results.
- Understood and supported at all levels within the practice.
- Very little is published about health screening in cats and dogs.
- Current consensus opinion – some form of screening in some cats is appropriate so long as
  - The risk–benefit equation for the pet (of undertaking the test) and the owner (anxiety associated with the test and any abnormal parameters found) is taken into account.
  - The test results are available prior to anaesthesia.
  - The tests are selected individually.
  - An action plan is available should abnormal results be found.

Rationale
- Pre-anaesthetic screening determines whether the anaesthetic will be safe and/or whether modifications to the routine anaesthetic regime are required.
- Geriatric screening allows identification of sub-clinical disease and hence earlier management and improved outcome.

1.1.2 Which cats to screen and what screening tests to use
Options are as in Table 1.

Developing a screening plan
- All members of the practice need to be comfortable with the service that is offered.

Table 1 Patient and test selection for screening

Which patients?	Which tests?
*Recommend to all patients over a specific age	All patients get the same screening
Only screen patients prior to anaesthesia	Screening becomes more in-depth as the patient ages
Only screen at owner's request	
Actively discourage screening and manage clinically significant disease as it occurs	*Screening targeted based on historical information

*approach recommended by author

- Clear written guidelines should be available for all staff to follow.
- Clients need to be informed of
  - The existence of the plan.
  - What the plan offers – the pros and cons.
- Clear pricing of the various plans offered.
- Everyone must appreciate that screening can create anxiety for the owner if there are 'abnormal' results.
- Clear 'what if' guidelines should be developed:
  - Clients need to have any abnormalities discovered explained to them as to the significance and put into perspective.
  - If you measure a parameter such as blood urea you need to have developed a policy within the practice of an appropriate response if the result is abnormal.
  - Waiting is an acceptable response coupled with further screening at a time in the future; however, if the response is always to wait and rescreen and to do nothing interventional until the patient becomes unwell then what is the point of screening?
  - Changes in anaesthetic protocol should be defined and the costs involved made clear.

What tests to do?

- In the absence of evidence the 'best' tests to do in an outwardly healthy individual with no significant previous history is unknown:
- Traditional – urea, ALT, TP, glucose (creatinine, ALK-P).
- Less traditional but potentially valuable for pre-anaesthetic screening – USG and dipstick, PCV, electrolytes (with ALT, TP, urea).

Less traditional but potentially valuable for geriatric screening – USG and dipstick, PCV, calcium, cholesterol, BP (with ALT, TP, urea).

1.1.3 Interpreting the test results and developing an action plan

- Tests should be as sensitive and specific (Box 1) as possible to avoid false-positive and false-negative results that could initiate unnecessary, more invasive, risky and expensive further investigation.

Box 1   Sensitivity and specificity

Sensitivity = proportion of positives which are correctly identified, i.e. 258 abnormal livers of which 231 identified, therefore SENSITIVITY 231/258 = 90%.
Specificity = proportion of negatives which are correctly identified, i.e. 86 normal livers of which 54 identified, therefore SPECIFICITY 54/86 = 63%.

What to do when …
…the protein is low
Action point
- Total protein is >5 g/l (albumin >3 g/l) below the reference range.

NB – *Accurate measurement of albumin on in-house machines is difficult so a low albumin in the face of a normal total protein should be checked at an external laboratory.*

- With large falls in proteins, three main causes are likely; urinary loss, GIT loss and failure of liver production.
- Less common causes of hypoalbuminaemia – see Section 3.15
- Elevated albumin levels are due to dehydration.
- Elevated globulin due to dehydration, immune or inflammatory response or neoplasia.

Response
- Pre-anaesthetic – elective procedures should be delayed and investigation undertaken.
- Geriatric screen – monitor or investigate potential cause depending on general health and other abnormalities documented.

…the urea (± creatinine) is high
See Section 3.7.
- Consider whether cause is likely to be pre-, intra- or post-renal in origin.
- Most cases are likely to be pre- or intra-renal.
- Urea/creatinine will not rise until 75% of renal mass is lost.
- All cases should have urinalysis performed.

Response
- Pre-anaesthetic – fluid therapy and maintenance of renal blood flow during anaesthesia are important.
- Geriatric screen – assign to an IRIS stage if intrinsic renal disease with appropriate adjunctive tests.

…the ALT/ALP is high
- Increased liver enzymes are more likely to be pathologic in cats (see Section 3.12).

Response

- Pre-anaesthetic – low–moderate increases are unlikely to affect anaesthetic risk unless there is evidence to support reduced liver function that could affect drug metabolism.

- Geriatric screen:
  - Increases >200 iU should be monitored if the cat is healthy.
  - Increases >500 iU should be investigated further even if the cat appears healthy.

...the PCV is low

- Mild anaemia is not uncommon especially in older cats; it is often a reflection of systemic disease elsewhere.
- Pre-anaesthetic – mild anaemia (PCV >22%) is unlikely to affect anaesthetic risk or require a change in anaesthetic protocol.

- Geriatric screen:
  - Chronic, non-regenerative anaemia can be very slowly progressive and patients can have significant falls in PCV without obvious clinical signs.
  - The level of anaemia can be difficult to evaluate on physical examination with poor correlation between physical examination and measured PCV.
  - If the PCV is more than 2–3% below the reference range a full haematology including smear examination and reticulocyte count should be performed.

1.1.4 Screening for neoplasia

- Cancer is a major cause of death or euthanasia in older cats.
- If the tumour is advanced before clinical signs are apparent options for treatment, particularly curative therapy, are unlikely.
- Computed tomography and MRI are sensitive ways of looking for mass lesions associated with any type of tumour; however, in man, 90% of lumps identified on CT screening are non-neoplastic. The availability and cost of CT/MRI and the need for general anaesthesia make this method of screening inappropriate for the majority of cats.
- Radiography is significantly less sensitive and abdominal ultrasound time consuming and very operator dependent.
- Few blood or urine tests for early diagnosis are available (Table 2) and often sensitivity and specificity are poor with false-positive results creating anxiety in clients and necessitating further more invasive diagnostics or false negatives giving the client and clinician a false sense of security that may mean subsequent warning signs are missed or misinterpreted.

Table 2 Blood and urine screening tests for cancer in cats

Test	Target	Accuracy
Veterinary bladder tumour antigen	Transitional cell carcinoma	Not reported
Plasma/urine metadrenalines	Phaeochromocytoma	Not reported
Serum thymidine kinase	Haematopoietic neoplasms	Not reported
Serum biomarkers	Lymphoma	Sensitivity and specificity 85%

1.2 PREVENTATIVE MEDICINE

1.2.1 Vaccination

Initial vaccination

- Most manufacturers recommend an initial vaccination at 6–9 weeks of age and a second injection at 12–14 weeks.
  - This schedule is designed to begin vaccination as soon as a significant number of individuals have lost their maternally derived immunity and to give a second injection when almost all individuals will respond.
  - Despite this a percentage of individuals will not seroconvert to vaccination, making the first booster at 15 months of age important to ensure protection.
- Vaccination can be performed earlier than 6 weeks in high-risk groups, but should be as an additional immunisation and is outwith the manufacturer's recommendations. Killed, genetically engineered or subunit vaccines should be used.

Booster vaccination

- Frequency of booster vaccination is controversial and there is disagreement between the recommendations of the data sheets provided by manufacturers and guidelines produced by other organisations such as the American Association of Feline Practitioners.
  - Currently in the UK manufacturer recommendations for boosting of core vaccines are annual.
  - AAFP recommends re-vaccination of cats every 3 years following the use of modified live FPV, and respiratory virus vaccines after the first booster vaccination at 15 months of age.
  - Published literature is conflicting.
  - Vaccination outside the manufacturers' recommended schedule should be discussed with the client – if vaccine failure occur the veterinarian should

be able to demonstrate informed consent from the cat's owner.
  - The frequency of booster vaccination is further complicated by the production of multivalent vaccines with different components potentially having different recommendations for frequency of re-vaccination.
- Booster frequency should also be based on local disease prevalence, susceptibility of the individual to infectious disease, previous history of vaccine reactions, intercurrent disease (such as FIV) and current treatments (such as use of immunosuppressive drugs).
  - In areas of high disease prevalence, outdoor cats may well be receiving frequent challenge with field infection and therefore maintain high levels of immunity whereas in those areas cats that rarely go outside/meet other cats will be at higher risk of meeting the infectious agent if they do contact other cats and therefore need to have their vaccinal immunity maintained at a high level.
- Many owners feel that vaccination of older cats is unnecessary; however, as cats age immunity wanes and these individuals can be more susceptible to infectious disease and less able to mount an effective immune response should infection occur.
- Presence of antibodies predicts resistance to infection in FPV and FCV and in most (90%) of cats against FHV-1. Antibody levels are not predictive of resistance to FeLV infection.

Vaccine choice

- There are an increasing number of diseases for which vaccination is available.
- Attempts have been made to classify vaccination against some infectious diseases as essential (core vaccines) and others as optional (non-core) (see Table 3).
- Decisions should be based on regional disease incidence, household history and lifestyle of the kitten (indoor vs. outdoor).

Table 3 Core vs. non-core vaccines

Core	Non-core	Value controversial
FPV	FeLV	FIP
FHV-1	Chlamydophila	FIV
FCV	Bordetella	Giardia
Rabies[a]	bronchiseptica	

[a]Rabies endemic, travel to rabies-infected area likely, governmental policy.

Vaccine reactions

- Generally very rare and often associated with other vaccine components rather than the infectious agent itself.
  - Pedigree cats especially Burmese and semilong hair cats, e.g. Birman and Maine Coon, are overrepresented.
- Many cats and kittens will show mild signs following vaccination – this can be a good indicator of response to vaccination initiating an immune response.
- Significant illness that occurs post-vaccination should be reported to the manufacturer and investigated as far as possible to determine cause.

Injection site sarcomas

- Primarily associated with adjuvanted FeLV and rabies vaccination but have occurred following the use of other injectable preparations.
- Risk is approximately 1:10 000 cats.
- Locally invasive and moderate risk of metastasis.
- Vaccination on limbs/tail has been recommended as these sites are more amenable to radical surgery.
- Post-vaccination masses are common but should resolve within 4–6 weeks.
- Persistent masses should be investigated and should be removed if >20 mm with a wide surgical margin (including deep margin) with adjunctive radiation and chemotherapy considered.

Pre-vaccination testing for FeLV

- FeLV ELISA/RIM testing in healthy kittens where prevalence of FeLV is low has a high false-positive rate (>50% if prevalence <1%).
- Testing 'at risk' groups is of value.
- 'At risk' groups will depend on local knowledge of FeLV prevalence and distribution.
  - Feral and rescue cats are often considered 'high risk' but this is not supported by epidemiologic studies.
- Any positive result needs further confirmation.

1.2.2 Parasite control

- Regular endo and ectoparasite control is part of good husbandry as well as reducing public health risk.
- Frequency and type of parasite control will depend on
  - The life style of the cat.
  - Local disease prevalence and parasite resistance.
  - Individual sensitivity of the individual to parasitism, e.g. flea bite hypersensitivity.
  - Previous adverse reactions to specific compounds.
  - Specific disease issues that require treatment.
- Endoparasites can still be present in elderly indoor cats.

Available products

- A wide variety of products are available (see Table 4).
- Permethrin-based flea products for use in dogs are highly toxic to cats.
- Products for controlling larval stages of ectoparasites in the environment are also available.
- Some products also contain insect repellents, e.g. flumethrin, in combination with other parasiticides, e.g. imidacloprid.
- Over-the-counter products are also available as shampoos, tablets, spot-ons and collars:
  - Testing and efficacy of some of these products is limited.

Table 4 Active ingredients of parasiticides for use in cats

Active ingredient	Route	Taenia	Dipylidium	Echinococcus	Giardia	Angiostrongylus	Toxocara	Toxocara arrested larva	Uncinaria	Ancylostoma	Trichuris	Lungworm	Dirofilaria	Fleas	Flies	Ticks	Demodex	Sarcoptes	Otodectes	Lice	Combined with
1 Dichlorophen	O	X	X	X																	
2 Emodepside	T	X	X	X			X	X		X											17
3 Fenbendazole	O	X	x		X	X	X	X	X	X	X	X									
4 Fipronil	T													X		X			X	X	
5 Garlic	O	Efficacy is poorly established																			
6 Imidacloprid	T, C													X	X	X					
7 Ivermectin	I, T																X	X	X	X	
8 Lufenuron	I, O													X							12
9 Mebendazole	O	X		X		X	X	X	X	X	X										
10 Metaflumizone	T													X							
11 Methoprene	T													X		X					4
12 Milbemycin	O	X	X		X		X		X	X	X	X	X								17; 8
13 Moxidectin	T						X		X	X	X	X	X	X				X	X		6
14 Nitenpyram	O													X							
15 Piperazine	O						X		X												
16 Praziquantel	O, T	X	X	X																	Many
17 Pyrantel/oxantel	O						X		X	X											17
18 Selamectin	T					X	X	X	X	X	X	X	X	X				X	X	X	
19 Tiabendazole	ED																		X		

X – good efficacy; x – limited efficacy; C – collar; ED – ear drops; I – injectable; O – oral; T – topical.

1.3 PAEDIATRICS

1.3.1 Introduction
- Neonatal period covers the first 7–10 days of life.
- Characterised by poor neurological function, the progressive development of spinal reflexes and a total dependency on the dam.
- Followed by a transitional period (10–21 days of age) characterised by the development of a competent audio-visual system, further development of the neurological system and an increasing independence from the dam.
- Kittens enter a period of socialisation from 3 weeks of age lasting until around 3 months of age during which time feeding and sleeping occupy progressively less of the day, being replaced by social activity.
- There is maturation of the nervous system and hepatic and renal function.
- Kitten mortality is around 15–40% in the first 12 weeks of life with the majority of deaths occurring in the first week.

Definitions
- *Paediatric* – kitten hood covers the first 12 months of life but kittens have more or less adult physiology by 6 months of age.
- *Congenital* – defect present at birth, although it may not be clinically apparent on examination at this time. May or may not have a genetic basis.
- *Inherited* – defect has a genetic basis, may be no evidence at birth but will develop with age, e.g. PKD.

Is it inherited?
In general, inherited problems affect a proportion of the litter, unless the queen or stud cat is affected. The defect tends to be similar in all kittens. Congenital problems occurring due to an insult during pregnancy tend to affect all kittens but to varying degrees and sometimes different organs dependent on the exact stage of development at the time of the insult.

Major causes of kitten mortality
- Congenital anatomic or metabolic defect.
- Infectious disease.
- Inadequate/inappropriate nutrition.
- Trauma – dystocia, cannibalism, neglect.
- Neonatal isoerythrolysis.
- Low birth weight.

1.3.2 Evaluating the paediatric patient
Physiology
- Significant physiological changes occur during the first weeks of life that will directly affect the clinical signs shown, and the ability of the neonate to respond to disease.
- Separation of the placenta causes an increase in peripheral resistance and hypoxia develops rapidly inducing gasping respiration.
- Constriction of the umbilical vein squeezes significant quantities of blood from the placenta into the neonate and hence, where possible, should be left intact.
- In response to the increasing oxygen tension the ductus arteriosus narrows (complete closure in 1–2 days) and the pulmonary vessels dilate.
- Increased left-sided pressure results in the closure of the foramen ovale between the atria.
- Fetal pO_2 rises correcting the acidosis that develops in the newborn.
- Thermoregulation in the newborn is poor as the ability to shiver (develops by 6–8 days) and vasoconstrict in response to falling body temperature is limited.

Glucoregulation
- Newborn kittens have limited reserves of glycogen and poor hepatic gluconeogenic responses to low blood glucose.
- Able to maintain glucose levels for 24 hours if healthy.

Hepatic and renal function
- Hepatic microsomal enzymes which are involved in many metabolic functions including drug metabolism may not be fully functional until 4–5 months postpartum, though near-normal liver function is probably present from around 8 weeks of age.
- Albumin levels in neonates are significantly lower than in adults, which can result in increased circulating drug levels.
- Glomerular filtration rate is approximately one-fifth of adult levels and tubular secretion mechanisms do not mature until approximately 8 weeks of age. This means that glycosuria is common and urine specific gravity is low (1.006–1.007).
- Kittens have a limited ability to conserve fluid; hence fluid requirements are high at around 120–180 ml/kg/day.
- Urine production begins in the first 24 hours.
- Protein excretion increases to 12 weeks then falls, fractional excretion of calcium falls and phosphate rises with maturity.

Immune function
- Neonates possess a degree of immune competence, but do not have a fully matured spectrum of responses.
- Reduced activity of cells involved in non-specific immune responses, such as neutrophils, is likely.
- With a poorly functioning immune system in terms of speed, magnitude and breadth of response, good passively acquired immunity is crucial.

Passive immunity
- Greater than 90% of passive immunity is provided from colostral intake; however, the protection afforded depends on the immune status and exposure of the dam.
- Gut permeability to immunoglobulins begins to decline within 8 hours of birth and no further absorption is possible after 48–72 hours.
- Passive immune protection of the intestinal tract continues during the whole period of suckling as IgA antibodies resist gastric degradation and can bind potentially harmful pathogens in the gut lumen.
- Colostrum also contains cellular components though their precise role is unclear.
- Kittens should be born into the same environment as the one in which the dam has been housed.
- Plasma transfusion to colostrum-deprived kittens has not been shown to be of value.

Cardiovascular function
- Heart rates in newborn kittens may respond to hypoxia by falling rather than rising (a protective mechanism).

Neurological development
- Over the first 11–12 weeks of life, kittens develop normal adult reflexes and response.
- Until that time they display primitive reflexes which gradually disappear.
- Behaviour patterns tend to be much simpler, being driven by hunger and the search for warmth.
- Newborn kittens will sleep for more than 80% of their time and will tend to lie quietly when replete and warm.
- When stressed (for whatever reason) they will cry and crawl around making side-to-side head movements.

Baseline data and physical examination
- Reference ranges for haematological and biochemical parameters are different from adults, therefore results need to be interpreted according to the age of the kitten (Table 5).
- Rectal temperature of dry, healthy day-old kittens is around 35.5°C (±0.8) [96°F (±1.5)] rising gradually over the first week of life to around 37.8°C (100°F). Adult temperature is achieved by approximately 4 weeks of age. Reference range for physiologic values in kittens are given in Table 6.
- Circulating blood volume of kittens is small (25–40 ml in a 4-week-old kitten), hence repeated blood sampling can cause severe anaemia and should, therefore, be kept to a minimum.

Table 5 Reference ranges for haematological and biochemical values in kittens

Parameter Age	Kittens (mean or range)			
	0–3 days	2 weeks	4 weeks	6 weeks
PCV (%)	41.7	33.6–37.0	25.7–27.3	26.2–27.9
Hb (g/dl)	11.3	11.5–12.7	8.5–8.9	8.3–8.9
MCV (fl)	81.6	65.5–69.3	52.7–55.1	44.3–46.9
WBC ($\times 10^9$/l)	7.55	9.1–10.2	14.1–16.5	16.1–18.8
Age (weeks)	2 (range)		4 (range)	
Total protein (g/l)	40–52		46–52	
Albumin (g/l)	20–24		22–24	
Sodium (mmol/l)	ND		149–153	
Potassium (mmol/l)	ND		4.0–4.8	
Chloride (mmol/l)	ND		120–124	
Inorganic phosphate (mmol/l)	ND		2.03–2.41	
Calcium (mmol/l)	ND		2.35–3.24	
Urea (mmol/l)	<5		<5	
Creatinine (μmol/l)	ND		36–54	
Cholesterol (mmol/l)	4.29–11.59		0.58–11.36	
ALK-P (U/l)	68–269		90–135	
ALT (U/l)	11–24		14–26	
Creatinine kinase (U/l)	ND		ND	
Glucose (mmol/l)	6.08–10.32		7.92–8.96	
Bilirubin (μmol/l)	1.7–16.9		1.7–3.4	
Bile acids (μmol/l)	<10		<10	

Table 6 Physiological values in young kittens

Age (days)	Rectal temperature (°F) [°C]	Heart rate (bpm)	Respiratory rate (/minute)	Environmental temperature (°F) [°C]
0–7	96 ± 1.5 [35.5 ± 0.8]	200–250	15–35	85–90 [29.5 – 32.5]
8–14	100 [37.8]	70–220	15–35	80 [26.5]
15–28	–	70–220	15–35	80 [26.5]
29–35	Adult	70–220	15–35	70–75 [21 – 24]
>35	Adult	70–220	Adult	70 [21]

Clinical evaluation

Case history
- Basic information is essential to evaluate clinical and laboratory findings.
- Include a breeding history of the household, cattery management (hygiene, worming, vaccination, etc.), health of the queen during the pregnancy, the health of the remainder of the litter, age of the kitten and pattern of the illness to date.

Clinical examination
- Examination can be difficult.
- Neonates tend to show limited responses to disease, initially becoming agitated and crying, progressing to inactivity, hypothermia and loss of the suckling reflex.
- Changes can be very rapid; it is important that the owner is made aware of the potential significance of these signs to allow aggressive, early treatment.
- Weight gain can be a sensitive indicator of developing problems and can be easily measured by the owner. Failure to gain weight over any 24-hour period is worthy of further investigation.

External features
- Body weight; hair coat (amount, condition, parasites); state of hydration; signs of injury; appearance of umbilicus; discharge from nose; urine staining (patent urachus); diarrhoea/rectal patency; congenital malformation.

Eyes
- Swelling under lids indicates pus formation (often *Staphylococcus* spp., very rarely *Chlamydophila felis*); eyes open between 5 and 14 days, pupillary light response is usually present within 24 hours of the eyes opening, mild corneal cloudiness often present as eyes open.

Ears
- External auditory meatus closed at birth and opens between 6 and 14 days. Check for mites and middle ear infection (indicated by a bulging tympanum).

Mouth
- Mucous membrane colour; evidence of cleft palate.

Thorax
- Heart rate around 200–220 beats/minute; respiration 15–35 per minute; regular rhythm; heart murmurs may be functional (usually soft); lung sounds difficult to distinguish but should be present; check for symmetry and malformation of the thoracic cavity e.g. pectus.

Abdomen
- Should feel full, but not swollen or tight; liver and spleen not palpable; intestines soft, mobile and non-painful; urinary bladder freely movable.

Neurological assessment
- Alertness, response to stimulation, suckle reflex; other reflexes appropriate to age; gait (walking from around 4 weeks old); posture.
- Flexor and extensor dominance appears more variable in kittens than puppies.

1.3.3 Investigation of neonatal disease
- Routine biochemistry and haematology can be performed from a very early age on blood obtained by jugular puncture.
- Many infectious diseases develop too rapidly to obtain results quickly enough (especially bacterial culture and sensitivity) to be of value to that individual.
- As infections are frequently a litter problem, laboratory data can improve management and treatment of any subsequent cases.
- Radiographs can be difficult to evaluate in kittens as mineralisation of the skeleton is poor and they are easily over-exposed, but can provide useful information. The kV should be reduced by up to half that used for an adult of similar body thickness.
- Faecal examinations can be easily performed and are of particular value where protozoan parasites are suspected.
- Many cases will, however, end up at post-mortem. Maximum information can be obtained if the carcass is fresh and, if not immediately available for post-mortem, the body should be stored in the fridge and not the freezer. Use a systematic approach and record details.

1.3.4 Treatment of the paediatric patient
- Special consideration needs to be given when giving drugs or fluids to paediatric patients.

Drugs
- Absorption, distribution, metabolism and excretion of drugs can be significantly different from adults.
- Few drugs have had dose rates calculated for use in the neonate.
- Generally an increase in initial dose is required with a lengthening of the interval between doses.
  - Kittens have a high body surface area but reduced metabolic capacity.
- Great care should be taken when administering some types of antimicrobials orally because of the potentially adverse effects on the developing gut microflora.
- Subcutaneous and intramuscular absorption of drugs is slower and less reliable than in adults.
- Antibacterials administered to the dam do not reach therapeutic concentrations in the milk.
- Nutritional support either by naso-oesophageal or gastric intubation is important particularly in the face of sepsis.

Fluid therapy
- Fluid requirements are higher in neonates than adults, but total volumes can be low.
- Syringe driver can be of great value and can be significantly cheaper than fluid pumps; otherwise a burette with a paediatric giving set (60 drops/ml) will ensure that the kitten is not over-hydrated.
- Tend to be acidotic but reduced hepatic function can mean that they are less able to metabolise lactate into bicarbonate.

- Glucose can be replaced using a 5% dextrose solution mixed 50:50 with lactated Ringer's or by giving 1–2 ml of 10–25% glucose IV to a profoundly depressed kitten.

Methods of drug and fluid administration

Intravenous

- 23 or 25 g catheter can be placed in the cephalic vein of many small kittens.
- Short legs can make the catheter very positional and flow difficult to maintain.
  ○ Splinting the leg can help but is uncomfortable for the kitten.

Intraperitoneal

- Not ideal as absorption can be relatively slow, especially in the face of hypovolaemia, and is poorly suited to long-term fluid therapy.
- Risks of puncturing viscera are low.
- Aseptic technique is mandatory.
- Fluid requirements should be calculated and the volume divided to be given 2–3 times daily.

Intraosseous

- Where venous access is not possible.
- Cortical bone is sufficiently soft such that a hypodermic needle (18–19 g) can be placed.
- Surgically prepare area and the needle is placed in either the proximal tibia or proximal femur.
- Only one attempt should be made at each site because if the bone is already punctured it will result in fluid leaking out.
- Fluids, drugs or whole blood can be given at the same rates as for IV therapy.

1.3.5 Common infectious diseases of kittens

Ectoparasites

- Fleas – can cause serious anaemia in young kittens with a heavy burden.

- Ear mites – common but rarely a serious disease.
- Lice – indicator of poor husbandry.
- Demodex or sarcoptes – rare in kittens.
- Check suitability of parasiticide for use in kittens of that age/weight.

Protozoan parasites

- Coccidia – breeding establishments, acute diarrhoea may be haemorrhagic.
- Toxoplasma – anorexia, lethargy and hypothermia.
- Giardia – acute small intestinal diarrhoea.
- *Tritrichomonas foetus* – foul smelling watery diarrhoea
- Protozoan parasites will be minimised by good husbandry, hygiene, daily disposal of faeces and avoiding overcrowding.
- Potentiated sulphonamides need to be used with care in neonates due to their reduced hepatic metabolism.

Endoparasites

- *Toxocara* spp. and *Toxascaris leonina* are almost ubiquitous parasites of kittens being transmitted in the dam's milk.
- Heavy infestations are associated with unthriftiness, diarrhoea, poor coat condition and a 'pot-bellied' appearance.
- Rarely complete bowel obstruction is caused.
- Regular worming should be performed in all.
- Piperazine, though widely used, is potentially toxic particularly in kittens and overdose is common due to the size of the tablets.
- Benzimidazole group is more efficacious, safer and easily administered.
- Data sheets for other endoparasiticides should be checked to ensure they are suitable for the patient's age.

Bacterial infections

- Variety associated with neonatal septicaemia in kittens:
  - Commonly *Staphylococcus*, *Escherichia*, *Klebsiella*, *Enterobacter*, *Streptococcus*, *Enterococcus*, *Pseudomonas*, *Clostridium*, *Bacteroides*, *Fusobacterium* and *Salmonella* spp.
  - *Bordetella bronchiseptica* – fatal respiratory infections.
  - Gram-negative bacilli are found most frequently.
  - Haemoplasma – *M. haemofelis* seems most pathogenic causing depression, lethargy, severe anaemia.
- Death can occur suddenly with few clinical signs, but more commonly frequent crying, restlessness, hypothermia, diarrhoea, dyspnoea, haematuria and cyanosis are seen.
- More chronic disease – kittens fail to gain weight as expected.
- Diagnosis is based on history and clinical examination.
- Treatment needs to be aggressive with antibacterials, fluids, glucose and oxygen.
- Potentiated amoxicillin represents a logical first-choice drug in the absence of culture and sensitivity results.

Diarrhoea

- Common in neonates but the role of bacteria is less clear.
- Majority of cases are self-limiting and can be treated using dietary manipulation and fluid therapy.
- Antibacterials should be avoided if possible as they can further disrupt the developing bowel microflora.

Viral infections

- Uncommon in kittens until maternally derived immunity begins to wane at around 5–6 weeks.
- FIV, FeLV, FIP and FPV can infect kittens transplacentally as well as perinatally via body fluids and milk.
- Transplacental spread of FPV can be associated with the use of modified live vaccines in pregnant queens.

1.3.6 Neonatal isoerythrolysis

- Blood group A kittens born to a B-group queen – naturally occurring anti-A antibodies passed in the colostrum resulting in immune-mediated destruction of the kitten's red cells.
- Clinical signs – fading at a few days of age, haemoglobinuria, jaundice, tail tip necrosis.
- Mortality can be high even with aggressive treatment.
- Avoid mating an A-group tomcat to a B-group queen.
  - Where this occurs, kittens hand-reared for the first few days until gut closure has taken place.

1.3.7 Fading kitten syndrome

- Fading kittens is a syndrome that covers a multitude of infectious and non-infectious conditions of the neonate resulting in an animal that is born apparently healthy but gradually becomes inactive, loses the suckle reflex and dies in the first 2 weeks of life.
- Localising signs are usually absent.
- This condition represents a clinical description rather than a diagnosis and requires investigation as outlined above.

Causes

- Congenital abnormality.
- Teratogenic effects.
- Inadequate nutrition.
- Inadequate colostrums.
- Low birth weight.
- Trauma.

- Neonatal isoerythrolysis.
- Infectious disease.

Key history
- Breeding history of household.
- Disease status of household.
- Individual breeding history of queen.
- Number of kittens born alive and dead.
- Health of queen now and during pregnancy.
- Status of other litter members.
- Status of other kittens in the household.
- Recent arrivals/showing/mating.
- Pattern of illness to date.
- Health parameters noted by breeder, e.g. weight gain.
- Hygiene, worming, vaccination and flea control regimes.
- Has the kitten ever appeared normal?
- Did the kitten ever suckle normally?
- Has supplementary feeding been provided (risk aspiration)?
- Blood group of queen and stud cat (if known)?

Clinical examination
- Examine the kitten, available litter mates and the queen (page 16–17).
- Weight gain can be a sensitive indicator of declining health in kittens and will often occur before other signs of illness.
- External features
- Mouth – mucosal colour, cleft palate.
- Thoracic auscultation and abdominal palpation.
- Neurological assessment:
  - Alertness.
  - Suckle reflex.
  - Response to noxious stimuli.
  - Reflexes (not fully developed until 12 weeks).

Decision making
- Level of problem – household, litter or individual.

- Congenital vs. hereditary.
- Infectious vs. anatomic.
- Likelihood of trauma.
- Possibility of neonatal isoerythrolysis.

Diagnostic investigation
- Routine haematology and biochemistry.
- Faecal and urinalysis.
- Bacterial culture.
- Serology.
- Imaging studies.
- Biopsy/post-mortem.

NB1 – *Maximum information can be obtained at post-mortem if the carcass is fresh. If post-mortem is not immediately available the body should be stored in the fridge. NB2 – Serology for infectious disease in kittens under 5–6 weeks is of limited value due to the presence of maternally derived antibodies and/or the time required for a kitten to mount a detectable immune response.*

1.3.8 Pain relief
- It is extremely difficult to assess pain in neonates/paediatric patients.
- Better to assume pain is present.
- Opiates can be used to effect.

1.4 GERONTOLOGY

1.4.1 Introduction
Definition
- In people, there is no set age at which patients may be under the care of a geriatrician, the decision is determined by the individual patient's needs and the availability of a specialist.

When is a cat old?
- Changes in nutritional, behavioural and metabolic function can be demonstrated

as early as 7–8 years (approximately equivalent to a 50-year-old person).

- Cats are generally considered to be old (senior equivalent to a 60–65-year-old person) when they reach 11–12 years and geriatric (equivalent to an 80-year-old person) when they are over 15.

- Cats mature more quickly and then age more slowly when compared to the dog especially medium and large breeds.

1.4.2 Effects of ageing

- Relatively little information about physiological changes with ageing in cats.

See Table 7.

Table 7 Age-associated changes in major organ systems

GIT	Dental disease
	Decreased salivation and taste sensation
	Some evidence to suggest changes in gut function
	Loss of oesophageal muscle tone
	Atrophy and fibrosis of gastric mucosa
	Reduced colonic motility
	Reduced villous height and epithelial cell turnover
Kidneys and water balance	Decreased nephron numbers
	Increased sensitivity to dehydration
	Decreased sensitivity to thirst
Pulmonary	Loss of lung elasticity
	Increase in pulmonary fibrous tissue and decrease in alveolar numbers
Liver	Decreased numbers of hepatocytes
Endocrine and metabolism	Decreased growth hormone levels and adrenal function
	Slow decline in metabolic rate
	Loss of lean body mass
	Reduction in energy requirements by 30–40%
	Poor thermoregulation
Haematopoietic and immune system	Decreased haemoglobin concentration
	Reduced immune competence
	Bone marrow becomes pale and fatty
	Less resistant to disease
	Immune surveillance targeting potentially neoplastic cells declines
Skin	Thinning and loss of elasticity
Special senses	Reduced visual acuity and increased susceptibility to ocular damage
	Decreased sense of smell
Activity and behaviour	Decreased activity
	Increased time spent sleeping
	Reduced ability to react to sudden environmental change
	Loss of learned behaviour – grooming, excretory habit

1.4.3 Nutritional changes
- By changing diet in an older cat the aim is to maintain health, maximise longevity and reduce the risk of developing age-associated diseases.
- Limited evidence that feeding an older cat a senior diet will affect health, longevity or disease occurrence:
  - One study looking at addition of antioxidants and chicory root to the diet predicted modest increases in longevity of 11 months.

Nutritional needs
- Reduced activity and lean body mass, hence decreased basal metabolic rate.
- Reduced nutrient digestion and absorption.
- Decreased sensation from food – smell and taste.
- Decreased ability to adapt to change – older cats may not tolerate sudden changes in diet even if the new diet to be fed may have a beneficial effect in the long term.

Dietary changes

Energy
- Widely believed that older cats require less energy, associated with decreased resting metabolic rate and activity:
  - BUT caloric intake may need to be increased due to reduced gut function.

Protein
- Restriction in old cats is inappropriate, except in the face of other diseases such as chronic renal failure:
  - Higher protein diets also tend to be more palatable; this is important in older cats with reduced appetite secondary to sensory loss.

Fat
- Important for palatability and energy density.

- Sufficient fat must be given to provide essential fatty acids and fat-soluble vitamins.
- Increased levels of omega 3 polyunsaturated fatty acids (PUFAs) may be beneficial in the control of hypertension, maintenance of renal blood flow and reducing the level of deleterious cytokines which may be involved in weight loss in older cats.
- Excessive levels of PUFAs can lead to the accumulation of peroxidised fats increasing free radical damage.

Calcium and phosphorus
- Phosphate restriction on the basis of the likelihood of reduced renal function.

Potassium
- Increased requirement associated with CKD in which potassium wasting occurs secondary to polyuria and acidosis.
- Acidifying diets, such as those designed for management of urolithiasis, also cause potassium loss and are probably inappropriate in the majority of older cats as the risks of struvite urolithiasis are substantially reduced in older cats.

Magnesium
- Older cats may also require increases in dietary magnesium.

Texture
- Dental disease is the most common condition of old cats.
- Dry foods with softened texture or moist foods may improve palatability.

1.4.4 Common diseases of elderly cats
- Chronic kidney disease (16–30% of cats over 15 years old).
- Dental disease.
- Hyperthyroidism.
- Neoplasia.
- Weight loss.

1.4.5 Assessment of the elderly cat
- History and physical examination.
- ± Faecal and urinalysis.
- ± Haematology and biochemistry.
- Thyroid function.
- Blood pressure:
  - Hypertension relatively common associated with various diseases, e.g. CKD or hyperthyroidism.

Weight
- Significant decline in the number of obese cats over 12–13 years of age.
- Significant increase in underweight cats over 15–16 years of age; the important goal is to try and maintain a stable, optimal weight.
- Both obesity and cachexia are associated with a significant increase in mortality in cats over 8 years.

Intercurrent disease
- Higher likelihood that an older cat has other disease processes besides the presenting complaint.
- Important considerations when deciding on what and how an investigation is to be performed.
- May influence prognosis.
- May affect therapeutic decisions.

1.4.6 Therapeutic considerations
- Effect on drug absorption is probably minimal.
- Subcutaneous absorption is likely to be reduced due to
  - Less interstitial fluid.
  - Reduced vascularity.
  - Increased incidence of dehydration.
- Decreased lean body mass affects drug distribution and effective body weight.
- Decreased fat may affect drug distribution and increases effective body weight.

- Plasma half-life will tend to be increased due to decreased renal/hepatic function.
- Older cats will cope less well with sudden changes in drug dose rates.
  - Increased sensitivity to hypotensive agents.

1.5 SUPPORTIVE CARE – FLUID THERAPY AND ANALGESIA

1.5.1 General principles
Many cats will need symptomatic and supportive care when they present prior to investigation or specific therapy. This section will focus on two major elements of supportive care: fluid therapy and pain relief. Nutritional support is covered in Section 4.13.5.

Hospitalised sick cats also benefit from TLC that would include grooming, provision of toys, boxes to hide in or scratch, playing and being given space to move around, e.g. an empty consulting room.

1.5.2 Fluid therapy
- Routine treatment of sick cats.
- Fluid overdose can occur easily with gravity-fed systems and can be fatal.
- Essential to ensure system flushed through before connecting to the cat.
- Unless continuous warming facilities or rapid delivery, heating the fluid bag is of little value due to speed of delivery.
- Choice of fluid important – volume, colloidal osmotic pressure, oxygen-carrying capacity.

Rate of administration
Crystalloids
- Choice (see Table 8).
- Should be calculated on body surface area and age.

Table 8 Commonly used colloids and their composition

Crystalloids	Na^+	K^+	Cl^-	Ca^{2+}	HCO_3^-	Use
7.2% NaCl	1232	0	1232	0	0	Rapid volume expansion lasts 30–60 minutes 2–4 ml/kg
0.9% NaCl	150	0	150	0	0	General use, especially low Na^+, high K^+ or Ca^{2+} or alkalosis
Hartmann's	131	5	111	2	111	Standard maintenance, acidosis (with functional liver)
0.18% NaCl	30	0	30	0	0	Hyperosmolar states, high Na^+
5% dextrose	0	0	0	0	0	Hyperosmolar states, drug diluents, never as a bolus

Colloids	Na^+	K^+	Cl^-	MW	COP	Comments
Haemaccel	145	5	145	30	25–28	Primary use is to expand
Gelofusine	77	0	62.5	35	33	volume with better duration than crystalloids and
Pentastarch 6%	150	0	150	200	32	maintain IV COP. Gelatins last a few hours and have a poorer expansion than pentastarch (12–24 hours).

- For practical purposes 2 ml/kg/hour approximates to maintenance for adult cats.
  - Maintenance rates for kittens:
    - <12 weeks – 5–6 ml/kg/hour.
    - 12–24 weeks – 3–4 ml/kg/hour.
- Standard surgical rate is 5 × maintenance.
- Shock rates 40–70 ml/kg/hour.
- More careful consideration of fluid rates when
  - Acute renal failure may be present.
  - Suspected or known cardiac dysfunction.
  - Bradycardia is present.
  - Severe anaemia (PCV <10–12%) especially if dehydrated.
  - Severe hypokalaemia (K+ <2.5 mmol/l).

Colloids
- Up to 10 ml/kg as a slow IV bolus.
- Maintenance 1 ml/kg/hour.

- Bovine haemoglobin glutamer (Oxyglobin) has both colloidal and oxygen carrying capacity. Maximum dose 7ml/kg; potential to cause pulmonary oedema.

Blood transfusions
See section 4.11.6.

1.5.3 Analgesia
Choice of analgesic will depend on the likely underlying diagnosis, in the short term; if this is in doubt then opiates are much less likely to cause problems than NSAIDs. Where significant pain is present combination of pain relief, particularly NSAIDs and opiates given together, may be necessary.

- Assessing pain in cats can be difficult – if in doubt and it is safe give pain relief and observe cat for signs of improvement that indicate that pain was present.

- Signs suggestive of pain in cats:
  - Inability to rest/sleep.
  - Inappropriate activity level.
  - Sitting in the back of the kennel.
  - Mental attitude/demeanour (stupor or anxiety).
  - Changes in attitude/personality.
  - Poor hair coat.
  - Lack of comfort when palpated.
  - Facial expression, staring, fixed gaze, dilated pupils.
  - Lack of appetite and thirst.
  - Altered vocalisations.
  - Posture.
  - Tachycardia.
  - Tachypnoea.
  - Attempts to remove bandages are very focused on one area and *may* be due to pain.
  - Body temperature and blood pressure *may* be increased or decreased.

Opiates
See Table 9.
- Different opiates are appropriate for managing different levels of pain:
  - Only buprenorphine licensed for use in cats.
- Cats are more sensitive to opiate side effects than dogs.
- Appropriate for short- to medium-term pain relief.
- Suitable documentation essential according to the legal category of the opiate used.

CRI opiate-based pain relief
- CRI cocktails are intended to follow on from loading dose pain relief.
- Morphine, lidocaine and ketamine (MLK) – 60 mg M + 1000 mg L + 60 mg K/l (0.9% NaCl) @ 1–3 ml/kg/hour, protect bag from light.
- Fentanyl, lidocaine and ketamine (FLK) – fentanyl instead of morphine 1.2 mg/l (0.9% NaCl) @ 1–3 ml/kg/hour, protect bag from light.

NSAIDs
See Table 10.
- Very effective in managing pain and will provide further pain relief even when high-dose opiates have been given.
- Particularly suited for long-term pain relief.
- There is no current evidence that appropriate, long-term use of NSAIDs have negative consequences.
- Fewer NSAIDs are licensed and safe for use in cats due to reduced glucuronidation of some drugs within the liver:
  - This does not apply to all NSAIDs and in fact half-life for some is shorter in cats than dogs.
- Use of NSAIDs is generally contraindicated when
  - The cat is significantly dehydrated.
  - Renal function is compromised.
  - Gastrointestinal ulceration is suspected or likely to occur.
  - There is moderate–severe cardiac disease.
  - Glucocorticoids may be an essential part of therapy:
    - Glucocorticoids can be given no sooner than 24 hours after NSAIDs with suitable gastric protection.
    - Preferable wash-out period would be 4 days.
  - Glucocorticoids have been given within the last 48 hours.
    - Preferably not within last 4 days.

Misoprostol
- Where NSAID overdose is known or suspected to have occurred, misoprostol, a prostaglandin analogue, can be used to reduce likely side effects.
- Tablet size makes dosing cats problematic (200 µg tablets) – 5 µg/kg PO q8h.
- Misoprostol can cause diarrhoea, abdominal pain, vomiting and abortion.

Table 9 Selection of opiates suitable for use in cats

Generic name	Site of action	Route of administration	Dose rate (mg/kg)	Comments
Buprenorphine	Partial agonist OP3 receptor	IV, IM, SC, PO (0.3 mg/ml)	0.01–0.02 q6h	1, S3
Butorphanol	Primarily OP2 agonist, OP3 antagonist	IM, SC (10 mg/ml), PO (5 mg, 10 mg tablets)	0.2–0.5 q6–12h	POM-V
Codeine	Mechanism unclear, mu receptor?	PO (15, 30, 60 mg tablets; 5 mg/ml syrup)	0.5–2 q12h	2, POM-V
Fentanyl	Pure OP3 agonist	IV (0.05 mg/ml); patch (12, 25, 50, 75 µg/hour)	See pg 25; 12µg/hour patch suitable for most cats	S2
Methadone	Pure OP3 agonist	IV, IM, SC (10 mg/ml)	0.1–0.3 IM q4–6h	S2
Morphine	Pure OP3 agonist	IV; IM (10 mg/ml)[a]	0.1–0.4 q3–6h	3, S2
Pethidine	Pure OP3 agonist	IM, SC (10–50 mg/ml)	5–10 q1–2h	S2
Tramadol	All opioid receptors, esp. OP3	PO (50, 100, 200, 300 mg capsules, 5 mg/ml)	2–4 q12h	4, POM

Legal category: POM-V – prescription only medicine – veterinary, S2 – schedule 2; S3 – schedule 3. Pethidine = meperidine.
1. Absorbed orally in cats (oral pH different to man/dogs), use injectable solution rather than sublingual tablets.
2. Also use as cough suppressant and anti-diarrhoeal; analgesic effect is mild, injectable preparation is available.
3. Oral tablets, suppositories and syrups are available; will often cause vomiting.
4. Also inhibits noradrenalin and 5HT pathways providing alternative pathways for pain relief.
[a]NB – injectable morphine preparations 10, 15, 20 and 30 mg/ml – check concentration being given especially where practice also uses morphine in horses.

Table 10 NSAIDs for use in cats

Generic name	Trade name	COX selectivity	Route	Available preparations	Dose rate (mg/kg)	Comments
Aspirin	Various	Non-selective COX inhibitor	PO	75, 300 mg tablets	1–2 mg/kg q24h 10–25mg/cat q48–72hr	H, 1, 2
Ketoprofen	Ketofen	Non-selective COX inhibitor	IV, IM, SC, PO	1 mg/ml injectable 5 mg tablets	First dose 2 mg/kg then 5 d @ 1 mg/kg q24h	HR, 1, 2, 3
Meloxicam	Metacam[a]	Preferentially inhibits COX-2	SC, PO	2, 5 mg/ml injectable 0.5, 1.5 oral suspension 1, 2, 5 mg tablets	0.3 mg/kg (single) or first dose 0.1 mg/kg with long term 0.05 mg/kg q24h	H, 1, 3
Robenacoxib	Onsior	Preferentially inhibits COX-2	SC, PO	20 mg/ml injectable 5, 6, 10 mg tablets	First dose 2 mg/kg, long term 1 mg/kg q24h	HR, 1, 3
Tolfenamic acid	Tolfedine	COX selectivity uncertain	SC, PO	40 mg/ml injectable 6, 20 mg tablets	4 mg/kg q24h for 3 days	HR, 1, 2, 3

H – hepatic metabolism with biliary excretion, HR – hepatic metabolism with renal excretion; COX – cyclooxygenase.
1. Standard GI and hypotension, lowest effective dose, almost exclusively used as an anticoagulant in cat.
2. Anticoagulant dose or has anti-platelet action.
3. Small risk of precipitating CHF in patients with CV disease.
[a]Available under other trade names as well.

Other drugs

Medetomidine and dexmedetomidine
- Can be given as single dose at 5–20 µg/kg.

Gabapentin
- Used for neuropathic pain, mechanism of action is unknown.
- Dose up to 5–10 mg/kg PO q8–12h.
- Can cause mild sedation and ataxia.

Benzodiazepines
- Used as muscle relaxants.

Methocarbamol
- Skeletal muscle relaxant. Dose 20–45 mg/kg PO q8h.
- Side effects – salivation, vomiting, lethargy weakness, ataxia and CNS depression.

Amantadine
- N-Methyl-d-aspartate (NMDA) antagonist analgesic.
- May potentiate effects of other analgesics.
- 1–4 mg/kg q24h PO – start at lowest dose and increase slowly.

Amitriptyline
- NMDA antagonist analgesic.
- Also used for behavioural therapy, FLUTD and management of ureteroliths.

Non-drug modalities
- Consider physiotherapy, acupuncture and other therapies.

1.6 SEDATION AND ANAESTHESIA

1.6.1 Introduction
It is outside the scope of this text to present a detailed discussion of sedation and anaesthesia in cats. The purpose of this section is to present a selection of protocols for sedation and anaesthesia that are appropriate for undertaking medical procedures in cats with various levels of sedative/anaesthetic risk. Before sedating or anaesthetising a patient it is worth considering
- Whether the examination(s) can be undertaken without sedation/anaesthesia.
  - Does the risks of doing so outweigh the benefits of not sedating/anaesthetising.
- The effect the presenting signs and working diagnosis have on risk and choice of agent.
- All the procedures that would be appropriate to be undertaken to minimise the need for repeat sedation/anaesthesia.
  - What other procedures may be necessary should initial finding under sedation/anaesthesia redirect the investigation.
- Facilities that may be required to recover and monitor the cat following the sedation/anaesthetic.

1.6.2 Pre-procedure assessment
- All cases should have had a recent physical examination.
- (Dex)medetomidine should generally be avoided in hypotensive, hypovolaemic or senior (especially geriatric) cats but can be an effective in systemically well cats.
  - Lower-end premedication doses and minimum necessary induction agent should be given.
- Kittens under 12 weeks more susceptible to the sedative effects of opioids and benzodiazepines.
- Patient should be placed in one of the five American Society of Anaesthesiologists' (ASA) stages.

Stage
1. Normal healthy cat.
2. Cat with mild systemic disease.

3. Cat with severe systemic disease that is not incapacitating.
4. Cat with severe systemic disease that is a constant threat to life.
5. Moribund cat not expected to survive 24 hours with or without operation.

1.6.3 Sedative protocols

- Choice of sedative will depend on
  ○ Procedure to be undertaken – how painful, how long, how still does the cat need to be.
  ○ Experience of the clinician and type of equipment available.
  ○ Status of the cat.
  ○ Demeanour of the cat.
  ○ Whether the sedation is to be given IV, IM or SC.
- Following sedation the cat should be kept in a quiet environment with subdued lighting and monitored.
- Following IM or SC administration sufficient time should be allowed for sedation to become effective.

- If sedation is ineffective decide whether it is appropriate to
  ○ Increase the dose.
  ○ Add in another agent.
  ○ Proceed to anaesthesia.
  ○ Abandon the procedure and reconsider the approach.

Sedative protocols
See Table 11.

Reversal with atipamezole
- 2.5× mg dose for medetomidine (half the volume).
- 5× mg dose for dexmedetomidine (half the volume).

1.6.4 Anaesthetic protocols

Premedication
- Reduces the dose of anaesthetic required and smoothes induction.
- Allows catheter placement in fractious cats.

Table 11 Selected sedative protocols for cats

Agent	Dose rate	Route	Level of sedation and pain relief	Risks
Acepromazine + buprenorphine	0.02–0.03 mg/kg 0.01–0.02 mg/kg	SC, IM or IV	Mild	ASA 1–3
Acepromazine + butorphanol	0.02–0.03 mg/kg 0.2–0.3 mg/kg	SC, IM or IV	Mild	ASA 1–3
Acepromazine + methadone[a]	0.02–0.03 mg/kg 0.2–0.4 mg/kg	IM or IV	Mild–moderate	ASA 1–3
Medetomidine[b] + ACP + opiate	2.5–10 µg/kg Can be repeated once	IM or IV	Moderate	ASA 1–2 Normal CV function
Midazolam + ketamine	0.2–0.3 mg/kg 5–10 mg/kg	IM or IV	Moderate to marked	ASA 2–4 Not cats with HCM
Methadone[a]	0.2–0.3 mg/kg	IM	Variable	ASA 4–5

[a]Can substitute with morphine 0.2–0.4 mg/kg – must be given slowly IV, more likely to cause vomiting and transient excitement than methadone.
[b]Use half the dose rate for dexmedetomidine.

- ACP and an opiate are appropriate for most cases.
- NSAIDs should not form part of the routine premedicant; each patient should be assessed for potential contraindications to their use prior to inclusion.

Induction

See Table 12 for suggested intravenous induction protocols.
- Pre-oxygenate as appropriate.
- Induce in a calm quiet environment.
- Intramuscular protocols can be used, they are more difficult to titrate to effect and less applicable to cats undergoing medical investigation (as compared to routine procedures, e.g. neutering):
  - Medetomidine, morphine/buprenorphine/butorphanol and ketamine.
  - Xylazine and ketamine.

Intubation

- Generally required for most procedures.
- Cats can be difficult to intubate.
- Local anaesthetic sprayed onto the larynx is usually necessary.
- Aim to minimise attempts to intubate and associated laryngeal trauma.
- Using larger endotracheal tubes reduces dead space resistance:
  - A 4.5–5 mm uncuffed tube is suitable for most adult cats.
  - A small paediatric bronchoscope will fit down a 5 mm ET tube.
- The use of laryngeal masks is becoming more popular in cats as endotracheal intubation is not required. However, they do not protect the patient from aspiration.

Maintenance

- For most cases gaseous anaesthesia is appropriate using isoflurane or sevoflurane.

Table 12 Intravenous induction agents

Drug	Propofol	Alfaxalone
Use	Standard IV induction agent	Standard IV induction agent
Dose rate	Give 0.5–1 ml, wait for 1–2 minutes, then incrementally until intubation. With premedication 2–5 mg/kg[a]	Give slowly to effect. With premedicant up to 5 mg/kg (Has been given IM in cats)
Formulation	Shake well before using 10 mg/ml emulsion	Pregnane neurosteroid 10 mg/ml solution solubilised in cyclodextrin
Comments	Rapid induction causes apnoea, cyanosis, bradycardia and severe hypotension. Muscle rigidity, paradoxical movement and tremors on induction may worsen with further doses of propofol; wane with time. Repeat doses are associated with Heinz body anaemia.	Do not use in combination with other IV anaesthetic agents. Mild cardiorespiratory effects. Metabolised in liver and excreted via bile and kidneys. Half-life 45 minutes in cats. Longer recovery if CRI or top-up boluses used for maintenance.

[a]Dose can be reduced by using midazolam/diazemuls at 0.5 mg/kg IV given a few minutes before induction.

Circuit

- Humphrey ADE circuit without soda lime with free gas flow rate of 70–100 ml/kg/minute.
- Ayre's T-piece (± Jackson-Rees modification) with free gas flow rate of 250–300 ml/kg/minute.

Intravenous

- In some situations total intravenous anaesthesia is appropriate, e.g. bronchoscopy:
  - Propofol – 0.2 mg/kg/minute CRI or 2 mg/kg q5min to effect.
  - Propofol – 0.12–0.3 mg/kg/minute CRI + fentanyl – 0.1 mg/kg/minute CRI.
  - Alfaxan – 0.11–0.13 mg/kg/minute or 1.1–1.3 mg/kg q10 min to effect.

Monitoring

See Table 13.

- Appropriate for ASA stage and procedure being performed.

Recovery

- TPR should be monitored periodically.
- Monitoring should continue after extubation even if the cat is appearing alert:
  - Laryngeal oedema can occur obstructing the airway post extubation.
  - Post-anaesthetic deaths do occur after apparently and initial smooth recovery and extubation especially after nasal investigation.

Table 13 Monitoring of anaesthesia

	Pulse oximetry (SpO$_2$)	ECG	Capnography (ETCO$_2$)	Blood pressure (BP)
What does it tell you	Oxygen saturation of haemoglobin in arterial blood and pulse rate	Heart rate and rhythm	Partial pressure of CO$_2$ in expired gas	Systolic BP – Doppler; Systolic, diastolic + mean BP – oscillometric
Strengths	Simple and easy to use, can be placed at a variety of locations	Visual and numerical display. Essential to distinguish poor circulation due to arrhythmia vs. circulatory collapse	Reflects interaction of metabolism, ventilation and pulmonary circulation as well as functioning of anaesthetic equipment	Assessment of pulse rate and quality of output
Limitations	Vasoconstriction and movement reduce reliability. Oxygen dissociation curve is sigmoid so SpO$_2$ slow to respond to a fall in arterial oxygenation. Hypoventilation can exist with high SpO$_2$	No information about the quality of circulation If T waves are tall the machine will often double count	Limited value without capnographic curve. Experience required to interpret curve and decide upon appropriate action	Can be difficult to place particularly on sick patients that are vasoconstricted/ hypotensive with poor pulse pressures

1.7 EMERGENCY AND CRITICAL CARE ALGORITHMS

1.7.1 Introduction

This section is intended to provide basic information primarily as algorithms for managing common feline emergencies that will present in general practice.

Triage

Regardless of the presumed cause, basic triage is vital to prioritise further investigation and emergency intervention. It might also alter decisions as to which emergency drugs to use. The following should be assessed and subsequently monitored:

- Level of consciousness.
- Airway and breathing.
- Heart rate and rhythm.
- Perfusion parameters – pulse, mucous membrane colour and capillary refill time.
- Temperature.

Emergency blood panel

Focus on parameters that can cause sudden deterioration in a patient's status or affect drug use/therapy:

- PCV (and total solids).
- Glucose.
- Calcium.
- Electrolytes (potassium and sodium).
- Acid–base balance.
- Ammonia (bile acids) – if unavailable then ALT.
- Urea or creatinine.

Team organisation

- 3–4 people are required to manage a life-threatening emergency situation:
  - Clear role assignment improves efficiency and reduces the risk of something being left undone:
    1. Team leader – directs activity, makes decisions, primary case responsibility.

2. Drug/fluid administrator – placing IV lines, organising fluid and drug administration order by the team leader.
3. Monitor and recorder – placing of monitoring equipment, monitoring of vital parameters, recording changes, procedure performed and drugs administered.
4. Gopher – fetching and carrying, communication with owner.

1.7.2 Trauma/RTA

Basic approach

- Detailed history of the incident.
- How long ago?
- Is the patient improving, stable or deteriorating?
- Other medical problems/medication, e.g. NSAIDs?

Initial management

- Triage.
- Deal with life-threatening conditions:
  - AIRWAY → BREATHING → CIRCULATION.
- Place monitoring equipment and begin monitoring chart to evaluate trends:
  - Temperature, pulse, respiration.
  - Blood pressure and pulse oximetry.
  - Urine output.
  - PCV, TP, electrolytes, urea, blood gas.
- Establish IV access as soon as possible

Level of consciousness (LOC)

Declining

- Consider metabolic, hypoxia, hypotension, toxins, drugs, primary brain pathology.
- Hyperexcitability – manage as for seizures (section 1.7.6).
- Progression – alert → depressed → stupor → coma
  - Raise head and neck up to 20°.
  - Secure airway against aspiration.
  - Try and maintain end-tidal CO_2 @ 30–35 mmHg.

○ O$_2$ therapy – maintain saturation >99%; pO$_2$ >60%.
○ Avoid aggressive fluid therapy if possible – colloids preferred to crystalloids.
○ Glucocorticoids of no proven benefit.
○ Mannitol 0.25–1 g/kg as bolus over 20 minutes.

Heart rate and rhythm
- Tachycardia – usually extracardiac, e.g. blood loss.
- Bradycardia – pressor, e.g. dobutamine 5–10 mg/kg/minute CRI, atropine.

NB1 – *bradycardic cats do not cope well with aggressive fluid therapy.*
NB2 – *consider CNS injury.*

- Arrhythmia – only intervene if significant effect on output – most arrhythmias are better untreated.

Perfusion
- Pale, hypotensive, normal PCV – fluid resuscitate:
  ○ Bolus colloid (5 ml/kg over 30 minute).
  ○ Crystalloid up to 70 ml/kg in first hour.
- PCV low – blood or blood substitute.

Common injuries to consider
- Soft tissue trauma – diaphragmatic, body wall or bladder rupture.
- Damage to liver, spleen, pancreas.
- Bruising – can be severe and difficult to assess without shaving.
- Appendicular fractures.
- Spinal cord and cauda equina damage.
- Bleeding.
- Lung trauma causing pneumothorax (may include rib fractures).
- Shock.
- Mandibular fracture/luxation.

1.7.3 Dyspnoea

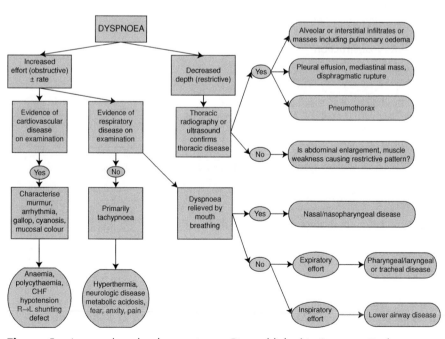

Figure 1 Approach to the dyspnoeic cat. First published in Sturgess: *Pocket Handbook of Small Animal Medicine* (Manson Publishing, 2012). Reproduced by permission of the publisher.

KEY TOPICS IN FELINE MEDICINE

1.7.4 Collapse

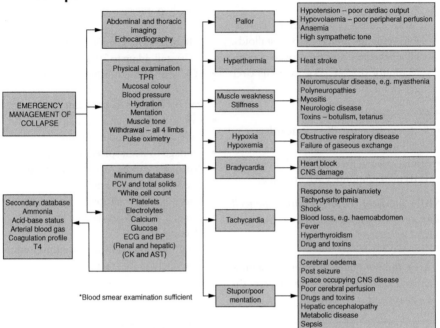

Figure 2   Approach to the collapsed cat. First published in Sturgess: *Pocket Handbook of Small Animal Medicine* (Manson Publishing, 2012). Reproduced by permission of the publisher.

1.7.5 Urinary obstruction

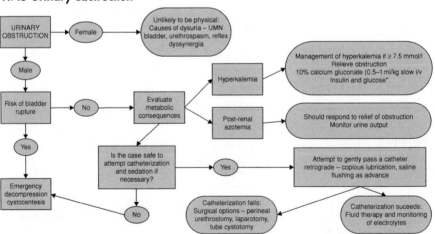

Figure 3   Approach to the obstructed cat. First published in Sturgess: *Pocket Handbook of Small Animal Medicine* (Manson Publishing, 2012). Reproduced by permission of the publisher.

*Insulin and glucose can potentially cause fatal hypoglycaemia; monitor blood glucose every 30–60 minutes for 3 hours and use neutral insulin

1.7.6 Seizures

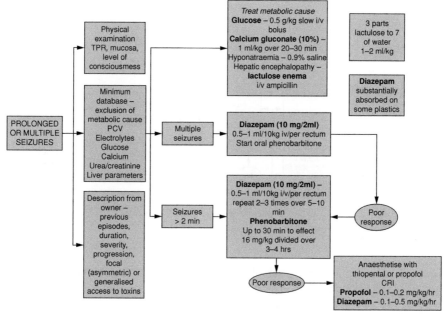

Figure 4   Approach to the seizuring cat. First published in Sturgess: *Pocket Handbook of Small Animal Medicine* (Manson Publishing, 2012). Reproduced by permission of the publisher.

1.7.7 CPCR

Personnel
- Ventilation and team leader.
- Cardiac compression.
- Administer fluids and drugs.
- Monitoring, record keeping.

Procedures
- Establish an airway using a cuffed endotracheal tube, if not possible then tracheostomy – allows controlled ventilation.
- Establish IV access.
- Maximise monitoring – pulse/heart rate and rhythm, respiration, temperature, mucosal colour, PLR, level of consciousness, ECG, pulse oximetry, end-tidal CO_2, electrolytes, blood gas and lactate.

KEY TOPICS IN FELINE MEDICINE

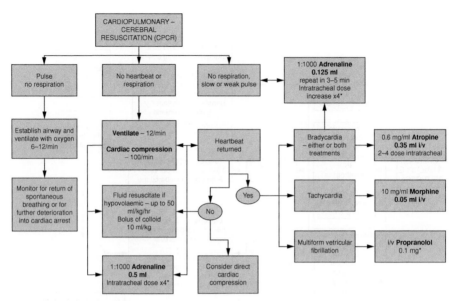

Figure 5 Cardiopulmonary cerebral resuscitation (CPCR). First published in Sturgess: *Pocket Handbook of Small Animal Medicine* (Manson Publishing, 2012). Reproduced by permission of the publisher.

NB – Volume based on a 5 kg cat
*Lidocaine can be used in cats but they are more sensitive to toxicity – 0.25–1 mg/kg slow IV followed by CRI @ 0.01–0.04 mg/kg/minute (place 10 ml of 20% lidocaine in a 100 ml bag of saline = 2 mg/ml for 5 kg cat given at 1.5–6 ml/hour)

SECTION 2

CLINICAL SIGNS

Notes on Feline Internal Medicine, Second Edition. Edited by Kit Sturgess. ©2013 John Wiley & Sons, Ltd.
Published 2013 by Blackwell Publishing Ltd.

CLINICAL SIGNS

INTRODUCTION

Section 2 focuses on the approach to a wide variety of common clinical presentations listed in alphabetical order. Each subsection is arranged to discuss causes of the presentation, key history that needs to be explored, which decisions need to be made to problem solve the case, diagnostic approach and therapy and management. A quick guide to appropriate diagnostic testing is provided in Table 14.

Differential lists contain some conditions that rarely cause the clinical sign or are rare in cats. These are included to aid the reader when dealing with cases for which initial diagnostics have not shown the sign to have been caused by one of the more common conditions.

Further details of specific conditions can be found in section 4 (organ systems) or 5 (infectious disease).

Table 14 sets out the general and specific tests and their priority for each condition. Further details of test specifics are in each subsection relating to that presenting sign. Depending on the history (age, breed, sex, foreign travel, worming history, trauma etc.) and physical examination findings, tests performed and particularly the order of testing may need to be modified.

2.1 ABDOMINAL ENLARGEMENT

2.1.1 Introduction
Abdominal enlargement can be associated with a wide variety of different organs, physiologic and pathologic processes. The prognosis for the patient is therefore hugely variable and warrants further investigation to define the cause of the enlargement and the underlying process involved.

2.1.2 Causes
- Fluid:
  - Free fluid (see ascites, Section 2.4).
  - Confined fluid – urine, cysts (rare), hydronephrosis, fluid in GIT, pyometra (common in older unspayed queens).
- Solid:
  - Organomegaly (including neoplasia).
  - Fat.
  - Pregnancy.
  - Faeces.
  - Abdominal muscle weakness associated with hyperadrenocorticism or severe cachexia/malnutrition; tearing of the abdominal wall.
- Gas:
  - Pneumoabdomen – GI rupture, spontaneous or post surgery.
  - Confined gas – gastric dilation, intestinal obstruction.

2.1.3 Key history
- How quickly has the abdomen become enlarged?
- Is the abdomen painful?
- Is there weakness, lethargy, dyspnoea or evidence of shock?
- Are there other clinical signs?
- Has the cat been seen to urinate/defaecate recently? Is there faecal or urinary tenesmus?
- Is the cat attempting to vomit?
- Is pregnancy possible?

2.1.4 Focus of physical examination
General physical examination with thorough abdominal palpation and thoracic percussion.

2.1.5 Decision making
- If physiologic processes (fat deposition or pregnancy) have been excluded, further investigation of cause is likely to be necessary.
- Generally, imaging will provide the most rapid way of locating the cause of the enlargement but is poorly sensitive as to the pathologic process.
- *If there is weakness, rapid and ongoing enlargement, lethargy, dyspnoea*

CLINICAL SIGNS

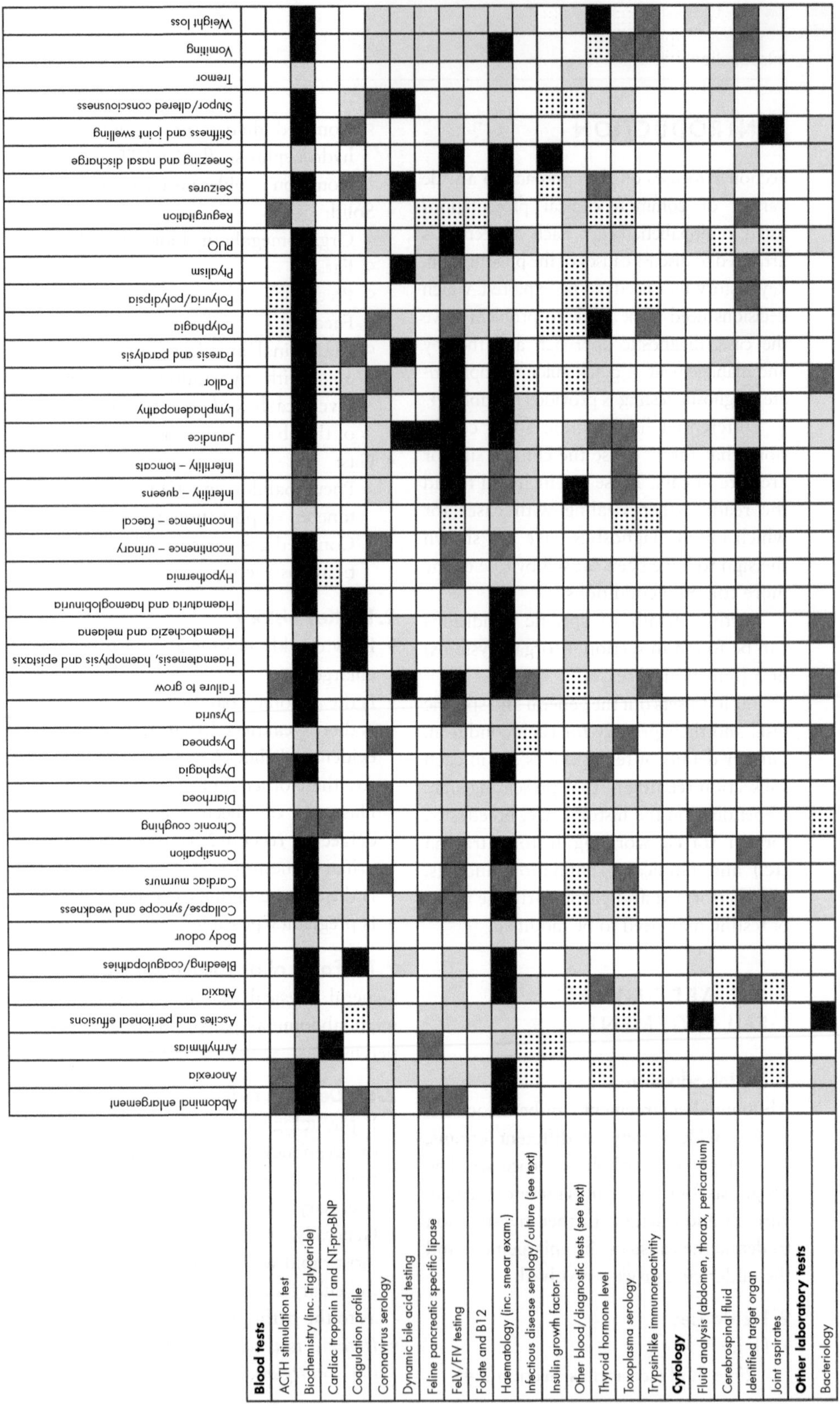

Clinical signs (column headings):

- Weight loss
- Vomiting
- Tremor
- Stupor/altered consciousness
- Stiffness and joint swelling
- Sneezing and nasal discharge
- Seizures
- Regurgitation
- PUO
- Ptyalism
- Polyuria/polydipsia
- Polyphagia
- Paresis and paralysis
- Pallor
- Lymphadenopathy
- Jaundice
- Infertility – tomcats
- Infertility – queens
- Incontinence – faecal
- Incontinence – urinary
- Hypothermia
- Haematuria and haemoglobinuria
- Haematochezia and melaena
- Haematemesis, haemoptysis and epistaxis
- Failure to grow
- Dysuria
- Dyspnoea
- Dysphagia
- Diarrhoea
- Chronic coughing
- Constipation
- Cardiac murmurs
- Collapse/syncope and weakness
- Body odour
- Bleeding/coagulopathies
- Ataxia
- Ascites and peritoneal effusions
- Arrhythmias
- Anorexia
- Abdominal enlargement

Tests (row headings):

Blood tests
- ACTH stimulation test
- Biochemistry (inc. triglyceride)
- Cardiac troponin I and NT-proBNP
- Coagulation profile
- Coronavirus serology
- Dynamic bile acid testing
- Feline pancreatic specific lipase
- FeLV/FIV testing
- Folate and B12
- Haematology (inc. smear exam.)
- Infectious disease serology/culture (see text)
- Insulin growth factor-1
- Other blood/diagnostic tests (see text)
- Thyroid hormone level
- Toxoplasma serology
- Trypsin-like immunoreactivity

Cytology
- Fluid analysis (abdomen, thorax, pericardium)
- Cerebrospinal fluid
- Identified target organ
- Joint aspirates

Other laboratory tests
- Bacteriology

| Faecal culture/parasitology |
| Toxicology |
| Urinalysis including UPC and culture |
| Urine SG and dipstick |
| **Imaging** |
| Echocardiography |
| Fluoroscopy |
| Radiographs – abdomen |
| Radiographs – appendicular skeleton |
| Radiographs – skull |
| Radiographs – thorax |
| Radiographs – vertebral column |
| Ultrasound – abdominal |
| Ultrasound – other |
| Ultrasound – thorax |
| CT/MRI |
| **Other tests** |
| Biopsy* of target organ |
| Blood pressure |
| Electrocardiography |
| Electrophysiology |
| Endoscopy/exploratory surgery |
| Holter/event monitoring |
| Oral examination (sedation/general anaesthetic) |
| Rectal examination |
| Trial therapy (drugs, diet, etc.) |

*Surgical, ultrasound guided, endoscopic or laproscopic/thoracoscopic as appropriate

Important screening test or high yield specific tests
May be necessary but test rarely diagnostic or condition rare or rarely causes the sign
Secondary tests dependent on results of history, physical examination and screening tests
May be required as a tertiary test

Table 14 Appropriate tests and order of testing by presenting clinical signs

or signs of shock, emergency stabilisation may need to precede further diagnostics.

NB – *The pathologic process can lie outside the abdomen, e.g. heart failure.*

2.1.6 Diagnostic approach
- History and physical examination.
- Presence of a fluid thrill.
- Percussion for gas.
- Palpable organomegaly.
- Radiography and/or ultrasound.

Interpretation of imaging
Radiography – look for displacement of stomach axis (hepatomegaly/microhepatica) or other organs (displaced away from mass). Displacement to the periphery suggests a central mass. 'Ground glass' appearance suggests free abdominal fluid.

Organomegaly
- Stomach filled with ingesta, air.
- Constipation (see Section 2.11).
- Urinary bladder distended (see Section 2.16).
- Small intestinal dilation.

Gastric dilation
- Overeaten – prey, dry food that has swollen.
- Aerophagia secondary to pain or dyspnoea.
- Gastric dilation/volvulus rare in cats.
- Gastric foreign bodies relatively uncommon and rarely cause abdominal enlargement.
- Failure of pylorus to relax and empty usually results in vomiting before palpable distension.

Small intestinal dilation
- Obstructive disease – foreign body, intussusception, parasites, neoplasia.
- Ileus.

Diffuse organomegaly
Usually associated with infiltrative disease (inflammatory or neoplastic), also consider splenic engorgement or torsion, peri-renal pseudocyst, hepatic lipidosis, amyloid, granulomatous disease.

Focal organomegaly
Neoplasia, abscess, cyst, granuloma, nodular hyperplasia, haematoma.

Multiple organ involvement
- Hepatosplenomegaly – common combination usually associated with disease of the reticuloendothelial system or extramedullary haematopoiesis.
- Acromegaly.
- Amyloidosis.
- Lymphoma.
- Lysosomal storage disease.

Other causes
- Lymphadenomegaly may be palpable but is less easy to identify on radiography, although it can usually be found on ultrasound.
- Pancreatic enlargement (rarely palpable in the cranial mid abdomen) may cause abdominal enlargement due to localised peritoneal effusion and sometimes organ displacement.
- Adrenomegaly is very rarely palpable.

2.1.7 Management and therapy
Will be highly dependent on cause but in ascitic patients, removal of 50% of the estimated fluid volume will relieve many of the clinical signs in the short term but fluid can reform rapidly worsening hypoproteinemia or causing hypovolaemia.

2.2 ANOREXIA

2.2.1 Introduction
Cats tend to be less food-driven than dogs; hence anorexia (inappetence) is an extremely common presenting sign.

Although it is often associated with other more organ-specific signs, it can be the only change (associated with weight loss (See section 2.43) in chronic cases) presented. Hyporexia refers to partial anorexia or reduced appetite.

2.2.2 Causes

Due to the frequency of anorexia, there is limited value in problem solving this clinical sign. However, the degree of anorexia is important as it can affect prognosis as well as require therapeutic intervention before a diagnosis has been reached. The differential diagnosis of anorexia needs to be considered when it is the first or only clinical sign shown. Some anorexic cats are actually dysphagic – see section 2.14.

2.2.3 Key history
- What is the cat's normal appetite like?
- Are other clinical signs present?
- How long has the cat been anorexic/inappetent?
- Did the anorexia precede or follow the onset of other signs?
- How much is the cat eating?
- How much weight loss has there been?
- What strategies to encourage eating have already been used?
- What is the cat's attitude to food?
  - Disinterested.
  - Will pick at new foods, table scraps.
  - Asks for food, but then only eats a few mouthfuls.
  - Keen to eat but backs away from food as soon as it starts eating (suggests oropharyngeal pain)*.
  - Tries to eat but drops food*.
- Is the cat bright and active or dull and lethargic?

2.2.4 Focus of physical examination
Mouth and GIT.

*indicates dysphagia

2.2.5 Decision making
- Accurate, serial weighing is essential when weight loss may be occurring.
- Healthy cats will lose 2–3% of bodyweight per week if starved completely. Weight loss greater than this suggests that anorexia alone is not responsible and there is an underlying disease preventing a reduction in BMR that is the normal response to starvation.
- Estimate the cat's caloric intake compared to requirement:
  - Resting energy requirements (RER) $(kcal/day) = 75 + [30 \times bodyweight (kg)]$.
  - Maintenance energy requirements $(kcal/day) = 1.4 \times RER$.
- Does the anorexia need treating as a primary problem?
- What feeding method is appropriate?

2.2.6 Diagnostic approach
In the absence of other clinical signs, anorexia is most likely to be associated with oral or GI disease. If there are other associated signs, investigation should be focused on these.

2.2.7 Management and therapy
No underlying cause identified after initial screening.
- Appetite stimulants – mirtazapine (3.75 mg/cat PO q72h), cyproheptadine (1–2 mg/cat PO q12–24h), oxazepam (1–2 mg/cat PO q24h).
- Methods of supplementary feeding (section 4.13):
  - Manual feeding may be successful – consider environment and associations of feeding.
  - Force feeding – can worsen anorexia and lead to learned taste aversion.
  - Chemical appetite stimulants.
  - Tube feeding.
  - Total or partial peripheral parenteral nutrition.
- Further diagnostics (see Table 14 page 40–41).

CLINICAL SIGNS

2.3 ARRHYTHMIAS

2.3.1 Introduction

Due to their faster heart rates, rhythm disturbances can be difficult to appreciate on auscultation. Cats do not normally have a sinus arrhythmia; hence any irregularity of rhythm is likely to be abnormal. Arrhythmias (synonymous with dysrhythmia) can present in a number of ways and be caused by a variety of different mechanisms.

Presentation
- Asymptomatic – discovered as part of routine physical examination.
- Cat is unwell but the arrhythmia is not contributing to the clinical signs; however, it is a reflection of underlying disease.
- Arrhythmia is responsible for clinical signs – lethargy and weakness progressing to ataxia and disorientation; collapse progressing to seizure and coma; sudden death.

2.3.2 Causes (Table 15)

2.3.3 Key history
- Age, breed, sex.
- e.g. Maine Coon predisposed to HCM and associated rhythm disturbance.
- Are there signs of heart disease – dyspnoea, decreased activity?
- Is the cat urinating?
- Are there signs of other systemic diseases?
- Is the cat on any form of drug therapy, nutritional or herbal supplement?
- Access to toxins.
- History or evidence of trauma.

2.3.4 Focus of physical examination
- Signs of other systemic diseases.
- Cardiac auscultation.
- Pulse rate, quality and synchrony with heart.
- Jugular distension or pulse.

NB – *A regular rhythm does not exclude the possibility of an arrhythmia, e.g. third-degree AV block.*

2.3.5 Decision making
- Is the arrhythmia incidental?
- Should I investigate further or monitor?

2.3.6 Diagnostic approach (Table 14 page 40–41)
- ECG – see Section 4.2.3 for tips on obtaining ECGs from cats:
  - 24-hour Holter monitoring if arrhythmia intermittent or when paper trace ECG felt to be non-representative.
  - ECG response to vagal manoeuvre or drugs (e.g. atropine).
- Cardiac troponin I (muscular damage) and NT-proBNP (volume loading).
- Thoracic radiography – cardiac vs. pulmonary disease.
- Exclude non-cardiogenic disease as a cause of the arrhythmia.
- Haematology, biochemistry, urinalysis.
- Echocardiography.

2.3.7 Management and therapy

Deciding when to treat an arrhythmia is not always clear-cut as the consequences of leaving the arrhythmia untreated and the effects of treatment are difficult to predict particularly as all anti-arrhythmic drugs are pro-arrhythmic too. Further, there are relatively few drugs for treating arrhythmias in cats that have been used with any frequency.

In general, treatment should be considered
- When the rhythm disturbance is causing significant clinical signs or haemodynamic instability:
  - Underlying disease such as an electrolyte disturbance should be treated and anti-arrhythmic drugs only used if the rhythm disturbance might cause circulatory collapse before treatment of the primary condition has had time to be effective.

Table 15 Common cardiac and non-cardiac causes of arrhythmias in cats

Cardiac	Hypoxic	Autonomic	Metabolic/endocrine	Electrolyte	Drugs/toxins
Cardiomyopathy	Anaemia	CNS neoplasia	Acid/base	Hypercalcaemia	Virtually anything
Endocarditis	Diaphragm dysfunction	Fever/hyperthermia	Hyperthyroidism	Hypocalcaemia	Electric shock
Mechanical irritation	Pulmonary parenchymal disease	Raised intracranial pressure	Hyperviscosity	Hyperkalaemia	
Ischemia	Pulmonary shunting	Pain, stress, fear	Hypothermia	Hypokalaemia	
Myocarditis	Hypotension	Vomiting	Pancreatitis	Hypomagnesaemia	
Neoplasia	Pleural disease	Dysautonomia	Diabetes mellitus		
Trauma	Shock		Sepsis		
Valvular disease	Thromboemboli		Splenic disease		
Fibrosis of conduction pathways	Upper respiratory tract obstruction		Uraemia		
Heartworm (not UK)					

CLINICAL SIGNS

- Where if left untreated the rhythm disturbance is likely to cause tachycardia-induced cardiomyopathy.
- Where the rhythm disturbance is intermittent but clinical signs are severe and potentially life-threatening when they occur.
- Where the patient is relatively unstable and the rhythm disturbance shows features that tend to be associated with deterioration such as multiform ventricular ectopic beats, R-on-T.

2.4 ASCITES AND PERITONEAL EFFUSIONS

2.4.1 Introduction

Peritoneal effusions describe the accumulation of fluid within the peritoneal space; ascites refers to the presence of a serous transudate usually of hepatic or cardiac origin. Some other causes of abdominal enlargement, e.g. organomegaly, can have features similar to free fluid (see Section 2.1).

2.4.2 Causes

- Transudate.
- Exudate.
- Chyle.
- Bile.
- Urine.
- Blood.

2.4.3 Key history

- Speed of onset.
- Other clinical signs.
- History of trauma.
- Ability to urinate/dysuria.
- Dyspnoea or tachypnoea.
- Petechiation or ecchymosis.
- Oedema.
- Changes in activity/exercise.

2.4.4 Focus of physical examination

Establish that abdominal enlargement is due to fluid.

Cardiovascular system especially jugular vein.

2.4.5 Decision making

Fluid suspected on history and physical examination with a positive fluid thrill on ballottement.

The presence of fluid generally demands further investigation. The speed with which this is appropriate will depend on the clinical status of the cat. Many cats with serous transudates appear remarkably well and investigations can proceed in a stepwise fashion.

2.4.6 Diagnostic approach

- Where the volume of fluid is relatively small, effusions can be a radiologic/ultrasonographic finding without discernible clinical signs.
- Diagnostic abdominocentesis (if there is no evidence for a coagulopathy):
  ○ Submit fluid for protein analysis (total proteins, albumin, globulin, A:G ratio), lipids (triglyceride and cholesterol), cytology and culture – see Table 16.
  ○ Urine suspected – creatinine level relative to plasma.
- In small-volume effusions, ultrasound guidance may be required or abdominal lavage (cytology and culture only) necessary:
  ○ Abdominal lavage – instil 20 ml/kg of warm saline, move gently around the abdomen and aspirate.
- Abdominal ultrasound usually more valuable than radiography. If there are moderate-to-large amounts of free fluid ultrasound interpretation can be more difficult.

Further diagnostics

- Thoracic radiography – there are far fewer conditions that cause a bi-cavity effusion making the diagnostic root more simple

- Routine haematology, biochemistry, urinalysis and retrovirus serology.
- Echocardiography – approximately 5% of cats with heart disease present with abdominal fluid.
- Exploratory laparotomy/guided biopsy.

2.4.7 Management and therapeutic approach

Will depend heavily on cause (see Section 2.3.7). In many cases, drainage will provide temporary relief (see also 2.1.7) but should generally be avoided if there is haemoabdomen.

2.4.8 Specific conditions

Uroabdomen

Usually occurs as a result of blunt trauma but can rarely occur secondarily to obstruction, neoplasia or ureteric rupture.

Iatrogenic
- Excess pressure during manual evacuation of the bladder.
- Following cystocentesis.
- Penetration of the bladder or transection of the ureter during abdominal surgery.

The urethra is retroperitoneal and will not cause uroabdomen; urethral rupture causes urine to leak subcutaneously and is usually associated with overlying skin necrosis.

NB – *Apparent urination does not exclude the possibility of uroabdomen.*

Clinical signs
- Relatively sudden onset of ascites.
- Cat usually systemically unwell – dull, depressed, lethargic.

Diagnosis
- Imaging ± contrast (retrograde urethrogram).

- Abdominocentesis – straw to bloody fluid, usually negative on culture, creatinine levels > blood and similar to urine but dependent on length of time the uroabdomen has been present.

Therapeutic approach
- Prognosis depends on degree of damage.
- If bladder is extensively damaged, euthanasia may be necessary.
- If a bladder present on imaging then
  ○ Appropriate fluid therapy.
  ○ Drain abdomen and lavage.
  ○ Place indwelling catheter.
  ○ Most cats can be managed conservatively; frequently the point of leakage is not evident on exploratory laparotomy.

Bile peritonitis
- Rare.
- Usually secondary to bile duct obstruction but can occur as a result of trauma.
- Bile sludging with cholangiohepatitis.
- Choleliths.
- Neoplasia – primary or pancreatic.
- Pancreatic inflammation.
- Bile duct stricture.
- Iatrogenic following bile sampling especially at laparotomy.

Clinical presentation
- Abdominal swelling.
- Pain.
- Jaundice.

Management
- Ultrasound to assess the gall bladder, bile duct and for evidence of neoplasia.
- Routine biochemistry.
- Thoracic radiography.
- Aggressive supportive care and usually surgical intervention is required.
- If neoplasia is present the prognosis is extremely poor.
- Post-surgical complications are common.

CLINICAL SIGNS

Haemoabdomen

There is usually no need to directly treat the haemoabdomen unless bleeding is continuing in which case coagulopathies should be ruled out and the patient stabilised prior to considering surgical exploration. In emergency situations, the peritoneal blood can be used for an auto-transfusion but lacks clotting factors. Abdominal bandaging may be helpful if there is continued slow bleeding.

Transudates, exudates and chyle (Table 16)

Pure transudate

Results from hypoalbuminaemia (see Section 3.15) or portal hypertension. Usually albumin is <12 g/l but effusions will occur at high levels if portal hypertension accompanies hypoalbuminaemia.

Modified transudate

These can result from a wide range of pathophysiologic processes but generally due to increased vascular permeability secondary to an inflammatory response or increased hydrostatic pressure.
- Portal hypertension.
- Abdominal neoplasia.
- Chylous effusions.
- Right-sided heart failure (including pericardial effusion).
- Inflammatory disease.
- Uroabdomen.
- Bile peritonitis.
- Idiopathic.
- Torsion.
- Pancreatitis.

Exudate

Result from vasculitis or severe inflammation.

Non-septic
- High protein content with relatively low cell numbers, degenerate neutrophils not a feature, no bacteria present.

NB – *Bacteria can be difficult to confidently exclude on cytology, so non-septic exudates should always be submitted for culture.*

- Feline infectious peritonitis (FIP).
- Lymphocytic cholangitis.
- Amyloidosis – can also cause haemoabdomen.

Septic
- High protein and cells, degenerate neutrophils, bacteria present.
- Penetrating wound.
- Intestinal perforation.
- Ruptured pyometra.
- Abscess.

Bi-cavity effusions

These suggest a systemic inflammatory process, most commonly associated with neoplasia.
- Neoplasia.
- FIP.
- Congestive heart failure.
- Eosinophilic disease.

Portal hypertension

Usually secondary to increased resistance to blood flow through the liver due to hepatocyte swelling or fibrosis, but can occur following a portal thromboembolus. Can be a pure or modified transudate depending on the site of pathology.

Diagnosis
- Biochemistry including dynamic bile acid testing.
- Ultrasound of liver and portal vein with Doppler.

Table 16 Characteristics of common peritoneal effusions

	Nucleated cells ($\times 10^9$/l)	Protein (g/l)	Cytology
Transudates			
Pure	<1.0	<25	Usually few present
Modified	0.5–5.0	25–50	Mixed population of mesothelial and red and white cells
Haemorrhagic	>1.0	>30	Similar to blood usually without platelets – compare fluid PCV with blood PCV
Chyle	Variable	>25	Milky with primarily mature lymphocytes; neutrophil and macrophage numbers increase with chronicity
Exudates			
Non-septic	>5.0	>30	Neutrophils and macrophages without bacteria. Depending on cause, neoplastic cells may be seen
Septic	>5.0	>30	Bacteria present, neutrophils often degenerate
Bile	>5.0	>30	As for non-septic often with bilirubin crystals in macrophages

CLINICAL SIGNS

2.5 ATAXIA

2.5.1 Introduction

Ataxia refers to a gross lack of coordination of muscle movements due to neurologic disease resulting in an abnormal gait; superficially, this can appear similar to muscular stiffness (see section 2.39) and weakness (paresis/paralysis [see section 2.31]). In reality, ataxia is often used to describe any uncoordinated gait regardless of origin as cause is unknown.

The list below is not exhaustive; the key objective is to define the site affected. Localisation of a lesion can be difficult as cats are often reluctant to walk in the consulting room and can provide conflicting neurological assessments on a day-to-day basis.

2.5.2 Causes

Non-neurologic causes
• Joint disease.
• Cardiorespiratory insufficiency.
• Anaemia.
• Hyperviscosity.

• Metabolic – hypokalaemia, hypocalcaemia, hypoglycaemia.
• Myopathies.
• Myasthenia gravis.
• Shock.
• Sedative drugs and intoxicants, e.g. cannabis.

Neurologic causes

Cerebral ataxia
Primarily abnormal posture but some gait abnormalities present.
• Degenerative – ischaemic encephalopathy.
• Space-occupying lesions – neoplasia.
• Trauma.

Vestibular ataxia
Circling, head tilt (unless bilateral), loss of balance, nystagmus.

Nystagmus
• Slow phase away from lesion.
• Vertical nystagmus indicates central vestibular disease, proprioceptive deficits usually present.

Causes of nystagmus
- Physiologic horizontal nystagmus is normal in Siamese.
- Congenital disease – reported Siamese and Burmese.
- Peripheral and central vestibular disease.

Peripheral vestibular disease
- Idiopathic (40%).
- Otitis media/interna (40%).
- Neoplasia.
- Ototoxicity – aminoglycosides, furosemide.

Acquired central vestibular disease
- Degenerative – thiamine.
- Inflammatory (45%) – FIP (10%), *Toxoplasma* (5%), Cryptococcosis, bacterial otitis interna (15%).
- Toxic – lead.
- Space-occupying lesion (30%).
- Vascular disease (10%).
- Trauma.
- Feline ischaemic encephalopathy.

Cerebellar ataxia
- Associated with intention tremor, dysmetria/hypermetria, wide-base stance and gait.
- Congenital hypoplasia – feline parvovirus (FPV).
- Acquired – as for central vestibular disease.

Spinal cord lesions
The cat is cranially normal, lesion localisable to spinal cord region. UMN signs – lesion is C1–C5; T3–L2. UMN ± root signs – lesion is C6–T2; L3–S3. Lesions cause proprioceptive ataxia.

Causes
- Degenerative – intervertebral disc, fibrocartilaginous embolus.
- Inflammatory.

- Toxic – organophosphate/chloride poisoning.
- Space-occupying – neoplasia, disc disease, haemorrhage, hypervitaminosis A causing exostoses, osteomyelitis.
- Trauma.

Peripheral neuropathies
- Exostoses secondary to hypervitaminosis A.
- Ischaemic neuropathy.
- Toxic.
- Multiple cartilaginous exostoses.
- Neoplasia.
- Trauma.
- Polyneuropathies.
- Botulism.

Progressive degenerative neuropathies in kittens
- See also Section 1.3.
- Large group of diseases, many are thought to have a hereditary basis.

2.5.3 Key history
- Diet.
- Access to toxins.
- Likelihood of trauma.
- Duration of clinical signs.
- Progression of disease.
- Mental status.

2.5.4 Focus of physical examination
Neurologic evaluation to decide on site of lesion.

Full ocular examination.

2.5.5 Decision making
- Based on the physical examination, what is the most likely site of the lesion?
- What further investigation is appropriate for the likely causes for that region?
- Have I excluded non-neurologic causes?

2.5.6 Diagnostic approach (see table 14 page 40–41)

Table 17   Suggested sequence of diagnostic tests

	Test	Rationale
Primary tests	Full haematology and biochemistry; Survey thoracic radiographs ± echocardiography	Rule out non-neurologic metabolic causes, anaemia and cardiovascular disease
Secondary tests	Radiography – bulla or spinal series Serology for retroviruses, coronavirus, *Cryptococcus*, *Toxoplasma*	Rule out peripheral vestibular disease or bony vertebral lesions and infectious causes of inflammation
Tertiary tests	Lead levels Myelography Cerebrospinal fluid, joint fluid analysis Advanced imaging CT or MRI Nerve/muscle biopsy Acetylcholine receptor antibody level	Tertiary diagnostics dependent on clinical presentation and results of physical examination and initial diagnostic testing

2.5.7 Management and therapy

Highly dependent on cause and many conditions are only amenable to palliative treatment.

2.5.8 Specific conditions

Idiopathic feline vestibular syndrome
Acquired syndrome of unknown cause, peracute onset, median age 4 years. Most commonly occurs in late summer and autumn. Lateralising lesion, the cat presents distressed, falling or rolling to that side (<10% cases are bilateral). Vocalisation is common. Horizontal or rotator nystagmus is present, which gradually resolves (over days). Treatment is ineffective, fluids may be required if the cat is unable to drink or eat, sedation may be appropriate in severely disorientated cases. Cases recover over 2–4 weeks although 25% have residual head tilt.

2.6 BEHAVIOURAL CHANGES

2.6.1 Introduction

It is outside the scope of this text to address behavioural problems in cats.

However, a number of systemic diseases can present as 'behavioural problems' and should be considered and ruled out prior to a behavioural approach.

2.6.2 Causes

Behavioural signs usually caused by organic disease
- Persistent circling.
- Aimless pacing.
- Head pressing/getting stuck.
- Inability to recognise owners and familiar objects.
- Dullness, depression and lethargy.
- Hiding.
- Sudden changes in appetite.
- Sudden onset of frequent urination.
- Faecal incontinence.
- Tremor.
- Apparent deafness.

Common medical conditions associated with behavioural changes
- Metabolic disease – uraemia, hepatic encephalopathy, DM.
- Electrolyte disturbances – sodium, potassium, calcium.
- Inflammatory disease.
- Infectious disease – FIP, FSE, rabies.

CLINICAL SIGNS

CLINICAL SIGNS

- Neoplasia.
- Hypertension.
- Hyperthyroidism
- Hypoxic states.
- Intoxicants – narcotics, carbon monoxide, ototoxic drugs.
- FLUTD (causing apparent inappropriate elimination).
- Dietary allergy.
- CNS disease – meningoencephalitis, neoplasia, epilepsy.

2.7 BLEEDING/ COAGULOPATHIES

2.7.1 Introduction
The ability to clot is a function of the vascular wall, platelets and coagulation cascade. Reserve capacity is large, hence cats presenting with a bleeding tendency will have severe compromise of one or more of these systems.

2.7.2 Causes
See Section 3.3.

2.7.3 Key history
- Was the bleeding spontaneous or did it follow trauma?
- Have previous episodes occurred?
- Has a bleeding tendency been noted during surgery?
- Access to toxins.
- Haematuria, melaena, haematemesis.
- Familial history.
- Breed.
- Is the bleeding localised or generalised?
- Other organ involvement.

2.7.4 Focus of physical examination
Mucous membranes and skin surface to evaluate evidence of bruising/bleeding.

Abdominal ballottement, thoracic auscultation and percussion to look for evidence of third spacing.

2.7.5 Decision making
- Is it bleeding from a single or multiple sites?
- Is the bleeding likely to be due to a localised problem, e.g. nasal tumour or a generalised coagulopathy, even though the bleeding may be localised at present?
- What type of bleeding is occurring – petechiation (usually platelets), ecchymosis or cavity bleeding (usually coagulation system)?
- Has the bleeding caused sufficient blood loss to require blood transfusion?
  - Is any form of surgical intervention appropriate/safe?

2.7.6 Diagnostic approach
- Full haematology including reticulocyte count.
- Biochemistry.
- Survey thoracic and abdominal radiographs.

NB – *A normal number of platelets does not rule out platelet problems (thrombocytopathy), which can be primary or more commonly acquired (due to coating of platelets, e.g. in myeloma, preventing them from functioning).*

- Spontaneous bleeding rarely occurs unless the platelet count is $<40 \times 10^9/l$, and usually much lower than this.
- Platelet count will fall as a result of haemorrhage, but rarely to a significant level. A mild thrombocytosis tends to occur following haemorrhage.
- Evaluation of haemostatic ability:
  - Whole blood clotting time – can be of limited value and tends to be unreliable.
  - Buccal mucosal bleeding time – a standardised test should be performed where possible. Care should be taken when blotting away bleeding not to disturb the clot being formed.

○ APTT – assess the intrinsic and final common pathway compared to a reference time – XII, XI, IX, VIII, X (V, II, I, XIII).
○ ACT – usually <65 seconds in cats; similar evaluation to APTT.
○ OSPT – extrinsic and final common pathway – VII, X (V, II, I, XIII).
○ Fibrin degradation products – evidence of activation of clotting cascade, DIC.
○ PIVKAs – proteins induced by vitamin K antagonists.
○ D-dimer – evidence of activation of clotting cascade, DIC.

2.7.7 Management and therapy
• Immediate care to replace lost circulating volume through cautious fluid resuscitation or blood transfusion:
○ All cats should have at least a type-matched transfusion.
○ Obtain diagnostic samples prior to giving fluids/blood products.
○ Vitamin K is rarely contraindicated.
○ If bleeding is localised then local intervention may be appropriate.
○ Consider pressure bandaging – rarely effective if there is a generalised coagulopathy.
• Long-term therapy requires diagnosis and disease-focused therapy where possible.

2.8 BODY ODOUR

2.8.1 Introduction
Since cats are generally fastidious about grooming, body odour is uncommon, but may be confused with halitosis or flatulence (see Section 2.18).

2.8.2 Causes
• Faecal or urine soiling.
• Odorous material on coat.
• Infected wound – cat bite abscess, open fracture, ulcerated neoplasm.

• Bacterial or fungal otitis externa.
• Pyoderma.
• Halitosis – primary oral disease, nasopharyngeal infection, e.g. foreign body, uraemia, ketoacidosis, bacterial bronchopneumonia, GI disease.

2.8.3 Key history
• How recently did the odour start?
• Was the onset acute or gradual?
• Is the cat well in itself with normal appetite, mastication and deglutition?
• Has the cat's grooming habits changed?
• Is water consumption normal?
• Has the owner noticed any lumps/bumps or areas the cat does not like having stroked?
• Is the cat coughing, sneezing, vomiting or has it a nasal discharge?
• Has the owner recently changed the cat's diet?
• Is the cat house soiling?

2.8.4 Focus of physical examination
• Evaluate breath for halitosis.
• Careful coat examination for surface chemical or soiling, abscesses and general level of grooming.
• Oral examination.

2.8.5 Decision making
• Where is the odour coming from – is the source easily identifiable?
• Is the odour localised or generalised?
• If there is a change in grooming habits, is this associated with an inability to groom (musculoskeletal disease) or lack of interest in grooming (systemically unwell, cognitive dysfunction, oral pain)?

2.8.6 Diagnostic approach
• Does bathing the cat remove the body odour and if so does it recur?
• Thorough surface examination including hair clipping if indicated.

CLINICAL SIGNS

- Oral and aural examination (may require sedation or anaesthesia) – include the nasopharynx if anaesthetised.

2.8.7 Management and therapy
- Bathing, clipping and lavage of superficial infection with appropriate antibacterial and/or antifungal use.
- Dietary change.
- Dental cleaning and prophylaxis.
- Management of other underlying diseases.

2.9 COLLAPSE, SYNCOPE AND WEAKNESS

2.9.1 Introduction
For an owner it may be difficult to distinguish these three conditions and they may form the progression of the clinical signs of a single disease process. Owners may also describe a cat that is weak as being lethargic. Collapse and weakness can be caused by a wide variety of disease processes whereas syncope (transient loss of consciousness) is usually due to inadequate cerebral oxygenation.

In many cases, collapse or weakness may be secondary to another clearly identified disease process, e.g. cardiovascular disease. This alternate root should be evaluated first to ascertain whether it is likely to cause the collapse seen or whether another, separate problem exists and the collapse needs to be investigated as a primary clinical sign.

Syncope is relatively rare in cats and usually due to a cardiac rhythm disturbance.

2.9.2 Causes
Broad categories of collapse are listed below but pain, stress and fever should also be considered. In geriatric cats, muscular weakness may be an age-related sign but may indicate underlying pathology such as osteoarthritic pain.

Cardiovascular
- Congestive failure.
- Thromboembolism.
- Rhythm disturbance – brady- or tachyarrhythmia.
- Obstruction to flow – aortic or pulmonic stenosis, severe LV outflow tract obstruction secondary to HCM.
- Pericardial tamponade.
- Hypertension.

Haematologic
- Anaemia.
- Major haemorrhage, e.g. trauma, coagulopathy.
- Hyperviscosity – polycythaemia, hypergammaglobulinaemia.

Musculoskeletal
- Fractures.
- Severe musculoskeletal pain, e.g. osteoarthritis.
- Myasthenia gravis.
- Luxating patella.
- Malnutrition causing severe cachexia and muscular weakness.

Metabolic
- Acid–base disorders.
- Hypovolaemia.
- Hypoglycaemia.
- Hypo- or hyperkalaemia.
- Hepatic encephalopathy.
- Hypocalcaemia.
- Phaeochromocytoma.

Neurologic
- Seizure.
- Intervertebral disc disease.
- Neurotoxins, e.g. organochloride.
- Narcolepsy.

Respiratory
- Allergic airway disease.
- Airway obstruction.
- Tracheal avulsion.
- Laryngeal paralysis.

Drugs

- Hypotensive agents, e.g. ACP, ACE inhibitors, beta-adrenergic blockers, diuretics.
- Pro-arrhythmic agents.
- Sedatives and anaesthetics (including non-prescribed drugs).

2.9.3 Key history

General

- Age of onset of clinical signs.
- Familial history.
- Drug use – flea sprays, wormers, herbal, etc.
- Access to toxins.

Specific – timing of episode

- Frequency.
- Duration.
- Are the episodes changing in frequency?
- Exercise status – on waking, at exercise.
- Association with eating – after fasting, on eating, after eating.
- What are the environmental conditions?

Specific – the episode itself

- Is there loss of consciousness?
- Does the cat choose to lie down (because of weakness) or does it fall over?
- Are there signs of respiratory distress?
- Are there any changes in the colour of the membranes?
- Is there muscular activity – tonic/clonic?

Specific – after the episode

- How long does it take for the cat to recover?
- Is the cat apparently completely normal immediately afterwards?
- Is there any 'postictal' behaviour?
- Is the cat normal between episodes?

2.9.4 Focus of physical examination

A full physical examination is mandatory with special attention being paid to the mucosal colour and cardiorespiratory and musculoskeletal systems. However, if the collapse is intermittent and the cat appears normal between episodes, then physical examination can be unrewarding when not collapsed. A full neurological examination should be carried out if routine findings are negative or unhelpful.

2.9.5 Decision making

Which is the most likely organ system to be involved?

- How can this best be investigated?
- Should more general tests be performed first (especially, if specific tests involve GA)?
- What is the likelihood of finding an answer?
- What is the likelihood of successful treatment?

2.9.6 Diagnostic approach

- Rule out metabolic and haematological causes.
- Survey thoracic and abdominal radiographs – mass lesions, cardiorespiratory disease, third-space fluid.
- Electrocardiography to look for a sustained rhythm disturbance or evidence of other cardiac diseases.
- If the collapse is intermittent, a 24-hour ambulatory ECG (Holter monitoring) may be helpful. Most devices are too heavy for cats to wear, so they need to be confined to a caged area, hence of limited value if the collapse is during exercise.
- Event monitors – most useful are implantable subcutaneous devices that can be externally interrogated following client activation and hold the ECG prior to and following collapse.
- Blood pressure.
- Skeletal radiographs – exclude severe osteoarthritis, fractures, destructive bone lesions.
- Arterial blood gas.

CLINICAL SIGNS

Specific tests
- Edrophonium (Tensilon) test – edrophonium can be difficult to obtain and results difficult to interpret.
- Acetylcholine receptor antibody for myasthenia.
- ACTH stimulation test – exclude hyper- and hypoadrenocorticism (both uncommon/rare in cats).
- Insulin measurement (when the cat is hypoglycaemic).
- EMG and muscle biopsy.

2.9.7 Management and therapy
- Management is very condition dependent.
- Few collapsing/syncopal cats will die when they collapse as generally collapse is a protective mechanism.
- Investigation of a single episode of collapse/syncope or weakness where the signs are no longer present is usually unrewarding.
- Low-grade but persistent signs of weakness should be investigated in a stepwise, logical fashion so that if progression occurs, baseline data are already available.

2.10 CARDIAC MURMURS

2.10.1 Introduction
Prevalence in healthy population is high largely due to HCM and the natural development of an increasing acute aortic angle with age that means murmurs can be created with firm stethoscope pressure. Approximately 0.2–1% of kittens are born with heart defects.

2.10.2 Causes
- Innocent – heard in kittens, intensity II/VI, early systolic ejection type, PMI mitral/aortic, radiate poorly, more pronounced during tachycardia.

- Functional (physiologic) usually high output states associated with marked sympathetic stimulation, soft low, grade early-mid systolic, ejection, PMI mitral/aortic valve:
  - Fever.
  - Anaemia.
  - Hyperthyroidism.
  - Portosystemic shunt.
- Congenital:
  - Mitral or tricuspid dysplasia.
  - VSD.
  - Aortic stenosis.
  - PDA.
  - Tetralogy of Fallot.
  - Persistent common AV canal.
- Acquired:
  - Hypertrophic cardiomyopathy due to LV outflow obstruction.
  - Arrhythmogenic right ventricular cardiomyopathy.
  - Papillary muscle enlargement.
  - Secondary to valvular incompetence (including dilated cardiomyopathy).
  - Dirofilaria.
  - Endocarditis.
- Respiratory.

2.10.3 Key history
Cats can hide the signs of cardiovascular disease; hence, careful questioning of the owner is essential with particular attention to levels of activity.
- Age, breed.
- When was the murmur detected?
- Murmurs in related cats.
- Travel abroad.
- Stature and growth.
- Signs of decompensated cardiac disease.
- Lethargy, inappetence, weight loss.
- Sleeping more.
- Dyspnoea.
- Collapse.
- Abdominal distension.

2.10.4 Focus of physical examination
Cardiac auscultation to define the murmur as accurately as possible.

Classification
- Intensity – grade 1–6.
- Point of maximum intensity.
- Radiation.
- Timing and duration.
- Pitch (frequency) and shape.
- Gallop (third heart sound S_3/S_4 combined).

NB1 – *In cats with tachycardic heart disease, timing, duration and shape can be difficult to define.*

NB2 – *Murmurs are often not valve associated (as in dogs), and loudest parasternally.*

NB3 – *Murmurs can be very rate responsive in cats varying considerably between examinations.*

- Pulse quality and synchrony.
- Heart rate and rhythm.
- Mucosal colour – pallor, cyanosis.
- Capillary refill time, warmth of extremities.
- Pulse quality and synchrony with heart rate.
- Respiratory rate, lung auscultation and percussion.
- Ascites or peripheral oedema.
- Hepatomegaly.
- Jugular pulse.
- Presence of goitre.

2.10.5 Decision making
- Is this likely to be an innocent murmur?
- Functional or primary cardiac?
- Likely cardiac structures involved?
- Is it a congenital defect?
- Is further investigation warranted – can I confidently tell how symptomatic the cat is and how quickly signs might progress?

- Is it a PDA (surgical option but rare)?
- Why does the client want to know?
- Why do I want to know?
- Are there signs of decompensated disease?

2.10.6 Diagnostic approach
- Haematology and biochemistry, particularly if extracardiac disease suspected:
  - Polycythaemia with right-to-left shunt.
  - Normoblasts – CHF without anaemia probably associated with erythropoietin stimulation due to mild hypoxia.
  - In significantly hypoproteinaemic cats, effusions may be non-cardiogenic.
  - Neutrophilia ± left shift, monocytosis, increased fibrinogen – suggest endocarditis.
  - Check renal function.
  - Increased liver enzymes due to congestion, hypoxia.
- BP
- Echocardiography.

NB – *Despite thorough echocardiography the source of a murmur in some cats can be elusive.*

- Angiography or other advanced imaging.
- Arterial blood gas analysis – difficult in conscious cats.

2.10.7 Management and therapy
Directed towards the underlying disease process where possible and the functional consequences of any cardiac pathology. There is no current evidence (but there have been no studies) demonstrating that early intervention in cats with asymptomatic murmurs associated with cardiac disease will delay the onset of clinical signs.

2.11 CONSTIPATION, TENESMUS AND DYSCHEZIA

2.11.1 Introduction

Definition
- *Constipation* – prolongation of intestinal transit time – faeces hard, dry and passed less frequently. Passage may be associated with tenesmus.
- *Obstipation* – intractable constipation – small amounts of liquid material may be passed around impacted faecal mass.
- *Megacolon* – dilated, hypomotile colon incapable of contracting and expelling faeces.
- *Tenesmus* – straining to pass faeces – needs to be differentiated from stranguria.
- *Dyschezia* – pain and difficulty when passing or attempting to pass faeces.

2.11.2 Causes

Table 18 Causes of constipation

Nutritional	Diet
	Ingestion of hair or small mammals/birds
	Pica – cat litter, wool
	Obesity
Behavioural – Environment causing failure to defaecate	Inclement weather
	Dirty litter tray or changes in cat litter
	Stressful surroundings
Pain	Pain/difficulty accessing litter tray/outdoors
	Orthopaedic disease – arthritis, trauma affecting spine, pelvis, hind limbs
Functional	Neuromuscular disease affecting colonic function
	Spinal or peripheral neuropathy
	Trauma – disc disease, 'tail pull'
	Dysautonomia
	Idiopathic megacolon (thought to be degenerative neuropathy)
Intraluminal obstruction	Colonic/rectal neoplasia
	Polyp
	Foreign body
	Stricture
Extraluminal obstruction	Narrowed pelvic canal
	Enlarged lymph nodes
	Anorectal/perianal abscess/swelling
	Perineal hernia
Metabolic	Hypokalaemia
	Hypocalcaemia
	Mixed
	Dehydration
Drug induced	Opiates
	Anticholinergics
	Aluminium/magnesium hydroxide, barium sulphate, sucralfate
	Antihistamines
	Adrenergic or calcium channel blockers
	Iron
	Benzodiazepines

CLINICAL SIGNS

Causes of constipation – Table 18
Causes of tenesmus and dyschezia

Similar to constipation in terms of luminal narrowing but also associated with inflammatory disease (colitis, IBD, proctitis, anal sacculitis) and perianal disease such as abscesses or fistulae.

2.11.3 Key history

- Duration.
- Is there tenesmus, dyschezia or haematochezia?
- Is the cat making any effort to defaecate?
- Recent changes in environment – moving house, new cats.
- History of trauma especially pelvic.
- Orthopaedic disease – lameness, pain on handling.
- Other clinical signs.
- Systemic disease causing dehydration, electrolyte imbalance.
- Other signs of dysautonomia – regurgitation, dilated pupils.
- Muscular weakness.
- What is the cat's diet? Is there pica?
- Previous hairball problems.
- Drug use.
- What do the faeces look like – thin, ribbon-like, small amounts of liquid both indicate obstruction?

2.11.4 Focus of physical examination

- Careful caudal abdominal palpation – degree of constipation, bladder size (rule-out urethral obstruction).
- Gait analysis, muscular tone, range of movement of joints and tail; symmetry of pelvis.
- Check for xerostomia (dry mouth) and tear production.
- Examination of the perianal region; kittens should always be checked to exclude atresia ani.

2.11.5 Decision making

- Severity of problem.
- Environmental changes necessary.

- Litter tray management
- Change in diet.

NB – *Diet cannot be used to treat constipation once it is present, but can be used to reduce recurrence once impacted faeces have been removed.*

- Is medical management appropriate – laxatives or enemas?

NB – *Toxicity of enemas – phosphate, glycerine.*

- Chronic laxative use, especially if paraffin-based, can lead to dietary deficiency especially fat-soluble vitamins.
- Is further investigation required?

2.11.6 Diagnostic approach (Table 14 page 40–41)

- Haematology, biochemistry, urinalysis:
  - Systemic disease, dehydration, electrolyte imbalance, renal function.
- Rectal examination.
- Imaging:
  - Plain radiography to identify extent of constipation.
  - An enema is often required to gain good detail of spine and pelvis, abdominal masses, etc.
  - Evidence for dysautonomia, e.g. megaoesophagus.
  - Contrast radiography:
    - Enema first.
    - Identify intraluminal obstruction.
  - Myelography, MRI, CT:
    - Suspected spinal disease.
- Endoscopy:
  - Proctoscopy/colonoscopy.
  - Good patient preparation essential – starve 24–48 hours, laxative (e.g. Klean prep), enema.
  - Rigid scopes fine for terminal colon.
  - Always biopsy.
  - Small intestinal endoscopy.
  - Some cases of IBD reported with megacolon.

CLINICAL SIGNS

- Intradermal histamine test – no reaction is supportive of dysautonomia.
- T_4/TSH stimulation test:
  - Hypothyroidism suspected, e.g. post-thyroidectomy, I^{131} treatment.

2.11.7 Management and therapy

Primary treatment of constipation will depend on the degree. Most cases require oral laxatives, enemas or manual evacuation.

Dietary decisions for preventing recurrence depend on cause with some cats responding better to low residue, single-source protein/hydrolysed diets rather than increasing fibre.

Resolving the underlying cause wherever possible carries the most favourable prognosis although some degree of colonic distension may remain.

Colectomy is not appropriate if obstructive causes are not managed first.

2.12 CHRONIC COUGHING

2.12.1 Introduction

Coughing is the sudden and often repetitive defence reflex, which helps to clear the large airways from excess secretions, irritants, foreign particles and microbes. Coughing is a protective, primitive reflex in healthy individuals. Chronic coughing is defined as a cough that is persistent or intermittent and of at least 3 weeks duration; frequently, there is poor response to symptomatic treatment.

A number of conditions can be mistaken for coughing by owners:

- Panting.
- Forced or laboured breathing.
- Wheezing.
- Reversed sneezing.
- Gagging.

- Retching.
- Attempts to vomit.

2.12.2 Causes

Coughing is generally caused by mechanical (foreign body or neoplasia), inflammatory or allergic disease.

- Nasopharyngeal:
  - Secretions draining backwards causing laryngeal/tracheal irritation.
  - Nasopharyngeal foreign body especially grass blades.
- Laryngeal:
  - Laryngospasm/oedema.
  - Paralysis.
  - Neoplasia – lymphoma is relatively common in cats.
- Tracheal (rare):
  - Foreign body.
  - Inflammatory mass.
  - Collapse.
  - Neoplasia.
- Small airways:
  - Airway inflammation and bronchoconstriction – allergic/inflammatory, eosinophilic.
  - Airway irritation.
  - Bronchopneumonia.
  - Bronchiectasis.
  - Parasitic infection (*Aelurostrongylus abstrusus*):
    - (Non-UK: *Eucoleus aerophilus*, paragonimiasis, *Troglostrongylus* sp., cuterebrosis, Capillaria – present in foxes in southern UK).
  - Fungal infection (*Cryptococcosis*):
    - (Non-UK: sporotrichosis, aspergillosis, histoplasmosis, blastomycosis, *Pneumocystis carinii*, coccidiodomycosis, *Paecilomyces lilacinus*).
  - Excessive airway secretion.
  - Ciliary abnormality (rare).
  - Dirofilaria *immitis* (heartworm: not UK).

NB – *Cats seem relatively insensitive to coughing associated with stimulation of pleural, mediastinal and pulmonary receptors; hence pleural effusions, masses in mediastinum (e.g. thymic lymphoma), megaoesophagus ± secondary aspiration pneumonia and cardiac disease rarely cause coughing.*

2.12.3 Key history
- Age, breed, sex:
  - Allergic airway disease in middle-aged Siamese cats.
  - Laryngeal paralysis more common in male cats.
- Duration of cough, is it becoming more frequent?
- Seasonality.
- Associated clinical signs – dyspnoea, lethargy, decreased exercise.
- Environment – exposure to chemicals, irritants, urban, rural, etc.
- Nature of cough:
  - Time of day.
  - Activity – at exercise, when stroking throat.
  - Single cough or paroxysmal.
  - Sound:
    - dry – inflammatory, allergic.
    - soft moist – pneumonia, allergic, parasitic.
  - Change in meow ⇒ laryngeal disease.
  - Terminal retching ⇒ inflammatory, allergic.
  - Productive – may bring up phlegm, but will often learn to swallow at the end of a coughing bout.

2.12.4 Focus of physical examination
Full evaluation of the upper and lower respiratory tract including presence of halitosis, tracheal pinch, thoracic auscultation, percussion and compression and nasal air flow.

2.12.5 Decision making
Based on the history and clinical findings, is the cough
- Primarily respiratory?
  - Airway disease (most common) or pulmonary (alveolar) disease?
- Secondary to other thoracic disease?
- Secondary to a systemic disease?

2.12.6 Diagnostic approach
- Owner diary and observation of pattern.
- Haematology – evidence of infection, eosinophilia.
- Biochemistry – low yield for cause; screening for older cats.
- Radiography:
  - Conscious/sedated first.
  - GA required for extubated larynx and inflated views.
  - VD, left and right lateral views.

NB1 – *VD view should be undertaken with great care in cats with respiratory compromise and in those cases, a DV view is safer.*
NB2 – *Artefact can be created if the cat has recently been in lateral recumbency prior to a VD/DV view.*

- Faecal flotation for parasites.
- Exclude FeLV/FIV as a contributing cause.
- Ultrasound of larynx.
- Examination of pharynx/larynx under anaesthesia.
- Bronchoscopy/examination of the oro- and nasopharynx:
  - Samples should always be taken – bronchoalveolar lavage, brushing submitted for cytology and culture. Biopsy for histopathology and electron microscopy.

○ Consider specialist culture/PCR for mycoplasma sp., fungal infection, mycobacteria, FHV-1.

NB1 – *Bacteria are rarely a primary cause of coughing in cats and usually occur secondary to another disease process. Exceptions include mycoplasma, mycobacterium,* Streptococcus equi subsp. zooepidemicus, Bordetella bronchiseptica.

NB2 – *Chlamydophila does very rarely cause respiratory infection and coughing.*

NB3 – *Biopsy of airway is usually unproductive unless for EM or a proliferative lesion is present.*

• CT or MRI, fluoroscopy if tracheal collapse suspected.

• Lung biopsy – Tru-cut, thoracoscopic or at thoracotomy.
• Arterial blood gas.
• Pulmonary function tests are currently being evaluated, but so far have been of limited clinical value.

2.12.7 Management and therapy

• Cough suppressants are rarely necessary or indicated, particularly if the cough is productive.
• Repeated attempts at symptomatic management are usually unsuccessful.
• Corticosteroids should be avoided until at least a working diagnosis has been established.

2.12.8 Approach to the coughing cat (Figure 6)

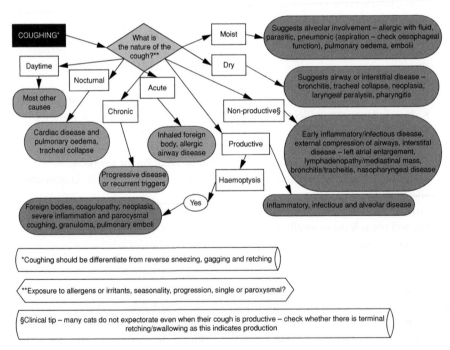

Figure 6 Approach to the coughing cat

2.13 DIARRHOEA

2.13.1 Introduction

Cats are less frequently presented with acute diarrhoea as they are less prone to scavenging; chronic diarrhoea may go unnoticed for sometime in cats that defaecate outside. Cats presenting for acute diarrhoea should be assessed and divided between those that are systemically well and likely to have self-limiting disease and those who are systemically unwell or have chronic diarrhoea and require further treatment/investigation.

2.13.2 Causes

- Diet:
  - Lactase deficiency.
  - Pharmacologically active ingredients in food, e.g. theophylline in chocolate.
  - Food preservatives and additives.
  - Food spoilage – bacteria or chemicals.
  - Preformed histamine in food (e.g. cheap canned fish).
  - Abrupt change in diet/dietary indiscretion.
  - Immediate-type dietary allergy.
  - Gluten-sensitive enteropathy.
  - Dietary hypersensitivity.
- Small bowel disease:
  - Inflammatory – lymphoplasmacytic, eosinophilic, granulomatous.
  - Viral infection – FPV, FeLV, FIV, FIP, rotavirus.
  - Parasitic – *Strongyloides* spp., *Toxocara* spp., *Toxascaris leonina*.
  - Protozoans – *Giardia lamblia*, *Toxoplasma gondii*, *Cryptosporidium* spp., *Isospora* spp., *Tritrichomonas*.
  - Foreign body especially partially obstructing linear.
  - Neoplastic – lymphoma, adenocarcinoma (plasmacytoma, leiomyoma, leiomyosarcoma, haemangiosarcoma).
  - Intussusception.
  - Bacterial infection – *Salmonella* spp., *Campylobacter jejuni*, *Clostridium difficile*.
  - Intestinal stricture, e.g. post-surgical, sharp foreign body.
  - Lymphangiectasia.
  - Intestinal volvulus.
  - Small intestinal bacterial dysbiosis – secondary to another disease.
- Large bowel diarrhoea:
  - Diet related.
  - Bacterial infection – see small intestinal causes.
  - Protozoan – *Giardia lamblia*.
  - Inflammatory – see small intestinal causes, ulcerative.
  - Neoplastic – see small intestinal causes.
  - Foreign body.
  - Intussusception – ileocolic, caecal.
- Altered bowel motility, e.g. nictitating membrane protrusion and diarrhoea syndrome.
- Non-gastrointestinal abdominal disease:
  - Pancreatitis.
  - Peritonitis.
  - (Exocrine pancreatic insufficiency).
- Congenital anomalies – short bowel syndrome:
- Post-surgical.
  - Extensive resection.
  - Adhesions.
  - Stricture.
  - Colectomy.
  - Loss of ileocolic valve.
- Toxicities:
  - Heavy metals.
  - Drugs.
  - Insecticides.
- Systemic disease:
  - Hyperthyroidism.
  - FIP.
  - Renal failure.
  - FeLV.
  - (Hypoadrenocorticism).

CLINICAL SIGNS

CLINICAL SIGNS

2.13.3 Key history
- Age, breed:
  - Young animals more likely to be infectious; IBD more common in middle-aged cats. Maine Coons over-represented with IBD.
- Acute or chronic signs.
- Is the cat vomiting?
- Vaccination and worming status.
- Diarrhoea in other pets, humans.
- Drug use.
- Access to outside – toxins, dietary indiscretion.
- Diet – general history and recent changes.
- Signs triggered by particular foodstuffs imply intolerance. *But* allergic disease is not associated with recent change in diet.
- Appetite – increased in malabsorption/maldigestion when cat is well, e.g. IBD, hyperthyroidism, EPI.
- Weight loss/poor growth.
- Does the diarrhoea respond to starvation?
- Character of stool:
  - Traditional characterisation into large and small bowel diarrhoea on frequency, volume, consistency, less useful in cats.
  - Enterocolitis common, giving mixed signs.
- Likelihood (previous history) of foreign body ingestion.
- Signs of systemic illness.

2.13.4 Focus of physical examination
Abdominal palpation and auscultation.

2.13.5 Decision making
- Is it primarily a GIT problem or is the diarrhoea associated with systemic disease?
- If the cat is systemically well, is the diarrhoea likely to be self-limiting?
- If there is weight loss, is it likely to be due to reduced intake (loss <1–2%/week)

or is there evidence of hypermetabolism/nutrient loss?
- Has previous symptomatic treatment been given (and failed) indicating further investigation necessary?
- Has the cat recently received appropriate anti-parasitic treatment?
- Has an appropriate dietary trial been conducted?

NB – *Some constipated cats with luminal obstruction will only produce small amounts of watery faeces that can be misinterpreted as the cat having diarrhoea.*

2.13.6 Diagnostic approach (Table 17 page 40–41)
Primary investigations
- Faecal culture and parasitology.
- Trial therapy with metronidazole, fenbendazole to exclude giardiasis.
- Dietary trial – exclusion or hypoallergenic diet.

NB – *Needs to be properly conducted with diet and water alone for a sufficient period of time. If there is no response within 2 weeks, dietary therapy is unlikely to be effective. If there is a partial response, a longer trial period may be needed.*

Secondary investigations
- Serology – FeLV, FIV, *Toxoplasma*.
- Biochemistry and haematology – to exclude systemic disease.
- T_4 estimation.
- Feline TLI test (NB – EPI is rare in cats) and pancreatic specific lipase.
- Folate and cobalamin (B_{12}) – interpretation less well established in cats, *but* if cobalamin is low, response to other therapies may be reduced.
- Survey thoracic and abdominal radiographs.
- Ultrasound of intestine, pancreas.

Tertiary investigations
- Biopsy – endoscopic, laparoscopic or full thickness at exploratory laparotomy.
- Other endocrine testing.
- Intestinal function tests – breath hydrogen, differential sugar absorption, duodenal juice culture, serum IgA estimation.

2.13.7 Management and therapy

Non-specific management – cat is bright and systemically well with a reasonably good appetite and the cause is likely to be self-limiting, e.g. sudden change of diet. Signs should resolve within 72–96 hours.
- *Watchful waiting* – effective in many cases but needs a clear time boundary if signs are not resolving and risks the owner deciding to self-medicate the cat.
- *Starvation* – frequently used but there is no clear evidence of value and a small risk that if the diarrhoea is recurrent the owner may use multiple periods of starvation that potentially cause significant weight loss and malnutrition.
- *Feeding a bland diet* – this should be small quantities of highly digestible low-fat food but has to be weighed against the potential negative effects of sudden dietary change.
- *Pro- and prebiotics* – potentially beneficial in shortening the period of diarrhoea and is an appropriate first-choice therapy in most cases.
- *Kaolin-based demulcents and absorbents* – no clear benefit or harm; can be difficult to administer in some cats.
- *Electrolytes* – unpalatable to many cats; if used, the cat should always have an alternative water source available to prevent dehydration worsening their condition.
- Vitamin supplements – no clear benefit or harm although some are beef-based and may cause problems if the diarrhoea is due to dietary hypersensitivity.
- *Avoid* – antimicrobials, glucocorticoids or NSAIDs unless specifically indicated.
- *Avoid* – unknown, untried or untested herbal and nutritional supplements.

For treatment and management of individual diseases see Section 4.3

2.14 DYSPHAGIA

2.14.1 Introduction

Dysphagia – difficulty in swallowing.

Three phases to swallowing – *oropharyngeal, pharyngeal* and *oesophageal* requiring coordinated muscular activity. Dysphagia can affect any one (or more than one) of these phases.

Oropharyngeal dysphagia

Oropharyngeal dysphagia are diseases affecting prehension of food, formation of a bolus and voluntary transfer to the oropharynx. Typical clinical signs include exaggerated chewing movements and quidding. Cats may adopt bizarre head positions. It is usually associated with an increase in appetite with weight loss.

Pharyngeal dysphagia

Pharyngeal dysphagia is the inability to coordinate swallowing to move the bolus of food into the oesophagus. Typical signs include repeated swallowing efforts, gagging and aspiration pneumonia. Initially most cats have an increased appetite but with time the appetite diminishes. Some cats will ask for food then back away as if it hurts once they try to eat.

Oesophageal dysphagia

Oesophageal function is abnormal so the bolus fails to move caudally into the stomach. Typical signs include regurgitation, discomfort after eating, increased appetite, an expanding soft mass at the thoracic inlet after eating and aspiration pneumonia.

CLINICAL SIGNS

2.14.2 Causes

Oral cavity disease – common:
- Dental/periodontal disease/pain.
- Gingivitis/stomatitis.
- Mandibular/maxillary pain or dysfunction.
- Eosinophilic granuloma.
- Neoplasia.
- Foreign body, e.g. embedded needle, linear material around the base of tongue.
- Retrobulbar masses.
- Cleft palate.
- Trauma causing a palate defect.

Disorders of the tongue – uncommon:
- Glossitis.
- Ulceration.
- Wound.
- (Neurologic (usually bilateral) – CN XII).
- (Neoplasia – squamous cell sarcoma).

Pharyngeal dysfunction – uncommon → rare:
- Polyps.
- Neoplasia.
- Lymphadenomegaly.
- Tonsillar enlargement.
- Salivary gland enlargement.
- Foreign body.
- (CN IX or X dysfunction).
- (Botulism).
- (Rabies).

Laryngeal disease – uncommon → rare:
- Paralysis.
- Inflammatory.
- Neoplasia – lymphoma.

Retropharyngeal disease – uncommon:
- Foreign body.
- Neoplasia.
- Lymphadenomegaly.
- Temporomandibular joint dysfunction/pain.
- Salivary gland disease.

Oesophageal disease – common:
- Megaoesophagus – uncommon:
  - Idiopathic.
  - Myopathy.
  - Dysautonomia.
  - Myasthenia gravis.
  - Myositis.
  - Oesophageal diverticulum.
  - Toxins.
  - (Endocrinopathy – hypoadrenocorticism, hypothyroidism).
- Oesophagitis – common:
  - Reflux.
  - Repeated vomiting.
  - Post-anaesthetic.
  - Drugs – doxycycline, NSAIDs, clindamycin.
  - Foreign body.
  - Toxic/irritant.
- Intraluminal obstruction – uncommon → rare:
  - Stricture – post-oesophagitis or surgery.
  - Foreign body.
  - (Inflammatory).
  - (Neoplasia).
- Extraluminal compression – uncommon → rare:
  - Mediastinal neoplasia mass.
  - Granulomas.
  - Lymphadenomegaly.
  - Cervical neoplasia mass.

Gastro-oesophageal junction – uncommon → rare:
- Hiatal hernia.
- Gastro-oesophageal intussusception.
- Neoplasia.

2.14.3 Key history
- Duration and progression.
- Associated clinical signs – retching, coughing, vomiting, regurgitation, ptyalism, nasal discharge, dyspnoea.
- Appetite especially at the start of signs.
- Describe eating behaviour – video.

- Is there a difference in ability to swallow solids vs. liquids?
- History of trauma, foreign body ingestion.
- Change in meow.
- Exercise tolerance/activity level.
- Weakness.
- Access to drugs/toxins/irritants.
- Constipation.

2.14.4 Focus of physical examination
- Oral examination.
- Head and neck.
- Thoracic palpation, auscultation and compression.
- Neurological and muscular examination.
- Observe the cat eating and drinking.

2.14.5 Decision making
- What type of dysphagia is present?
- Do I need to observe the cat eating before formulating a diagnostic plan?
- Is there evidence of aspiration pneumonia or dyspnoea that requires treatment?
- If fluoroscopy is indicated will it be possible and do I need to refer?

2.14.6 Diagnostic approach
- Haematology, biochemistry:
  ○ Rule out systemic disease.
  ○ Evidence for inflammation, infection or intercurrent disease.
  ○ Toxicology – lead, acetylcholine esterase activity (reduced if organophosphate poisoning).
- Serology – retrovirus, endocrine function, acetylcholine receptor antibody.
- Neurologic examination with advanced imaging if appropriate.
- Radiography – sedated for thorax, anaesthetise for head, neck and pharynx.
- Ultrasound – structures of head and neck, larynx, mediastinum.
- Laryngoscopy.
- Fluoroscopy – liquid and food.
- Endoscopic examination and biopsy.

- Dietary trial – consider the following factors:
  ○ Consistency.
  ○ Food type – kibble, liquid.
  ○ Feed from height.

NB – *Great care needs to be taken when anaesthetising or heavily sedating a cat with a known or suspected megaoesophagus due to the risks of reflux and aspiration.*

2.14.7 Management and therapy
- Directed towards primary cause if this is treatable.
- Dependent on the site and severity of the condition.
- During the workup and initial treatment, it is important to ensure adequate hydration and nutrition
  ○ appropriate diet type and consistency, feeding position.
  ○ may necessitate placement of a feeding tube – site of tube dependent on whether dysphagia is oral, pharyngeal or oesophageal.
- Educating owners as to the signs associated with aspiration pneumonia.
- Prognosis for many conditions listed in Section 2.14.2 is guarded to poor.

2.15 DYSPNOEA (RESPIRATORY DISTRESS)

2.15.1 Introduction
Common emergency presentation in cats with a very varied prognosis dependent on cause. Dyspnoeic cats are physiologically unstable and should be very carefully handled to minimise stress.
- *Dyspnoea* – sensation of breathlessness (difficult to evaluate in animals) seen as an increased respiratory effort and distress, i.e. laboured breathing.
- *Tachypnoea* – increased respiratory rate.

CLINICAL SIGNS

CLINICAL SIGNS

- *Hyperpnoea* – increased rate and depth of breathing (but not to the point of dyspnoea).
- *Orthopnoea* – dyspnoea associated with abnormal posture – sternal recumbency, elbows abducted, neck extended and mouth breathing.
- *Restrictive pattern* – rapid shallow breathing often with considerable abdominal effort suggests thoracic wall pain/trauma, pleural disease.

NB – *Cats do not tend to mouth breathe until they have severe respiratory compromise.*

Dyspnoea results from either a decreased ventilatory capacity or an increased ventilatory demand (e.g. hypoxia, acidosis, hypercapnia).

2.15.2 Causes

Causes of dyspnoea can be divided into three major (patho)physiologic groups or by underlying cause:
- *Physiologic dyspnoea* – occurs at exercise.
- *Pulmonary dyspnoea* – due to decreased effective lung volume or decreased functional capacity (e.g. fibrosis).
- *Circulatory dyspnoea* – inadequate oxygen delivery from the lungs to the tissues including anaemia.

Underlying cause

Non-respiratory:
- Cardiovascular disease:
  - Anaemia.
  - Polycythaemia.
  - Congestive heart failure.
  - Hypotension (shock).
  - Right-to-left shunting cardiovascular defect.
- Abdominal enlargement.
- Hyperthermia.
- Metabolic acidosis.

- Severe pain – usually tachypnoeic unless the pain is associated with thoracic wall structures.
- Muscle weakness, affecting diaphragm and/or intercostals, i.e. myopathy/ neuropathy.
- (Fear/anxiety – tachypnoea).

Upper respiratory tract disease:
- Rhinitis – infectious or inflammatory.
- Foreign body.
- Nasopharyngeal polyps.
- Neoplasia.
- Laryngeal paralysis/neoplasia/oedema (uncommon).
- Congenital/acquired disease of the nares.
- Tracheal disease (rare) – foreign body, oedema, neoplasia.

Lower respiratory tract disease:
- Bronchial disease:
  - Chronic bronchitis.
  - Feline 'asthma'.
- Diseases of the lungs:
  - Bronchopneumonia.
  - Neoplasia.
  - Pulmonary contusion (trauma).
  - Inflammatory lung disease.
  - Atelectasis.
  - Pulmonary emphysema.
  - Pulmonary embolus.
  - Idiopathic fibrosis (uncommon).
- Parasitic – *Aelurostrongylus abstrusus* (relatively common, but of low pathogenicity).
- Toxins, e.g. paraquat (rare).

Thoracic cavity disease:
- Pneumothorax.
- Thoracic effusion:
  - Pyothorax (thoracic empyema).
  - FIP-exudative pleurisy.
  - Haemothorax.
  - Chylothorax.
  - Hydrothorax, e.g. hypoproteinaemia, heart failure.

- Ruptured diaphragm.
- Pericardioperitoneal diaphragmatic hernia (uncommon).
- Mediastinal disease:
  - Neoplasia (lymphosarcoma/thymoma, etc.).
  - Pneumomediastinum (uncommon).
- Thoracic wall abnormality:
  - Pectus excavatum (common but rarely clinically significant).
  - Flat chest (common in some breeds, e.g. Burmese).
  - Neoplasia affecting soft tissue or ribs (rare).
- Thoracic wall trauma:
  - Pain.
  - Fractured ribs.
  - Torn intercostal muscles.
  - Flail chest.

2.15.3 Key history

- Age and breed, e.g. flat-chested Burmese kittens.
- Travel abroad (rule out heartworm, babesiosis).
- Duration, onset and progression of signs.
- History of trauma.
- Previous episodes of cardiorespiratory disease.
- Associated signs or pre-existing medical problems.
- Coughing.
- Change in meow.
- Stridor.
- Exposure to toxins, irritants, allergens, electrical wires.
- Respiratory signs in other animals/ people in the household.

2.15.4 Focus of physical examination

- Observation of respiratory pattern from a distance – stance, mouth breathing, characteristics of breathing pattern.
- Listen to the cat's breathing – stridor, snoring, snuffles, rattles (indicates nasal, nasopharyngeal or laryngeal disease).
- Mucous membrane colour and oral examination.
- Palpation of nares, trachea and larynx, thorax.
- Check airflow through nostrils onto a glass slide/moving a tiny piece of cotton wool.
- Thoracic auscultation, percussion and compression.
- Evidence of non-respiratory disease, e.g. trauma, goitre, ascites.

NB – *As cats do not mouth breathe readily, nasal disease can cause significant dyspnoea.*

2.15.5 Decision making (Figure 7)

- Is the dyspnoea respiratory or non-respiratory?
- If the dyspnoea is respiratory is it upper (nares → main bronchi) or lower (smaller airways → alveoli)?
- Is the dyspnoea being caused by pleural space disease?
- If URT, is the dyspnoea relieved on open-mouth breathing?
- How unstable is the cat?
- Should rest and oxygen be given immediately?
- How safe are further diagnostic tests?
- How am I going to perform further diagnostics?

2.15.6 Diagnostic approach

- Radiography – thoracic radiographs are mandatory at an early stage of investigation.

NB1 – *Great care needs to be taken when handling dyspnoeic cats as they often have very little respiratory reserve. If demand is significantly increased (due to stress of handling, examination, procedures), sudden death can occur.*

NB2 – *VD projections should be avoided in very dyspnoeic animals.*

CLINICAL SIGNS

CLINICAL SIGNS

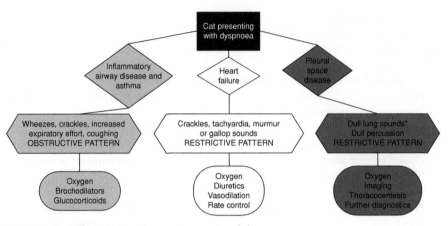

Figure 7 Differentiating the major causes of dyspnoea
*except if pneumothorax

- Thoracocentesis – diagnostic and therapeutic.
- Test of pulmonary function:
  - Pulse oximetry.
  - End tidal capnography.
  - Arterial blood gas analysis (difficult).
- Tests of cardiac function:
  - Blood pressure.
  - Cardiac troponin I and proBNP.
- Haematology, biochemistry and urinalysis to exclude systemic disease.
- Serology – FeLV, FIV, coronavirus, toxoplasmosis.
- Ultrasound of thorax – heart, pleural space (if effusion), non-aerated lung (collapse, mass).
- Laryngoscopy, laryngeal ultrasound.
- Computed tomography provides significantly improved sensitivity and three-dimensional sense.
- Bronchoscopy/rhinoscopy with lavage, cytology brushing, biopsy, culture.

2.15.7 Management and therapy
Management of acutely dyspnoeic cat:
- Cage rest and oxygen.
- Pleural effusion suspected – blind or ultrasound-guided thoracocentesis.

- Warming and blood pressure support (care if in CHF).
- Assess need for pain relief – opiates generally indicated.
- Drug treatment directed towards cause – diuretics, bronchodilation, blood transfusion.

2.15.8 Approach to the dyspnoeic cat
(See figure 1)

2.16 DYSURIA

2.16.1 Introduction
Key decision – Are the cat's clinical signs associated with obstruction or not?
- *Dysuria* – painful or difficult urination.
- *Pollakiuria* – passing frequent, small quantities of urine.
- *Stranguria* – straining or hesitancy prior to, during or after urination.

2.16.2 Causes
Inflammatory:
- Infectious – bacteria, *Candida*, *Capillaria feliscati*, (viral).
- Chemical – cyclophosphamide, Walpole's solution.
- Immune-mediated – granulomatous urethritis.

Table 19 Prevalence of various causes of LUTD

iFLUTD (%)	Urethral obstruction (%)	Urethral plug (%)	Uroliths (%)	Behavioural (%)	Incontinence (%)	UTI (%)	Anatomic (%)	Neoplasia (%)
55–64	19–58	10–21	12–22	0–9	0–4	1–15	0–11	0–2

Obstructive:
- Trauma.
- Reflex dyssynergia.
- UMN damage.
- Urolithiasis.
- Urethral plug.
- Iatrogenic – post-catheterisation, strictured urethrostomy.
- Foreign body.
- Compression from prostate or uterus (rare).

Anatomic (uncommon):
- Urachal anomalies.
- Ureterocoele.
- Urethral stricture.
- Phimosis.

Neoplastic:
- Transitional cell carcinoma.
- Other – squamous cell carcinoma, adenocarcinoma, leiomyoma, leiomyosarcoma, haemangiosarcoma.

Idiopathic:
- iFLUTD, (feline idiopathic cystitis [FIC]).

2.16.3 Key history
- Age, breed, sex.
- General lifestyle – recent stressor (e.g. house move, indoor/outdoor, other cats in household).
- Urinary history – use of litter tray, how many trays, access to outside.
- Diet (recent and current).
- Previous history of dysuria.
- Other clinical signs – pollakiuria, haematuria, periuria.
- Evidence of behavioural issues.
- Is the cat systemically unwell?
- Duration of clinical signs.
- History or evidence of trauma.

2.16.4 Focus of physical examination
- Is the urethra patent?
- Preferably observe urination.
- Non-observed urine production does not exclude passive overflow or bladder rupture.
- Abdominal palpation – particularly feel of bladder and response of cat to bladder palpation.

NB – *The bladder should be palpated with great care as it may rupture if grossly distended.*

- Examination of the external genitalia.
- Neurological examination.

2.16.5 Decision making
- What is the most likely cause (table 19)?
- Is the cat obstructed?
- Is emergency decompression required (catheterise or cystocentesis)?
- Is the cat hyperkalaemic?
- Is further investigation likely to produce a diagnosis?
- For a therapeutic trial, what are the criteria for success?

2.16.6 Diagnostic approach (Table 14 page 40–41)
Diagnostic approach (non-obstructed cats):
- Full urinalysis including sediment examination, UPC and culture.
- Haematology and biochemistry if
  - history of systemic illness.
  - calcium-containing uroliths suspected.
  - associated renal failure.

CLINICAL SIGNS

- Ultrasound – bladder and kidneys can usually be imaged (e.g. pyelonephritis, masses or uroliths within bladder).
- Diagnostic imaging:
  - Plain survey radiographs.
  - Double contrast cystogram.
  - Urethrogram.
  - Intravenous excretory urography.
- Dietary trial if uroliths present or iFLUTD suspected.
- Tissue sampling:
  - Catheter biopsy.
  - FNA/Tru-cut of mass.

NB – *Small risk of disseminating a tumour along the needle track through body wall.*

  - Cystoscopy and biopsy.
- Urolith analysis.
- Cystotomy for biopsy/urolith removal.

2.16.7 Management and therapy
A single episode may require little or no treatment or management change; the owner should be encouraged to record the episode (date, time, circumstances) in case further episodes occur. For repeat episodes increasing efforts to obtain a diagnosis should be made, multimodal therapy (diet, nutraceuticals, behavioural therapy and drugs) is recommended.

2.17 FAILURE TO GROW

2.17.1 Introduction
Growth is influenced by genetic, hormonal and metabolic factors. Failure to grow (stunting) can be proportionate or disproportionate and associated with normal or poor body condition.

2.17.2 Causes
- Abnormality of bone growth:
  - Chondrodystrophy.
- Deficient nutrient intake:
  - Inadequate or inappropriate diet.

- GI parasitism.
  - Persistent vomiting or regurgitation, e.g. vascular ring anomaly.
  - Maldigestion/malabsorption.
- Increased caloric demand:
  - Fever.
  - Chronic infectious or inflammatory disease.
  - Major trauma.
- Increased caloric loss:
  - Protein-losing enteropathy.
  - Protein-losing nephropathy.
  - Urine nutrient loss, e.g. juvenile-onset DM, renal glycosuria.
- Major organ defect:
  - Hepatic – portosystemic shunt, glycogen storage disease.
  - Renal – dysplasia, pyelonephritis.
  - Congenital cardiac anomaly.
  - Lysosomal storage disease.
- Endocrinopathy:
  - Hypothyroidism.
  - Hyposomatotropism.
  - Juvenile-onset DM.

2.17.3 Key history
- When was the growth problem first noticed?
  - Slow since birth ⇒ congenital defect.
  - Normal and then suddenly stopped ⇒ acquired disease.
- Stature of other members of the litter and parents.
- Diet, appetite and food intake.

NB – *Dietary imbalances can cause significant growth retardation, e.g. all meat diet despite an adequate calorie intake.*

- Could this be intentional, e.g. Munchkin kittens?
- Concurrent clinical signs, e.g. regurgitation, diarrhoea, polyuria, seizures, exercise intolerance, mental dullness/behavioural abnormalities.

2.17.4 Focus of physical examination
- Proportionate or disproportionate.
- Good or poor body condition – good condition associated with hypothyroidism, hyposomatotropism and chondrodysplasia.
- Mentation – dull with hepatic encephalopathy, hypothyroidism, abiotrophy.
- Skeletal proportions, angular limb deformity.
- Hair coat – alopecia, persistence of kitten coat.
- Presence of cortical blindness – portosystemic shunt.
- Oral examination.
- Cardiac murmur.
- Bowel wall thickness.

2.17.5 Decision making
- Nutritional adequacy.
- Congenital abnormality (if so which organ) vs. acquired disease.
- Hormonal disease.
- Acquired diseases tend to be infectious.

2.17.6 Diagnostic approach
- Ensure adequate and appropriate nutrition.
- Ensure adequate worming.
- Haematology, biochemistry, urinalysis and imaging to assess major organ disease:
  - Include hepatic function tests (bile acids).
  - Radiography – include appendicular skeleton.
  - Ultrasound should include echocardiography.
- Retrovirus serology + other infectious disease as appropriate.
- Hormonal tests – thyroid, IGF-1.
- Fibroblast culture, urinalysis for lysosomal storage disease.

2.17.7 Management and therapy
Many congenital abnormalities are not directly treatable but can be medically managed, e.g. hormonal replacement. Treatment of acquired disease requires accurate diagnosis and appropriate therapy, but the prognosis is often good with a compensatory growth phase occurring following treatment such that little, if any, difference in adult size is evident.

2.18 FLATULENCE

2.18.1 Introduction
Flatulence is a mixture of malodorous volatile gases (ammonia, hydrogen sulphide, mercaptans, short-chain fatty acids) resulting from aerophagia or bacterial fermentation. Flatulence needs to be distinguished from perianal faecal residue causing malodour, e.g. Tritrichomonas diarrhoea.

2.18.2 Causes
- Aerophagia.
- High-legume diet.
- Spoiled diet.
- Diet high in fats or poorly digestible proteins.
- Lactase deficiency.
- Malassimilation/malabsorption secondary to GIT disease.

2.18.3 Key history
- Chronic worsening problem or recent issue.
- General stress/anxiety levels.
- Recent changes in diet.
- Appetite.
- Faecal consistency and odour if known.
- Associated vomiting/diarrhoea.

2.18.4 Focus of physical examination
- GIT.
- Perianal area.

CLINICAL SIGNS

CLINICAL SIGNS

2.18.5 Decision making
- Is this a primary diet, disease or stress/behavioural issue?

2.18.6 Diagnostic approach
- Dietary change.
- Investigation of GI disease (see Section 4.3).

2.18.7 Management and therapy
Aerophagia should be reduced by avoiding stressful situations as far as possible. A highly digestible, moderate fat, lactose-free diet low in legumes should be given. Therapeutically no products have any evidence base and many need to be given multiple times in the day to be effective and some are difficult to administer to cats such as activated charcoal and bismuth subsalicylate. Other products that have been used include simethicone (25 mg q6h), *Yucca schidigera*, alpha-galactosidase, pancreatic enzyme supplements (but these can cause unpleasant body odour) and homeopathic remedies.

By preference, a probiotic paste would be the author's first choice with appropriate dietary change.

2.19 HAEMATEMESIS, HAEMOPTYSIS AND EPISTAXIS

2.19.1 Introduction
- *Haematemesis* – vomiting blood.
- *Haemoptysis* – coughing and expectorating blood – bright red and usually mixed with white, bubbly froth.
- *Epistaxis* – haemorrhage originating from the nose.

Haematemesis or haemoptysis are always worrying signs for owners often prompting an urgent request to be seen despite relatively small amounts of blood loss. The blood produced can come from a number of sources:
- Nasal philtrum.
- Nasopharynx.
- Oral cavity.
- Oesophagus.
- Stomach (usually 'coffee ground').
- Respiratory tract – blood either swallowed and then vomited back or expectorated after coughing.

2.19.2 Causes
- Bleeding disorder (see section 2.7).
- Trauma.
- Ulceration, e.g. oesophagitis, gastric ulceration.
- Foreign body.
- Dental disease.
- Neoplasia.
- Primary nasopharyngeal disease – ulcerative, neoplastic
- Primary lung disease – thromboembolism, hypertension, destructive pulmonary infection.
- Cardiogenic pulmonary oedema (rare in cats and usually terminal event).
- Hypertension.

2.19.3 Key history
- Age, breed.
- Duration and progression of clinical signs.
- Access to toxins especially anticoagulants and caustic chemicals.
- Drugs being given, especially NSAIDs.
- Appetite.
- Weight loss.
- Evidence or history of trauma or foreign travel.
- Volume of blood being produced – drops, teaspoonful, constant.
- Nature of blood – fresh, coffee grounds, clots.
- Unilateral or bilateral epistaxis.
- Recent anaesthesia and intubation that may have caused trauma.

- Associated clinical signs – coughing/retching implies nasopharyngeal or respiratory tract in origin.
- Other clinical signs – bleeding from other sites, weakness, pallor.

2.19.4 Focus of physical examination
- Mucosal colour.
- Petechiation or ecchymosis.
- Facial symmetry and/or pain.
- Depigmentation of hair over nasal bones.
- Nasal airflow.
- Oral examination.
- Cervical oesophagus.
- Auscultation and percussion of lung fields.
- Cranial abdominal pain.
- Neurologic examination if CNS signs (extension nasal tumour, hyperviscosity).

2.19.5 Decision making
- Has a significant amount of blood been lost – is emergency replacement required?
- Is there evidence of a bleeding disorder?
- From where is the blood originating – which organ system should I investigate?
- Is gastric protection required?

2.19.6 Diagnostic approach
- Haematology – full including smear examination.
- Assessment for bleeding disorder.
- Biochemistry – causes of ulceration, e.g. uraemia.
- Urinalysis – dipstick and SG.
- Blood pressure.
- Iron and iron-binding protein if PCV low and poorly regenerative.
- FeLV/FIV serology, (heartworm).
- Examination of oropharynx, nasopharynx, trachea, stomach and oesophagus under sedation/anaesthesia.

- Investigation of organ system involved with imaging, endoscopy and tissue sampling.

2.19.7 Management and therapy
Management depends on whether the problem is local or systemic.

Blood or blood products may be urgently required.

Light sedation may be appropriate in anxious and distressed cats, e.g. opiate + diazepam.

If epistaxis is severe, ligation of the carotid artery may be necessary whilst further diagnostics are undertaken; in less severe cases, ice packing the nose or intranasal, cold adrenaline (1:100 000) can be used.

An airway should be established and oxygen therapy given if the bleeding is associated with cardiorespiratory disease; suctioning of the trachea or oropharynx may be necessary.

2.20 HAEMATOCHEZIA AND MELAENA

2.20.1 Introduction
- *Haematochezia* – presence of fresh, undigested blood in faeces (usually in the absence of diarrhoea) usually from the colon.
- *Melaena* – black, tarry stools resulting from blood being digested in the small intestine.

These signs generally indicate GIT disease. It is important when asking a client about faecal colour and consistency that they are encouraged to describe it themselves, otherwise dark stools can be misrepresented as melaena.

2.20.2 Causes
Haematochezia:
- Colitis – inflammatory, parasitic, infectious.

- Proctitis.
- Ruptured anal sac abscess.
- Penetrating trauma to anus/rectum.
- Neoplasia.
- Bleeding disorder.
- Polyps.
- Rectal prolapse.
- Haemorrhagic gastroenteritis.

Melaena:
- Swallowed blood (see causes of haemoptysis).
- Oesophageal or gastric disease (see causes of haematemesis).
- Small intestinal disease.
- Inflammation or erosion.
- Neoplasia.
- Foreign body.
- Ischaemic bowel disease – intussusception, infarction, volvulus, severe hypovolaemic shock.
- Trauma.
- Infectious disease, e.g. parvovirus.
- Bleeding disorder and DIC.
- Severe acute pancreatitis.
- Drugs especially NSAIDs, glucocorticoids.
- Pancreatitis.
- Hepatorenal disease.

2.20.3 Key history
- Age, breed.
- Duration and progression of clinical signs.
- Access to foreign bodies or toxins especially anticoagulants and caustic chemicals.
- Drugs being given especially NSAIDs.
- Appetite.
- Weight loss.
- Evidence or history of trauma.
- Volume of blood being produced.
- Is the blood round the stool, throughout the stool or unassociated with defaecation?
- Presence of tenesmus.

- Associated clinical signs – diarrhoea, vomiting.
- Other clinical signs – bleeding from other sites, weakness, pallor.

2.20.4 Focus of physical examination
- Examination of GIT.
- Evidence of systemic coagulopathy – petechiation or ecchymosis.
- Evidence of respiratory, oral or nasal bleeding with the blood being swallowed.
- Examination of anus, anal glands and perianal area.
- Presence of perineal hernia.

2.20.5 Decision making
- Has a significant amount of blood been lost?
- Is there evidence of a bleeding disorder?
- Where is the blood originating from?
- Is there really melaena?

Differential diagnosis of dark faeces:
- Diet – especially if high in iron or iron supplemented.
- Drugs – salicylates, bismuth, charcoal.
- Biliverdin, not blood.

2.20.6 Diagnostic approach
Haematochezia and melaena:
- Rectal examination (may require sedation).
- Faecal examination.
- Haematology.
- Assessment for bleeding disorders.

Haematochezia:
- Rectal cytology.
- Rectal biopsy.
- Radiography of small intestine and colon – plain and contrast studies (may require enema).
- Ultrasound – abdominal and perineal view.

- Proctoscopy.
- Rigid or flexible colonoscopy and biopsy.

Melaena (assuming oral and respiratory causes excluded):
- Biochemistry – causes of ulceration, e.g. uraemia.
- Urinalysis.
- Blood pressure.
- Thoracic radiography to assess oesophagus.
- Abdominal imaging – plain, contrast and ultrasound.
- Upper and lower GI endoscopy and biopsy.
- Laparoscopy/laparotomy and biopsy.

2.20.7 Management and therapy

Haematochezia presenting without additional signs or physical findings will often respond to broad-spectrum anthelmintics, metronidazole and a novel protein, low-fat, low-residue diet.

Melaenic patients should always be provided with gastric protection until a diagnosis is achieved.

2.21 HAEMATURIA AND HAEMOGLOBINURIA

2.21.1 Introduction

Haematuria is often associated with dysuria (see section 2.16) and pollakiuria. It is important to distinguish haematuria/haemoglobinuria from other causes of urine discoloration prior to proceeding with an in-depth workup (Figure 8). Haemoglobinuria occurs as a result of lysis of red cells in dilute urine (red cell ghosts present on sediment) or loss of haemoglobin through glomerular filtration.

2.21.2 Causes

Renal (uncommon → rare):
- Acute pyelonephritis (presence of pyuria).
- Glomerulopathy (presence of proteinuria).
- Neoplasia (not lymphoma).
- Idiopathic.
- Polycystic disease.
- Nephrolithiasis.
- Infarction.
- Trauma.
- Vascular anomalies, e.g. AV fistula.

Lower urinary tract haematuria (common):
- FLUTD.
- Trauma.
- Calculi.
- Urinary tract infection.
- Retention cystitis.
- Neoplasia.
- Drugs, e.g. cyclophosphamide.
- Polyps or diverticuli.

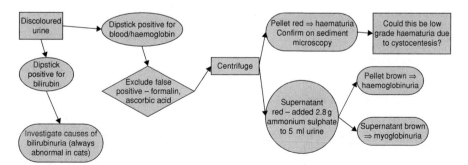

Figure 8 Laboratory differentiation of discoloured urine

CLINICAL SIGNS

Bleeding from genital tract, vagina, uterus, penis or prostate (uncommon → rare):
• Neoplasia.
• Trauma.
• Infection.
• Inflammation.

Haematuria/haemoglobinuria secondary to systemic disease (uncommon):
• Haemolytic anaemia.
• Bleeding disorder.
• Hyperthermia.
• Exercise.
• Microangiopathic disease.
• Transfusion reactions.
• Use of haemoglobin glutamer (Oxyglobin).

Sampling (common):
• Microscopic haematuria common in cystocentesis samples.

2.21.3 Key history
• Is the cat neutered – recent oestrus or parturition?
• Is there previous history of haematuria?
• When does the blood appear during urination?
• Is blood present every time the cat urinates?
• Is there bleeding from the prepuce/vulva unassociated with urination?
• Has there been haemorrhage from any other sites?
• Other urinary signs – dysuria, stranguria, pollakiuria, periuria.
• What is the faecal colour?
• History of trauma.
• Exposure to drugs or toxins.

2.21.4 Focus of physical examination
• Mucosal colour.
• Petechiation or ecchymosis.
• Palpation of the abdomen particularly bladder and kidneys.
• Examine external genitalia.

2.21.5 Decision making
• Is this haematuria/haemoglobinuria?
• Has a significant amount of blood been lost?
• Is there evidence of a bleeding disorder?
• From where is the blood originating?
• Is there evidence of trauma?
• Are there localising signs to a part of the urinary tract?

2.21.6 Diagnostic approach (Table 14 page 40–41)
• Urinalysis:
  ○ Compare urinalysis from voided versus cystocentesis sample.
  ○ Biochemistry.
  ○ Sediment analysis – confirm presence of red cells (or red cell ghosts).
  ○ Red cell casts ⇒ glomerulonephritis, vasculitis, renal infarction, renal tumour, severe glomerular disease, haemorrhage into tubules.
  ○ White cell casts and bacteria.
  ○ Neoplastic epithelial cells.
  ○ Culture and sensitivity.
• Assessment for bleeding disorders.
• Examination of the penis/vagina.
• Radiograph and ultrasound of bladder, kidneys and accessory organs:
  ○ Double contrast cystogram.
  ○ Retrograde urethrogram.
  ○ Excretory urography.
• Cystoscopy and biopsy.
• Exploratory surgery.
• Idiopathic renal haemorrhage suspected (rare), image ureters cystoscopically or catheterise ureters separately via bladder to collect urine from each kidney.

2.21.7 Management and therapy
The patient should be assessed for severity of blood loss and need for transfusion. Otherwise emergency treatment is not usually required. Differentiation between

systemic and local disease causing the haematuria/haemoglobinuria is a key first step followed by management of the underlying condition if required.

2.22 HYPOTHERMIA

2.22.1 Introduction

Body temperature is maintained by the hypothalamus that matches heat production (muscular activity and metabolism) with heat loss (from the skin, mucous membranes, respiratory tract [increased by panting], urine and faeces).

Heat loss is minimised by seeking shelter, piloerection, vasoconstriction and shivering.

Routine rectal temperature assessment does not measure core temperature, so the hypothermia recorded may be peripheral rather than central.

Classification – mild hypothermia >34°C; moderate 28–34°C; severe <28°C.

2.22.2 Causes

Iatrogenic:
- Anaesthesia.
- Surgery.
- Overzealous treatment of hyperthermia.

Systemic disease:
- Cardiac.
- Sepsis.
- Chronic renal failure.
- Severe malnutrition.
- Hypoglycaemia.
- Neurologic:
  ○ Head trauma.
  ○ Neoplasia.
  ○ Cerebrovascular accident.

Environmental:
- Exposure.
- Trauma.
- Hypothyroidism.

2.22.3 Key history

- Anaesthesia within past 24 hours.
- Concurrent illness:
  ○ Weight loss.
  ○ Diet and appetite.
  ○ PU/PD.
- Likelihood of exposure.
- History of trauma.
- Likelihood of sepsis.

2.22.4 Focus of physical examination

- Assessment of peripheral and core temperature.
- Peripheral pulse quality, capillary refill time and hydration status.
- Body condition score.
- Hair coat quality.
- Neurologic status and level of consciousness.

2.22.5 Decision making

- Is the hypothermia due to exposure or recent anaesthesia/surgery?
- Is there evidence of trauma?
- Is this systemic disease; if so which organ system(s) are involved?

2.22.6 Diagnostic approach

- T_4 level.
- Blood pressure.
- Imaging of target organ(s) if systemic disease indicated.

2.22.7 Management and therapy

Careful restoration of core body temperature.

External re-warming, e.g. wrapping in blankets/insulating material, hot-water bottles (care thermal burns), heat pads, Bair Hugger, etc., is appropriate to mild-to-moderate hypothermic cats.

Severe hypothermia may require internal or core warming – warmed intravenous fluids, peritoneal dialysis with fluid at 43°C (10–20 ml/kg exchanged every

CLINICAL SIGNS

30 minutes), colonic/gastric lavage with warm saline.

As warming occurs, there is a shift of cold peripheral blood to central circulation as peripheral vasodilation occurs as well as increased peripheral cooling of core blood that can cause 'afterdrop' (further decrease in temperature during initial warming period).

Intensive nursing is important in moderate-to-severe hypothermic patients. Metabolic acidosis, electrolyte, glucose levels, urine output and neurologic status should be monitored and managed and a continuous ECG recorded as cardiac arrhythmias are common.

When treating underlying disease remember that drug metabolism is slowed.

2.23 INCONTINENCE (URINARY)

2.23.1 Introduction
Incontinence – involuntary escape of urine during the storage phase.

Incontinence needs to be distinguished from inappropriate urination due to behavioural causes, associated with fear/stress and lack of access to the outside/litter tray often compounded by PD that decreases the inter-urination period.

Compared to dogs, urinary incontinence is uncommon in cats and most often associated with neurologic dysfunction.

2.23.2 Causes
Congenital abnormalities (rare):
• Ectopic ureter(s).
• Urethral sphincter mechanism incompetence (USMI) – rare as cats have relatively long urethras for their size.
• Pervious urachus.
• Bladder hypoplasia.
• Urethrorectal fistula.

• Spinal dysraphism causing vesicourethral dysfunction, e.g. Manx cats.

Acquired disease:
• Neoplasia (rare).
• Urethrovaginal fistula following surgery.
• Neurogenic bladder/urethral dysfunction.
• Detrusor hyperspasticity (urge incontinence) commonly seen in FLUTD.

2.23.3 Key history
• Age, breed and sex.
• Has there ever been normal urination?
• Is the mixture of voluntary urination and incontinence?
• Thirst.
• History of trauma.
• Tail function.
• Hindlimb gait abnormalities or faecal incontinence.
• Recent abdominal surgery.

2.23.4 Focus of physical examination
• Palpation of the bladder.
• Perineal examination.
• Neurologic examination:
  ○ Anal tone.
  ○ Tail function.
  ○ Hindlimb gait.

2.23.5 Decision making
• Is the bladder large or small?
• Is it easy to express urine?
  ○ Mid-large sized bladder easily expressible ⇒ LMN damage.
  ○ Large bladder, difficult to express UMN damage.
  ○ Small bladder ⇒ USMI or ectopic ureters.
• Do findings on bladder palpation match the neurologic findings?

2.23.6 Diagnostic approach
• Evaluation of kidney function.
• Imaging (ultrasound, (vagino)urethrography, double contrast cystography or

cystoscopy) to evaluate bladder shape and position, ureteric position and kidneys.

- Imaging of spinal cord – MRI or myelography.

2.23.7 Management and therapy
Surgical management of ectopic ureters and fistulae are possible.

Palliative management for several weeks of neurologic bladder dysfunction is indicated in the hope that vesicourethral function will recover. Cases should have their bladders regularly (three to four times per day) emptied manually or via catheter (UMN), accompanied by frequent urinalysis with culture.

Continence in LMN damage may be improved with bethanechol (1.25 mg q8h PO). Skeletal and smooth muscle relaxants (midazolam/diazepam, prazosin, dantrolene, phenoxybenzamine) may be helpful in aiding bladder expression in UMN damage by reducing urethral tone or spasm.

2.24 INCONTINENCE (FAECAL)

2.24.1 Introduction
Faecal incontinence – inability to retain faeces until defaecation appropriate with loss of conscious control.

Fifty per cent of cats presenting with faecal incontinence are euthanized within days of presentation.

2.24.2 Causes
Non-neurogenic sphincter incompetence:
- Neoplasia.
- Constipation.
- Diarrhoea.

Neurogenic sphincter incompetence:
- Confusion and disorientation.
- Old age.

- Spinal or cauda equina trauma.
- Spinal dysraphism and taillessness.
- Lumbosacral instability.
- Peripheral neuropathy – polyneuropathy, dysautonomia.
- Cauda equina syndromes.
- CNS disease.
- Damage to anal sphincter:
  - Laceration.
  - Anal gland, perianal or sphincter surgery.

Reservoir incontinence (reduced capacity of rectum) – ability to control defaecation overwhelmed by inflammatory colorectal disease, decreased storage capacity or increased faecal volume:
- Proctitis.
- Colitis.
- Diarrhoea.
- Constipation.
- Colonic obstruction – foreign body, neoplasia, polyp.
- Perineal hernia.

2.24.3 Key history
- Onset, duration and progression.
- Posturing to defaecate.
- Faecal consistence.
- Attempting to get to litter tray/outside ⇒ reservoir incontinence.
- Recent trauma or surgery.
- Hindlimb gait.
- Urinary continence.
- Tail carriage and function.
- General levels of mentation and activity.

2.24.4 Focus of physical examination
- Abdominal palpation – faecal presence and consistency in colon.
- Presence of caudal abdominal mass lesions.
- Palpation of bladder – size, position, ease of urine expression.
- Perianal examination.
- Rectal examination.

- Pain on palpation of lumbar spine, sacrum and pelvis.
- Neurologic examination:
  - Tail sensation and tone.
  - Hindlimb tone, postural responses, myotatic reflexes and gait.
  - Anal tone and reflex.

2.24.5 Decision making

- Is this true incontinence or a behavioural problem (middening) or an inability to access outside or the litter tray e.g. severe osteoarthritis?
- What type of incontinence is it – does it involve the sphincter or reservoir function?
- Is there likely to be treatable underlying pathology?

2.24.6 Diagnostic approach

- Many incontinent cats are elderly or have suffered trauma, so routine haematology, biochemistry and urinalysis is appropriate.
- Full faecal analysis if there is diarrhoea.
- Caudal abdominal ultrasound or radiography.
- Colonoscopy and biopsy for reservoir incontinence cases.
- Imaging of spinal cord – MRI or myelography.

2.24.7 Management and therapy

Resolution of the underlying cause is likely to be the only realistic way of managing faecal incontinence. Some improvement can be gained by reducing faecal bulk (low-residue diets) and water content together with slowing transit time with loperamide (0.04–0.2 mg/kg PO q8–12h) that also act to improve sphincter tone or phenylpropanolamine (1 mg/kg PO q8h) that increases the tone of the internal anal sphincter. In addition, dedicated nursing care and induction of defaecation may be required. Cats will rarely tolerate wearing nappies!

2.25 INFERTILITY – QUEENS

2.25.1 Introduction

Basic physiology (Figure 9)

- Seasonally polyoestrous.
- Cycling occurs as daylight hours lengthen.
- Induced ovulator.
- In the absence of mating, cats will cycle every 2–4 weeks (spring, summer and autumn).

2.25.2 Causes

Failure of oestrus:

- Not reached puberty:
  - Puberty usually at 2.3–2.5 kg around 6–9 months of age, but can be as early as 4 months and as late

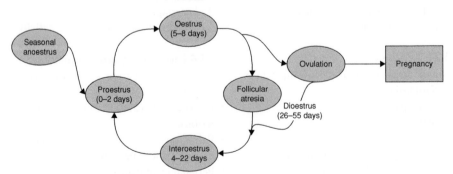

Figure 9 Reproductive cycle of the queen

as 21 months – affected by season and breed.
  ○ Onset seasonally influenced.
- 'Split heats' – proestrus signs occur and then subside:
  ○ usually due to inadequate follicular development and tends to resolve with maturity.
- Ovarian aplasia/hypoplasia.
- Abnormalities of sexual differentiation, e.g. XO or hermaphrodite.
- Ovariectomy/ovariohysterectomy has been performed previously.
- Oestrus interrupted:
  ○ Pseudopregnancy – ovulation has been stimulated (often by a neutered tomcat).
- Prolonged oestrus:
  ○ Overlapping ovarian follicles.
  ○ Behavioural oestrus during interoestrous period.
  ○ Functional ovarian follicular cyst.
  ○ Functional ovarian neoplasm.
- Pregnancy – queens introduced to toms in interoestrous period may not show signs of oestrus although subsequent pregnancy confirms oestrus and mating to have occurred.
- Lactational/post-lactational anoestrus.
- Silent oestrous:
  ○ Queen maintained in isolation may not show oestrous behaviour.
  ○ Oestrus inhibited in timid and subordinate queens.
- Intercurrent disease.
- Old age.

Unwillingness to mate:
- Stress associated with travel and introduction to stud cat.

Failure of ovulation:
- Queen and tomcat insufficient opportunities to mate.
- Failure of coitus.

Failure of fertilisation, implantation or early embryonic death:
- Anatomical abnormality of reproductive tract.
- Inadequate number of matings to stimulate ovulation.
- Stress.
- Uterine tumours or polyps.

Reabsorption and abortion:

NB – *Reabsorption is more common than abortion, but is sometimes confused with abortion due to the presence of a bloody vaginal discharge leading to the false assumption that the queen has eaten the aborted foetuses.*

Nutritional factors:
- Generally needs to be gross dietary inadequacies.
- Taurine deficiency.

Hormonal factors:
- Progesterone deficiency – premature regression of corpora lutea.
- Previous hormonal treatment designed to inhibit oestrus may have a prolonged effect.

Infectious disease:
- FPV.
- FeLV.
- FCV causing *in utero* deaths.
- *Chlamydophila felis* (*Chlamydia psittaci*).
- *Toxoplasma*.
- *E. coli* placentitis.
- Q fever

Chronic endometritis:
- Sterile endometrial cystic hyperplasia (>85% of queens over 5 years).
- Chronic bacterial infection (usually secondary to cystic endometritis).

CLINICAL SIGNS

CLINICAL SIGNS

2.25.3 Key history
- Age, breed:
  - Oriental breeds (Siamese, Burmese) achieve puberty earlier than long-haired breeds (Persians).
- Diet.
- Has oestrus ever been observed?
- Has the stud cat used been proven?
- Number of cats in the household and queen's position in that group?
- Length of ownership – is the queen known to be entire?
- Description of oestrus duration and behaviour.
- Observed mating behaviour and frequency.
- Intercurrent disease and vaccination status.
- Previous drug use.
- Fertility of siblings.
- Was the pregnancy confirmed?
- How long since last litter?
- Has more than one (unrelated) stud cat been tried?

2.25.4 Focus of physical examination
- Stage of maturity, growth and body weight.
- Video of oestrous behaviour and mating.
- Palpation of reproductive tract.
- Examination of external genitalia.
- Presence of vaginal discharge.
- Presence of milk.
- Evidence of intercurrent disease.

2.25.5 Decision making
- At what stage of the oestrous cycle is the infertility occurring?
- Is the infertility anatomic, hormonal, behavioural or disease-related?
  - Is the queen ever likely to become pregnant?
- Is the owner expecting too much?
- Is the queen already pregnant?
- Is investigation necessary at this stage?

2.25.6 Diagnostic approach (Table 14 page 40–41)
- Retrovirus, chlamydophila, toxoplasma serology.
- Vaginoscopy.
- Vaginal cytology.
- Vaginal microbiology.
- Imaging of uterus.
- Vaginourethrogram.
- Plasma progesterone assay:
  - Estimate time of ovulation – high levels occur following ovulation, low levels suggest non-ovulating queen.
  - Failure of maintenance of pregnancy.
- Laparotomy/laparoscopy:
  - Presence of uterus and ovaries.
  - State of ovaries.
  - Uterine biopsy.
- Karyotyping.
- Check fertility of stud cat.

2.25.7 Management and therapy
Some cases may be resolved simply with environmental changes and better observation of oestrus. Certain specific conditions may be surgically amenable. Pyometra can be successfully treated in some queens using a combination of antimicrobials and prostaglandin therapy. Although possible, oestrous induction, artificial insemination and embryo transfer are rarely appropriate in cats.

2.26 INFERTILITY – TOMCATS

2.26.1 Introduction
Infertile tomcats are rarely presented; investigation should focus on whether they have been a proven breeder, if not, anatomic causes of infertility need also to be considered. Relevant literature is sparse.

2.26.2 Causes
- Intersex.
- Failure of development of sexual organs:
  - Testicular hypoplasia.

○ Persistent frenulum.
○ Cryptorchidism.
○ Hypospadia.
- Abnormal sperm:
  ○ Low number.
  ○ Poor motility.
  ○ Abnormal morphology.
  ○ Testicular neoplasia.
- Pain on coitus.
- Orchitis (associated with FIP, tuberculosis), epididymitis, prostatitis.
- Urethral obstruction.
- Ring of hair around glans penis from previous mating.
- Trauma to penis or testes:
  ○ Priapism, phimosis and paraphimosis.
- Systemic illness.
- Loss of libido:
  ○ Unfamiliar surroundings.
  ○ Aggressive queen.
  ○ Malnourishment.
  ○ Obesity.
- Failure of mating to induce ovulation.
- Retrograde ejaculation.
- Overuse.

2.26.3 Key history
- Confirmed sire of previous pregnancies.
- Changes in mating routine.
- Changes in mating behaviour.
- Abnormal urination.
- Signs of systemic illness.
- Frequency of use.
- Preputial discharge.

2.26.4 Focus of physical examination
- Evidence of systemic disease.
- Abdominal palpation.
- Orthopaedic/spinal pain.
- Examination of testicles.
- Examination of prepuce.
- Examination of penis.

2.26.5 Decision making
- Behavioural problem.
- Anatomic abnormality.

- Quality of sperm.
- Acquired disease – FeLV, FIV serology.

2.26.6 Diagnostic approach
- Video of mating behaviour.
- Imaging of abdomen and testicles.
- Retrograde urethrogram.
- Cytology and culture of preputial discharge.
- Obtain sperm sample:
  ○ Train cat to use artificial vagina (low success rate).
  ○ Electroejaculation under general anaesthesia.
  ○ In some cats sufficient sperm is present in the urine after mating to allow evaluation.
- Examination of sperm sample:
  ○ pH.
  ○ Volume.
  ○ Sperm count.
  ○ Motility.
  ○ Abnormal spermatozoa.
- Check for chromosomal disorder.

2.26.7 Management and therapy
Non-reproductive disease, e.g. pain, should be managed accordingly. Ensure that diet is optimal and that more than one calling queen has been presented to the tomcat for mating. Poor libido is perhaps the most common cause of infertility associated with stressful surroundings that should be addressed. Rarely infertility is surgically amenable.

2.27 JAUNDICE (ICTERUS)

2.27.1 Introduction
Jaundice is caused by excess bilirubin levels in the blood; clinically apparent jaundice will not be evident until bilirubin exceeds around 40–50 μmol/l (reference range <10–15 μmol/l). Once bilirubin

CLINICAL SIGNS

CLINICAL SIGNS

enters the tissues it will persist longer than hyperbilirubinaemia.

Basic physiology
- 70–80% of bilirubin derived from destruction of senescent red cells.
- Bilirubin is produced by reduction of the porphyrin ring that carries the iron in the haem component of haemoglobin in the liver.
- Unconjugated (free; indirect) bilirubin is insoluble and bound to albumin, if bilirubin production exceeds albumin binding, bilirubin enters tissues:
  - Decreased binding occurs with
    - low plasma albumin.
    - binding sites already occupied, e.g. diazepam, sulphonamides, thyroxin.
    - acidosis (decreases affinity).
- Bilirubin is conjugated (glucuronyl transferase) in the liver, making it water soluble and excreted in bile.
- Conjugated bilirubin can be deconjugated and released back into the circulation if the liver is unable to excrete the conjugated bilirubin. This means that measurement of conjugated (indicating extra-hepatic disease) vs. deconjugated (indicating hepatic disease) bilirubin is of limited value except in the very early stages of disease.
- Some of the bilirubin excreted into the duodenum is deconjugated by gut microflora and oxidised to stercobilin (giving faeces their coloration), the remainder is reabsorbed (enterohepatic circulation).
- The presence of bilirubin in the urine is abnormal in cats.
  - Urobilinogen is produced in the gut, reabsorbed and excreted in the urine.
- Cats have a relative inability to glucuronidate and excrete the majority of their bile conjugated to taurine rather than glycine.

2.27.2 Causes of hyperbilirubinaemia
Pre-hepatic – increased production of bilirubin.

NB – *Haemolysis has to be rapid to exceed the liver's ability to conjugate.*

- Secondary immune-mediated haemolysis:
  - Haemoplasma (feline infectious anaemia).
  - FeLV-associated haemolysis.
  - Bacteraemia and septicaemia (hepatic component as well).
  - Heinz-body haemolysis, e.g. paracetamol poisoning, onions.
  - Paraneoplastic disease.
  - Breed related.
- DIC.
- Primary immune-mediated haemolytic anaemia (uncommon).
- Neonatal isoerythrolysis.

Hepatic – decreased hepatic uptake and conjugation.
- Cholangiohepatitis.
- Lymphocytic cholangitis.
- FIP.
- Hyperthyroidism.
- Hepatic neoplasia.
- Drug induced – benzodiazepine, tetracycline, glipizide.
- Hepatic fibrosis.
- Hepatic lipidosis.

Post-hepatic – decreased excretion.
- Intra-hepatic biliary compression:
  - Hepatocyte swelling.
  - Cholangitis.
- Traumatic rupture of gall bladder or bile duct causing bile peritonitis.
- Extra-hepatic obstruction:
  - Cholelithiasis.
  - Neoplasia.
  - Pancreatitis.
  - Pancreatic cyst or abscess.

○ Fibrous/inflammatory pancreatic nodule.

○ Sludging of bile.

2.27.3 Key history

- Age and breed.
- Health of litter mates.
- Diet.
- Drug, herbal, supplement use.
- Behavioural change.
- CNS signs – seizures, stupor, disorientation, ptyalism.
- Irritability/hyperactivity.
- Associated clinical signs.
- Anorexia.
- Weight loss.
- Weakness/collapse.
- Pallor.
- Vomiting/diarrhoea.
- PU/PD.
- Evidence of external bleeding.
- Faecal colour:
  ○ Melaena – GIT haemorrhage.
  ○ Pale, fatty faeces – biliary obstruction.
- Colour of urine:
  ○ Port wine – haemoglobinuria.
- History of foreign travel.

2.27.4 Focus of physical examination

- Confirm jaundice.
- Mucous membrane examination:
  ○ Pallor of associated anaemia.
  ○ Petechiation or ecchymosis.
- Abdominal palpation:
  ○ Hepatomegaly.
  ○ Ascites.
  ○ Cranial abdominal pain – liver, pancreas.
- Temperature.
- Ocular examination for uveitis (FIP).

2.27.5 Decision making

- Are any current medications/supplements likely to be responsible?
- Is the jaundice pre-, intra-, or post-hepatic?

- Is hepatic lipidosis likely?
- Associated coagulopathy
- Are there other signs suggestive of FIP?
- Is the cat encephalopathic?
- Is transfusion likely to be necessary – blood group/cross match?

2.27.6 Diagnostic approach

- Full haematology including reticulocytes.
- Biochemistry ± ammonia.

NB1 – *Bile acid estimation is unreliable in the face of high bilirubin levels.*
NB2 – *Amylase and lipase are unreliable indicators of pancreatic involvement.*
NB3 – *Gamma-GT tends to be normal in hepatic lipidosis.*

- Urinalysis – bilirubinuria, haemoglobinuria.
- Serology for FeLV.
- Feline pancreatic-specific lipase.
- PCR for Haemoplasma.
- Abdominal imaging:
  ○ Ultrasound is particularly valuable to distinguish intra- and post-hepatic jaundice as well as assessing the pancreas *but* cats with obstructive jaundice do not always have marked gall bladder and biliary dilation.
- Coagulation profile.
- Liver and gallbladder aspirate or biopsy.
- T_4 level.

2.27.7 Management and therapy

Most cats will be dull, depressed, dehydrated and anorexic; many will be painful. Fluid therapy (after blood samples have been obtained) and pain relief with opioids should be commenced. Appropriate nutrition is essential and method(s) of feeding considered. Immunosuppressive therapy should be reserved until a diagnosis has been reached. Mortality following biliary surgery in cats is high (up to 50%).

CLINICAL SIGNS

2.28 LYMPHADENOPATHY

2.28.1 Introduction
Mild lymphadenopathy will occur in response to systemic or regional inflammation/infection as a normal response to antigens present in the lymph passing through the node.
- *Lymphadenopathy* – disease of the lymph nodes.
- *Lymphadenitis* – inflammation of lymph nodes.
- *Lymphadenomegaly* (*lymphadenectasis*) – enlargement of lymph nodes.

NB – *For the purposes of this text lymphadenopathy will be used in most cases; lymph nodes will usually be enlarged, as this is the indicator that pathological changes are occurring.*

2.28.2 Causes
- Reactive:
  - Infection in adjacent tissue.
  - Septicaemia/bacteraemia.
  - Viraemia, e.g. FeLV, post-vaccination.
  - Inflammatory, e.g. dermatitis, periodontal disease, trauma.
  - Immune-mediated disease, e.g. polyarthropathy, hypereosinophilic syndromes.
  - Mycobacterium.
  - Ehrlichiosis.
- Abscessation of node.
- Lymphadenitis.
- Lymphoma.
- Primary haematopoietic neoplasm.
- Metastatic neoplasia.
- Haemorrhage.
- Foreign body.

2.28.3 Key history
- Age and breed – predilection for lymphoma.
- History of recent travel, vaccination or trauma (fight wounds etc.).
- History of surgical excision of suspected tumours.
- Is the cat systemically unwell?
- Associated clinical signs – why was the cat presented?
- Evidence of bleeding in urine, faeces.
- Rate of growth – in many cases the owner will not have noticed the lymphadenopathy, so duration of problem is unclear (except duration of any associated clinical signs).

2.28.4 Focus of physical examination
- Number and distribution of lymph nodes involved:
  - Are they regional?
  - If regional – is there evidence of a penetrating wound, trauma or inflammatory disease?
  - If multicentric – check joints, muscles.
- Degree of enlargement.
- Pain or heat on palpation.
- Evidence of respiratory distress ⇒ tracheobronchial lymph node enlargement.
- Enlargement of abdominal lymph nodes (abdominal nodes not normally palpable in cats).
- Pallor.
- Evidence of bleeding disorder.

2.28.5 Decision making
- Is the primary pathology within the lymph node, or does the lymph node enlargement reflect a systemic or localised disease?

NB – *FNA and biopsy are more likely to be diagnostic if the node is the site of primary pathology; where possible aspiration of submandibular nodes should be avoided (as they are frequently reactive) unless these are the only ones enlarged.*

- Is the disease process localised or generalised?

2.28.6 Diagnostic approach

- PCR for other infectious disease, e.g. Ehrlichia, Bartonella.
- Blood culture.
- Arthrocentesis.
- Biopsy of lymph node – FNA, wedge, excisional:
  - Submit part of lymph node for culture.
  - Retain some frozen in case other tests are required, e.g. immunohistochemistry, culture for tuberculosis.
- Bone marrow aspirate/core biopsy.

2.28.7 Management and therapy

Initial management should be symptomatic and supportive ensuring hydration and pain relief is adequate. Corticosteroids and antibacterials should be avoided until a (working) diagnosis has been established and all samples likely to be required have been taken. This is particularly important if lymphoma is suspected.

2.29 OCULAR CHANGES CAUSED BY SYSTEMIC DISEASE

2.29.1 Introduction

Ocular changes can be associated with a number of systemic diseases in cats; ocular examination can therefore be an important part of the physical examination particularly in cats that are hypertensive or suspected to have some types of infectious or inflammatory disease.

2.29.2 Causes

- Eyelids:
  - Mucocutaneous disease – pemphigus or SLE.
  - Altered lid position – Horner's syndrome.
  - Copper and zinc deficiency.
  - Nictitating gland – diarrhoea complex.
- Altered pupil size or globe deviation:
  - CN III, IV, VI or VII deficit.
- Conjunctiva:
  - FHV-1.
  - Chlamydophila.
  - Changes reflected in other mucosal sites.
- Cornea and sclera:
  - Lymphoma.
  - Hyperlipidaemia.
  - Decreased tear production – keratoconjunctivitis sicca (rare), dysautonomia.
- Hyphaema:
  - Hypertension.
  - Coagulopathy.
  - Trauma.
  - Lymphoma.
  - Metastatic neoplasia.
  - (Rickettsial disease).
- Uveitis:
  - FIP.
  - FeLV.
  - Toxoplasmosis.
  - Systemic fungal or algal infection.
  - Metastatic neoplasia.
  - Lymphoma.
  - Trauma.
  - Coagulopathy.
- Iris:
  - Portosystemic shunts – copper colouration.
  - Albinism – pink irises.
  - Blue eyes associated with deafness in white cats.
  - FeLV-associated spastic pupil syndrome.
- Lens (cataracts):
  - Nutritional.
  - Hypocalcaemia.
  - DM (uncommon).
  - Electric shock.
- Optic nerve and retina:
  - Optic neuritis/retinitis ± uveitis.
  - Inflammatory CNS disease.
  - Taurine deficiency.

CLINICAL SIGNS

○ Hypertension.
○ Papilloedema reflecting raised intracranial pressure.
• Vasculature:
  ○ Hyperlipidaemia.
  ○ Hypertension.

2.29.3 History, physical examination, decision making and diagnosis

Will depend on the region of the eye affected and should be directed towards looking for other evidence of systemic disease that will help to refine the differential list prior to performing diagnostic testing.

2.29.4 Management and therapy

Whilst topical therapy may be valuable to manage local signs, as these diseases are also systemic, additional systemic therapy will be necessary to address the underlying cause.

2.30 PALLOR

2.30.1 Introduction

Pallor can be caused by two different processes, anaemia and decreased tissue perfusion that can coexist in some cases, e.g. an RTA case with bleeding and multiple trauma.

2.30.2 Causes (Figure 10)

2.30.3 Key history

• Are signs acute or chronic in onset and are they progressive?
• Current and recent diet and medication.
• Is there any history of trauma or neoplasia?
• Has the cat been recently vaccinated or travelled abroad?
• Any history of littermates?
• Parasite control regime.
• Fluid intake and loss (e.g. diarrhoea, vomiting).
• External evidence of bleeding, melaena or haematuria.
• Exercise tolerance.
• Coughing or dyspnoea.
• Pica.
• Previous blood transfusion (potential transfer of parasites or delayed transfusion reaction).

2.30.4 Focus of physical examination

• Capillary refill time.
• Pulse quality – reduced (shock) vs. hyperkinetic (anaemia).
• Mucosal changes – jaundice, cyanosis, petechiation.
• Rectal temperature – can be low in hypovolaemia or shock and raised in

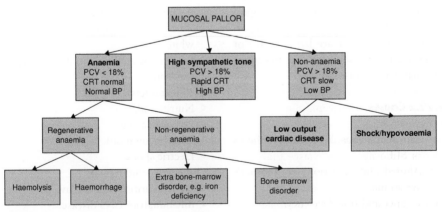

Figure 10 Approach to mucosal pallor

inflammatory, immune-mediated or neoplastic disease.
- Hydration status.
- Cardiac auscultation – presence of murmur, rate and rhythm.
- Respiratory rate, character and effort.
- Evidence of bleeding or a coagulopathy.
- Mentation.

2.30.5 Decision making
- Is there evidence of shock/collapse that requires urgent intervention?
  ○ Is fluid therapy required, if so at what rate?
- Is blood transfusion likely to be required?
- Is there evidence of cardiac disease?

2.30.6 Diagnostic approach
- A PCV/haematocrit should be measured:
  ○ PCV low – pursue causes of anaemia.

For anaemia to cause overt pallor, PCV is usually <18%.
- PCV normal:
  ○ Assess cardiac function – blood pressure, ECG, thoracic radiograph, echocardiography.
  ○ Look for causes of hypovolaemia or shock – full haematology, biochemistry, blood pressure, blood gas analysis, imaging.

2.30.7 Management and therapy
Fluid therapy (colloid vs. crystalloid vs. blood products) should be given to ensure adequate perfusion but beware of overload in cardiovascular disease and dilutional effects in anaemia. Pain relief is often necessary. Cases that are chronically anaemic may not require any immediate treatment but do require investigation to establish a diagnosis.

2.31 PARESIS AND PARALYSIS

2.31.1 Introduction
Mild limb weakness is not uncommon in sick cats; more significant weakness or paralysis requires further evaluation.
- *Paresis* – weakness.
- *Plegia* – paralysis.
- *Mono* – single.
- *Quadri* – all four limbs.
- *Para* – hindlimbs.
- *Hemi* – both limbs on one side.

2.31.2 Causes
The majority of cats with limb weakness or paralysis will have disease that affects neurologic function. Particularly in cats that are quadriplegic/paretic, it is important to also consider muscular or neuromuscular disease as the cause as well as the possibility of generalised LMN disease. Severe orthopaedic pain can mimic paresis in some cases.

General causes of weakness/paralysis:
- Transection of cord.
- Compression:
  ○ Static.
  ○ Dynamic.
- Concussion.
- Degeneration.
- Vascular disease.
- Infection.
- Inflammation.
- Neoplasia.

Causes of monoparesis/plegia:
- Root signs associated with lateralising lesion at the plexus.
- LMN damage.
- Thrombus.

Causes of hemiparesis/plegia – rare:
- Neoplasia.
- Vascular disease.
- Intracranial lesion.
- Trauma.

CLINICAL SIGNS

Causes of paraparesis/plegia:
- Congenital spinal malformation:
  ○ Spina bifida.
  ○ Hemivertebra.
- Disc disease:
  ○ Prolapse.
  ○ Discospondylitis.
- Infectious:
  ○ Spinal abscess.
  ○ Toxoplasma.
  ○ FIP.
- Trauma:
  ○ Fracture below T2.
  ○ Subluxation below T2.
- Ascending myelomalacia.
- Neoplasia:
  ○ Lymphoma.
  ○ Primary intra- or extramedullary.
  ○ Metastatic.
  ○ Nerve root.
- Vascular:
  ○ Aortic thromboembolism.
  ○ Fibrocartilaginous embolus.
- Nutritional:
  ○ Hypervitaminosis A.
  ○ Folding fracture secondary to nutritional hyperparathyroidism.
- Lysosomal storage disease.
- Demyelinating disease.

Causes of quadriplegia/paresis:
- Anatomic cervical lesions (C1–C4):
  ○ Vertebral malformation.
  ○ Vertebral fracture/subluxation.
  ○ Intervertebral disc.
- Inflammatory disease:
  ○ Meningitis.
  ○ Granulomatous meningoencephalitis (very rare).
- Infection:
  ○ FIP.
  ○ Toxoplasma.
  ○ Discospondylitis.
  ○ Abscessation.
  ○ Rabies.

- Neoplasia:
  ○ Lymphoma.
  ○ Primary intra- or extramedullary.
  ○ Metastatic.
- Vascular:
  ○ Aortic thromboembolism.
  ○ Fibrocartilaginous embolus.
- Nutritional:
  ○ Hypervitaminosis A.
  ○ Folding fracture secondary to nutritional hyperparathyroidism.
- Demyelinating disease.
- Ascending/descending myelomalacia.
- Lysosomal storage disease.

Causes of generalised LMN disease:
- *Toxoplasma.*
- Polyradiculoneuritis.
- Idiopathic polymyositis.
- Myasthenia.
- Polyneuropathy associated with DM.
- Botulism.
- Toxic – vincristine, coccidiostat.

2.31.3 Key history
- Age and breed.
- Diet.
- Lifestyle – free access outside:
  ○ Trauma.
  ○ Toxins.
- Acute onset or slowly progressive.
- If acute is it progressive?
- Difficulty jumping.
- Is there pain?
  ○ Neck pain.
  ○ Pain/discomfort on stroking or lifting.
  ○ Abdominal guarding ⇒ spinal pain.
- Other neurological signs – disorientation, seizure.
- Evidence of systemic disease.
- Faecal and urinary continence.
- Tail carriage and function.

2.31.4 Focus of physical examination
- Evidence of systemic disease.
- Localisation of neurologic lesion (Table 20).

Table 20 Localisation of spinal lesions

Site of lesion	C1–C5	C6–T2	T3–L3	L4–S3
Forelimb	UMN	LMN	Normal	Normal
Hindlimb	UMN	UMN	UMN	LMN

2.31.5 Decision making
- Is the disease primarily neurological?
- Is it focal or diffuse?
- Is it painful?
- Is it surgical or is conservative management appropriate?
- How intensive is management likely need to be?
- Is it likely to be treatable?

2.31.6 Diagnostic approach
- Radiography:
  - Plain.
  - Myelogram.
- CSF analysis.
- MRI or CT.
- Electrophysiology:
  - Electromyography.
  - Nerve conduction velocity.
- Biopsy:
  - Muscle.
  - Peripheral nerve.
  - (Brain).

2.31.7 Management and therapy
Initial management is centred on immediate needs of the patient for pain relief, respiratory support, bladder management and fluid therapy. Once stable, achieving a diagnosis is crucial particularly in terms of the likely or potential need for surgical intervention. Prognosis for these cases is highly dependent on underlying cause and for more severely affected cases the costs of intensive support and nursing that may be required for weeks.

2.32 POLYPHAGIA

2.32.1 Introduction
Polyphagia is consumption of food in excess of the normal caloric need. Rarely this is primarily associated with disease affecting the satiety centre. Cats generally regulate their caloric intake better than dogs but boredom and highly palatable, energy-dense diets can lead to polyphagia and obesity.

2.32.2 Causes of secondary polyphagia
- Hyperthyroidism.
- DM.
- Malabsorption/maldigestion:
  - Inflammatory or infiltrative intestinal disease.
  - Parasitism.
  - Lymphangiectasia.
  - Pancreatic insufficiency (rare).
- Repeated vomiting/regurgitation.
- Drugs:
  - Corticosteroids.
  - Benzodiazepines.
  - Cyproheptadine.
  - Mirtazapine.
  - Anticonvulsants.
  - Progestins.
  - Antihistamines.
- Lymphocytic cholangitis.
- Acromegaly.
- Hyperadrenocorticism.
- Hypoglycaemia.
- FIP – some cases.
- Feline spongiform encephalopathy.
- Disseminated *M. avium* infection – some cases.

2.32.3 Key history
- Duration, speed of onset and progression.
- Is behaviour normal?
- What is the normal appetite like?
- Are all foods or only specific types over-eaten?

CLINICAL SIGNS

- Is the cat continually worrying for food, does it eat excessively when fed or has its *ad lib* consumption risen?
- Has there been a change of body weight associated with polyphagia?
  - Has there been changes in body shape ⇒ acromegaly?
- PU/PD noted.
- Vomiting or diarrhoea?
  - Faecal consistency, colour, odour.
- Does the cat have episodes of weakness (hypoglycaemia)?
- Other systemic signs?

2.32.4 Focus of physical examination
- Exclusion of pregnancy or lactation as a cause.
- Mucosal colour – jaundice.
- Examination of GIT.
- Other evidence of endocrine disease, e.g. goitre, hair coat and skin changes.
- Neurologic examination if primary polyphagia suspected.

2.32.5 Decision making
- Is the cat actually polyphagic or dysphagic?
- Is there a physiologic cause of polyphagia, e.g. pregnancy, lactation, increased exercise?
- Is the polyphagia behavioural (or psychogenic)?
- Is the polyphagia primary (unlikely)?
- Is current medication likely to be the cause?
- Is it pica rather than polyphagia?
- Is it endocrine or intestinal?

2.32.6 Diagnostic approach
- Faecal parasitology.
- Imaging – thoracic radiography and abdominal ultrasound.
- Coronavirus serology.
- Endocrine testing – thyroxin, IGF-1, ACTH stimulation test.
- Folate, cobalamin and TLI.

- Endoscopy and intestinal biopsy to try and exclude maldigestion/malabsorption.

2.32.7 Management and therapy
The majority of cases will respond to management of the underlying disease process. Endoparasiticide use in cases without an overt diagnosis is the appropriate first therapy. Dietary restriction should be considered if polyphagia is associated with weight gain preferably in combination with environmental enrichment.

2.33 POLYURIA/POLYDIPSIA

2.33.1 Introduction
In virtually all cases of PU/PD, the driving force is polyuria; hence polydipsic cats should *never* be water restricted. Despite their polydipsia, some cats will still be dehydrated as their intake is not meeting their loss.

2.33.2 Causes
Common causes:
- Chronic renal failure.
- Hyperthyroidism.
- DM.
- Inflammatory bowel disease.
- Hepatopathy.
- Diet – recent change to dry food.
- Sepsis.
- Hypercalcaemia.
- Drug associated, e.g. furosemide.

Uncommon and rare causes:
- Hypocalcaemia.
- Acromegaly (and secondary DM).
- DI – central and nephrogenic.
- Hyperviscosity disease – polycythaemia, hyperglobulinemia.
- Hyperadrenocorticism.
- Renal tubular disease – Fanconi's or primary renal glycosuria.
- Feline spongiform encephalopathy (FSE).

- EPI.
- Hypoadrenocorticism.
- Psychogenic.

2.33.3 Key history
- Age.
- Intact or neutered.
- General health.
- Appetite and diet (recent change onto dry food).
- Weight loss.
- Behavioural or neurological signs.
- Changes in household.
- Trauma.
- Recent drug use.
- Changes in urine or urinary habits.
- How much is the cat drinking?
- What are the sources?
  - Water bowl.
  - Milk.
  - Insides – sink, bath, toilet.
  - Outside – puddles, water butt.

2.33.4 Focus of physical examination
- General demeanour.
- Face shape – acromegaly.
- Hydration status.
- Mucosal colour – polycythaemia.
- Palpable thyroid mass.
- Peripheral lymph nodes.
- Thorax – tachycardia.
- Abdomen:
  - Kidney – size, shape, pain.
  - Liver palpable.
- Cataracts (uncommon in cats with DM).
- Peripheral neuropathy – plantigrade stance.
- External evidence of endocrinopathy:
  - Hair loss.
  - Thin inelastic skin.
  - Cutaneous asthenia.
- External evidence of infection:
  - Abscesses.
  - Mastitis.
  - Vaginal discharge.

2.33.5 Decision making
- Major organ failure – systemically unwell.
- Endocrinopathy or early CRD – often systemically well.

2.33.6 Diagnostic approach
It is important that diagnostic tests are undertaken in a logical order and as far as possible before any treatment is given.
- Haematology and biochemistry including dynamic bile acids.
- Full urinalysis including culture and urine protein:creatinine ratio.
- Retrovirus serology.
- Thyroxin level.
- Imaging:
  - Thoracic and abdominal radiography.
  - Ultrasound – kidney, liver, adrenal, uterus.
  - Scintigraphy – hyperthyroidism.
  - MRI/CT – CNS or adrenal mass.
- ACTH response test – the protocol is different from dogs see section 4.7.4.
- Endogenous hormone tests:
  - ACTH.
  - PTH and PTHrP (PTH related protein).
  - ADH measurement (human laboratory).
- Glomerular filtration rate estimation.
- Desmopressin response test.
- Modified water deprivation test:
  - Must be performed correctly otherwise results are uninterpretable.
  - Potentially dangerous as can precipitate acute renal failure.

2.33.7 Management and therapy
So long as hydration status is good, although PU/PD may lead to loss of water-soluble vitamins, increased susceptibility to urinary tract infections and possibly medullary washout, it has little pathologic consequences. Many of the underlying disease processes, however,

CLINICAL SIGNS

CLINICAL SIGNS

do and need identification and treatment where possible.

2.34 PTYALISM

2.34.1 Introduction

Cats will frequently salivate (dribble) when stroked or associated with food; this is a normal physiologic response.

- *Ptyalism (hypersalivation)* – excessive secretion of saliva due to overproduction by one or more of the salivary glands.
- *Pseudoptyalism* – dribbling of saliva caused by an inability to swallow the saliva produced due to pain or obstruction or paralysis of the lips (see also section 2.14).

2.34.2 Causes

- Oral cavity disease:
  - Dental disease.
  - Gingivitis/stomatitis.
  - Neoplasia.
  - Cleft palate.
  - Trauma – Temporomandibular joint (TMJ) or mandibular fracture.
  - Caustic/irritant toxins.
  - FCV.
- Tongue inflammation, neoplasia.
- Salivary gland disease:
  - Sialoadenitis.
  - Salivary gland necrosis.
- Retropharyngeal lymphadenopathy.
- Dysphagia.
- Regurgitation.
- Nausea/vomiting.
- Hepatic or renal encephalopathy.
- Oesophageal disease:
  - Oesophagitis.
  - Megaoesophagus.
  - Oesophageal obstruction/stricture:
    - Foreign body.
    - Vascular ring.
    - Mediastinal mass.
    - Neoplasia.
- Gastric disease:
  - Ulceration.
  - Hernia.
  - Neoplasia.
  - Intussusception.
- Neurological disease:
  - CN IX, X or XII dysfunction.
  - Toxins, e.g. organophosphates.
  - Rabies.
  - Botulism.
  - Tetanus.
  - Seizures.

2.34.3 Key history

- Age and breed.
- Is there associated dysphagia or regurgitation?
- Is the ptyalism persistent or intermittent?
- Appetite.
- Lifestyle:
  - Access to toxins.
  - Access to irritants.
  - Likelihood of trauma.
- Duration and progression of signs.
- Order signs developed, e.g. ptyalism before anorexia or after.
- Other clinical signs:
  - Neurological signs.
  - Vomiting.
  - Weight loss.
- Blood in saliva.
- Does (did) the cat attempt to swallow the excess saliva?
- Halitosis.
- Recent general anaesthetic.
- Recent medication – doxycycline, clindamycin.
- Burns or ulcers on pads.

2.34.4 Focus of physical examination

- Thorough oral examination – may require sedation/GA, check under tongue.
- Neurological examination.
- Ability to open and close mouth and chew.

- Evidence of generalised muscular weakness.
- Palpate pharynx, larynx, retropharyngeal lymph nodes, salivary glands.
- Abdominal palpation – cranial abdominal mass, liver size.
- Cardiac auscultation – murmur with PSS.

2.34.5 Decision making

- Is it excess production, or an inability to swallow?
- Primarily a disease of the head and neck.
- GIT-associated disease.
- Systemic disease.

2.34.6 Diagnostic approach

- Dynamic bile acids.
- Virus isolation (FCV).
- Imaging:
  - Radiography of pharynx, thorax and abdomen.
  - Ultrasound – liver, retropharyngeal structures.
  - Fluoroscopy – swallowing.
- Oral examination UGA.
- Endoscopy and biopsy of upper intestinal tract.
- Acetylcholine receptor antibody.
- Acetylcholine esterase activity.
- Cranial MRI.

2.34.7 Management and therapy

Fluid and nutritional support is required for many cases. With some disease processes, chronic support may be necessary. If tube feeding is required, consideration should be given to the level at which disease is occurring so that a feeding tube can be placed distal to the point of dysfunction.

In the short term, the overall flow of saliva can be decreased using atropine or propantheline (0.25 mg/kg q8–12h), but these drugs have other potential adverse antimuscarinic effects.

2.35 PYREXIA (FEVER) OF UNKNOWN ORIGIN – PUO (FUO)

2.35.1 Introduction

PUO is defined as persistent (on several occasions over a number of days) or recurrent elevation in temperature >39.5°C (103°F) associated with non-specific clinical signs.

- Typically present with anorexia, lethargy ± weight loss.
- Persistent fever above 41.5°C (107°F) is associated with a significant risk of permanent organ damage.

2.35.2 Causes

- Excessive heat input:
  - Exposure.
  - Enclosed vehicle.
  - Tumble dryers.
  - Excessively hot environment in hospital.
- Excessive heat production:
  - Infection – localised or systemic, viral and systemic.
  - Inflammation.
  - Neoplasia.
  - Muscular activity – exercise, seizures.
  - Hypermetabolism, e.g. hyperthyroidism.
  - Stress.
  - Drug reactions.
- Inability to waste heat:
  - Dehydration.
  - Obesity.
  - Severe cardiovascular disease.
  - Drugs that inhibit skin vasodilatation, e.g. ACP.
  - Young and old cats.
- Hypothalamic disease affecting regulatory centres.
- Malignant hyperthermia.

2.35.3 Key history

- Age and breed.
- Neutered.

CLINICAL SIGNS

CLINICAL SIGNS

- Diet – pansteatitis on all fish diet.
- Lifestyle – fighting, retrovirus infection.
- Foreign travel.
- Trauma.
- Drug, supplement or herbal use.
- Recent illness or surgery.
- Lameness or pain.
- Duration of illness.

2.35.4 Focus of physical examination
- Degree of pyrexia.
- Lymphadenopathy.
- Abdominal palpation – pain, enlargement of liver, kidney.
- Petechiation, ecchymosis.
- Cardiac murmur, especially if soft.
- Localised muscular or orthopaedic pain.
- Joint swelling or effusion.
- Ophthalmic examination.

2.35.5 Decision making
- Could the pyrexia be stress related?
- Are there any localising signs?
- Is the pyrexia high enough (≥41°C [(105°F]) that immediate efforts to lower body temperature are required?

2.35.6 Diagnostic approach
- Full haematology, biochemistry, urinalysis and faecal examination.
- Thyroxin estimation.
- Survey thoracic, abdominal and skeletal radiographs.
- Echocardiography.
- Serum protein electrophoresis even if proteins are within reference range.
- Serology for infectious agents:
  - Retrovirus.
  - *Toxoplasma.*
  - *Cryptococcus.*
  - *Haemoplasma.*
  - *Bartonella.*
  - *Ehrlichia.*
  - *Borrelia.*
- Blood culture.

- Rheumatoid factor and ANA generally of very low diagnostic yield.
- Coombs' test.
- Synovial fluid aspirate, synovial biopsy.
- CSF analysis.
- Bone marrow aspirate biopsy.
- Trial therapy with NSAIDs.
- MRI for inflammatory, neoplastic or hypothalamic lesions.
- White cell labelling techniques or scintigraphy.
- Endoscopy and/or exploratory surgery.

2.35.7 Management and therapy
- Severely pyrexic animals:
  - Give NSAIDs ± phenothiazines.
  - If life threatening, use fans or cold water soaked towels but
    - this may increase metabolic rate if the hypothalamus is driving a hyperthermic response.
    - skin vasoconstriction may worsen the cat's ability to waste core heat.
- Management of PUO on initial presentation is better achieved with NSAIDs rather than antimicrobials.
- Inflammatory conditions are more common causes of PUO than bacterial infection. Hence corticosteroids are a better choice trial therapy than antibacterials in idiopathic cases. Monotherapy rather than polypharmacy should be given so that the effect of each drug on the pyrexia can be assessed.

2.36 REGURGITATION

2.36.1 Introduction
Oral regurgitation is the passive expelling of food, fluid or saliva from the oesophagus or stomach. Some cats will both vomit and regurgitate especially if chronic vomiting has resulted in oesophagitis.

Differentiation from vomiting:

- Passive return of food – often sausage shaped.
- Little discomfort unless associated with oesophagitis.
- No signs of salivation, nausea or active contraction of abdominal muscle.
- Appears undigested.
- No bile.
- Often re-eaten.
- Material produced usually alkaline as productive gastric regurgitation is uncommon

2.36.2 Causes

- Pharyngeal obstruction.
- Oesophagitis:
  - Reflux.
  - Toxic/irritant.
  - Infectious.
- Muscular oesophageal disease:
  - Megaoesophagus.
  - Dysautonomia.
  - Myasthenia gravis.
  - Myositis.
  - Myopathy.
  - Toxins – botulism, tetanus, acetylcholine esterase, lead.
- Oesophageal obstruction:
  - Intraluminal:
    - Oesophageal stricture.
    - Oesophageal neoplasia.
    - Granulomatous mass.
    - Foreign body.
  - Extraluminal:
    - Mediastinal mass.
    - Cervical mass.
    - Vascular ring anomaly.
- Oesophageal diverticulum.
- CNS disease – cerebellar and brainstem lesions.
- Peripheral neuropathy.
- Gastro-oesophageal junction:
  - Hiatal hernia.
  - Intussusception.
  - Neoplasia.

2.36.3 Key history

- Age and breed.
- Appetite.
- Weight loss.
- Character of regurgitated material:
  - Food, liquids, both.
  - Does it smell – diverticulum?
  - Blood.
- Is it at a consistent time after eating?
- Recent anaesthesia (weeks) or medication.
- Duration and progression.
- Change in meow.
- Activity.
- Generalised weakness.
- Signs of respiratory disease.
- Possibility of foreign body.
- Exposure to irritants or toxins.
- Constipation.

2.36.4 Focus of physical examination

- Oropharyngeal examination including under the tongue.
- Palpate cervical oesophagus.
- Thoracic auscultation, percussion and compression.
- Neuromuscular examination.
- Watch cat eat/drink (video).
- Constipation, reduced tear production and xerostomia suggest dysautonomia.

2.36.5 Decision making

- Is it regurgitation – differentiation from vomiting, expectoration and retching?
- Site at which food progression is failing:
  - Oropharyngeal.
  - Cervical oesophagus.
  - Gastro-oesophageal junction.
- Foreign body possible.
- Is a stricture likely?
- Evidence of generalised neuromuscular disease.

2.36.6 Diagnostic approach

Resolution of megaoesophagus requires early diagnosis and treatment.

CLINICAL SIGNS

- pH of material regurgitated
- Haematology and biochemistry if systemically unwell.
- Retrovirus serology.
- (TSH stimulation test).
- Schirmer tear test, pilocarpine or histamine response for dysautonomia.
- Imaging:
  - Plain, lightly sedated thorax.
  - Barium swallow (with care as risk of aspiration).
  - Fluoroscopy – contraindicated if possible oesophageal tear.
- AcCh receptor antibody level.
- Lead levels.
- Endoscopic examination ± biopsy.

2.36.7 Management and therapy

Megaoesophagus and oesophagitis are the two most common causes of regurgitation. If demulcents are given for oesophagitis these needs to be administered very frequently (q2–4h) and should be combined with H_2-blockers or proton-pump inhibitors to minimise further damage due to acid reflux. Megaoesophagus may not resolve following appropriate treatment of the primary disease, so long-term dietary change and feeding support with prokinetics ± a gastrostomy tube may be necessary.

2.37 SEIZURES

2.37.1 Introduction

Seizures and epilepsy are less commonly encountered in cats than in dogs. They are, however, the most common manifestation of forebrain disease in cats.

Seizures are usually associated with structural brain disease; idiopathic seizuring is rare.

- *Seizure (convulsion, ictus, fit)* – an involuntary paroxysmal disturbance of the brain usually manifesting as uncontrollable muscle activity.

- *Epilepsy* – recurrent seizures.
- *Preictal (aura, prodromal)* – the change in character (e.g. nervousness, attention seeking) or motor function (e.g. head turning) that occurs prior to a fit.
- *Postictal* – variable signs, e.g. sleepiness, pacing, depression, excitement, polydipsia, polyphagia, that may persist for 24–48 hours after a fit. Care must be taken when interpreting the severity of clinical signs or neurological deficits in this period.
- *Generalised seizures (grand mal)* – tonic–clonic movements, opisthotonos, limb rigidity, paddling/running movements and mass response (defaecation/urination).
- *Status epilepticus* – continuous fitting.
- *Partial seizures (focal).*
- Motor – contralateral tonic–clonic movement that may generalise in seconds usually indicates an acquired cortical or subcortical lesion.
- Psychomotor – behavioural changes secondary to acquired lesions in the temporolimbic system, e.g. tail chasing, biting at imaginary objects, aggression (rare in cats).
- *Absence seizures (petit mal)* – rarely recognised in animals, usually genetic (in man).
- *Non-motor* – loss of consciousness and transient collapse (very rare).

2.37.2 Causes

Extracranial:
- Metabolic:
  - Hepatic encephalopathy – especially associated with portosystemic shunts.
  - Hypoglycaemic – insulinoma, insulin overdose.
  - Azotaemia.
  - Hypocalcaemia – primary hypoparathyroidism, post-hyperthyroid surgery, pregnancy toxaemia.
  - Hypophosphataemia (rare), ketoacidotic diabetic cat.

- Toxins:
  - Organophosphates/carbamates.
  - Organochlorides.
  - Lead.
  - Ethylene glycol.
  - Dieldrin (wood preservative).
  - Strychnine.
  - Bromethalin.
  - Theobromide (in chocolate).
  - Thallium.
  - Alpha-chloralose.
  - Metaldehyde.
- Medications:
  - Potentially anything.
  - Piperazine.
  - Metronidazole.
  - ACP.
  - Flea sprays (fenvalerate and DEET).
  - Rapid reduction in anti-seizure medication.
- Hypoxia:
  - Cardiovascular disease.
  - Respiratory disease/obstruction.
  - Anaemia.
  - Post-anaesthetic.
- Hyperviscosity:
  - Polycythaemia.
  - Multiple myeloma.
- Acromegaly.
- Acute pancreatitis.
- Feline precursor porphyria.

Intracranial:
- Idiopathic epilepsy.
- Neoplasia:
  - Meningioma.
  - Lymphoma.
  - Astrocytoma.
- Infectious/inflammatory disease:
  - FIP.
  - Toxoplasmosis.
  - Cryptococcus.
  - Aujesky's disease.
  - Feline spongiform encephalopathy.
- Meningitis (bacterial meningitis is very rare).
- Encephalitis.
- Meningoencephalitis.
- Aberrant parasitic migration/*Coenurus* cysts.
- Ischaemic encephalopathy.
- Lysosomal storage disease.
- Trauma (seizuring can occur months later due to scarring).
- Haemorrhage.
- Thiamine deficiency.
- Hydrocephalus.

2.37.3 Key history
- Age, breed, sex:
  - Age of onset of seizures.
- History of littermates.
- History of trauma.
- Previous infectious disease (FIP, FeLV) diagnosed.
- Previous endocrine disorder diagnosed.
- Drug, herbal, supplement use.
- Diet – raw fish?
- Access to toxins.
- Chronicity – i.e. are the seizures intermittent or has the cat suddenly developed multiple or frequent seizures?
- Frequency, multiplicity of seizures.
- Association of seizures, i.e. asleep, excitement, feeding.
- Progression.
- Description of seizures (video).
- Is the cat normal between seizures?
- How quickly is the cat apparently back to normal?
- Other signs of systemic disease.

2.37.4 Focus of physical examination
- Face and head shape.
- Mucosal colour and capillary refill time.
- Cardiac auscultation.
- Abdominal palpation.
- Ophthalmic examination:
  - Evidence of papilloedema, cortical blindness, FIP, *Toxoplasma*, Cryptococcosis.
- Neurological examination.

NB – *An abnormal neurological examination within 24 hours of a seizure may be due to the seizure and not an underlying disease.*

2.37.5 Decision making
- Are these genuine seizures? (cf. collapse/syncope section 2.9).
- What is the likelihood of finding a cause?
- Is the disease process likely to be intra- or extracranial?

2.37.6 Diagnostic approach
Rule out extracranial disease.
- Haematology, biochemistry and urinalysis:
  - If hypoglycaemia suspected, the cat should be starved for at least 8 hours prior to sampling.
- Retrovirus serology.
- Blood pressure.
- Survey imaging.
- *Toxoplasma* and *Cryptococcus* serology.
- T$_4$, PTH and IGF-1.
- Fibroblast culture and urinalysis (for lysosomal storage disease).

Intracranial disease:
- CSF analysis.
- Electroencephalography.
- Cranial MRI or CT ± biopsy.

2.37.7 Management and therapy
For multiple seizures, diazepam (0.5–1 mg/kg) i/v or per rectum (repeated up to three times at 10 minute intervals if there has been no response) is the first choice treatment. If this is ineffective, then i/v phenobarbital to a maximum of 16 mg/kg divided over 3–4 hours.

Note: Phenobarbital takes 20 minutes for full CNS effects to occur.

For recurrent seizures, oral phenobarbitone initially at 2.5 mg/kg q12h remains the drug of choice with ongoing monitoring of seizure frequency and serum levels.

Long-term treatment of the primary cause offers the best prognosis.

Potassium bromide is poorly effective and toxic to cats causing an allergic pneumonitis.

2.38 SNEEZING AND NASAL DISCHARGE

2.38.1 Introduction
Sneezing and nasal discharge can be the chronic sequelae to respiratory virus infection or due to allergic/inflammatory rhinitis – both causes can be frustrating to manage. The best outcome for the cat is when specific, treatable disease is identified.
- *Sneezing* – deep inspiration followed by forced expiration against a narrow/closed pharynx/glottis. Sneeze created when glottis/pharynx opens and air is expelled through the nose and mouth.
- *Reverse sneezing* – violent, paroxysmal inspiratory effort caused by repeated diaphragmatic and intercostal muscle contraction designed to remove secretion and foreign material from naso- to oropharynx, so they can be swallowed.
- *Chronic nasal discharge* – there is no precise definition as to what constitutes chronic, but in line with other disease states this would encompass discharge lasting for over 3 weeks or 2 or more episodes in less than 12 months.

2.38.2 Causes
- Infectious agents:
  - Viral – FHV-1, FCV.
  - Fungal – Aspergillosis, Cryptococcus in UK but other fungal agents have been described.
  - Parasites – Capillaria, which is present in foxes in southern UK but not yet reported in cats or dogs.

- Protozoan infection.
- Bacterial – 1° causes include *B. bronchiseptica* and *Streptococcus equi* subsp. *Zooepidemicus*.
- Chronic rhinitis/rhinosinusitis.
- Inflammatory disease.
- Polyp.
- Nasopharyngeal disease/stenosis.
- Allergic disease.
- Foreign body – especially grass blades.
- Dental disease.
- Irritant/allergens.
- Neoplasia.
- Sinus disease.
- Cleft palate.
- Acquired oronasal fistula.
- Ciliary dyskinesia.
- Extranasal disease:
  - Pneumonia.
  - Regurgitation.
  - Dysphagia.

2.38.3 Key history
- Age and vaccinal status.
- Onset of signs:
  - Acute, chronic, recurrent, seasonality.
- Environment:
  - Exposure to irritants, e.g. are the owners smokers?
- History or respiratory virus infection and health of other cats/dogs in house.
- Is the patient systemically unwell, if so, what other body system(s) are likely to be involved?
- Signs:
  - Sneezing.
  - Nasal discharge.
  - ± abnormal respiratory noises.
- Nasal discharge:
  - Uni- or bilateral.
  - Mucoid or purulent.
  - Blood – alone or mixed with secretion.
- Other:
  - Halitosis.
  - Pawing at face.

- Change in face shape or point colour.
- Ocular signs.

2.38.4 Focus of physical examination
- Regional lymphadenopathy.
- Palpation of head and neck.
- Tracheal pinch.
- Percussion of frontal sinuses:
  - Difficult in cats – need cooperative patient with short facial hair.
- Aural examination.
- Oral examination.
- Fundoscopy.
- Thoracic auscultation.
- Nasal airflow testing:
  - Glass slide or fine piece of cotton wool.

2.38.5 Decision making
- Was the onset of clinical signs sudden or gradual and are the signs progressive?
- Is the nasal discharge uni- or bilateral?
- What is the likely localisation of the lesion?
- Is it chronic, relapsing and antibacterial responsive?
- Is the patient systemically unwell?
- Is there evidence of bony involvement – facial pain or asymmetry?

2.38.6 Diagnostic approach
- FCV/FHV-1 isolation or PCR.
- Selective bacterial culture:
  - Limited value with culture results tending to isolate faecal or respiratory commensals.
  - Role of mycoplasma in chronic nasal discharge and sneezing is unclear.
- Fungal serology, cytology and fungal culture of the nasal discharge.
- Oral nasopharyngeal and aural examination under sedation/GA.
- Radiography – head and neck.
- Coagulation profile.
- Nasal flushing.
- Antegrade and retrograde rhinoscopy with biopsy.

CLINICAL SIGNS

- Advanced imaging – CT and/or MRI.
- Exploratory rhinotomy.

2.38.7 Management and therapy

Where underlying cause is not found or untreatable, managing chronic rhinitis usually involves antibacterials for purulent disease or corticosteroid for inflammatory disease. Depending on the response, additional therapy with antihistamines, decongestants and environmental management may be required.

2.39 STIFFNESS

2.39.1 Introduction

Stiffness usually presents as reluctance to move, exercise or jump on to surfaces; it can be mistaken by the owner for lethargy (listlessness or apathy). A degree of stiffness is not uncommon as part of the ageing process but should have a gradual onset and slow progression.

2.39.2 Causes

- Polyarthropathy:
  - Degenerative – osteoarthritis.
  - Immune-mediated.
  - Infectious, e.g. *Borrelia*.
  - Post-vaccinal (FCV vaccine).
- Myositis:
  - Hypokalaemic polymyopathy.
  - Chronic renal failure.
  - Drug induced – methimazole.
  - Immune-mediated.
  - Eosinophilic.
- Abdominal guarding.
- Infectious:
  - *Toxoplasma*.
  - Tetanus.
- Pyrexia.
- Pansteatitis.
- Generalised orthopaedic pain.
- Myoclonus.
- Spinal pain.

2.39.3 Key history

- Age, breed.
- Onset and progression:
  - Acute vs. chronic.
  - Duration.
  - Slow or rapid progression.
  - Signs persistent, intermittent, cyclical.
- Appetite.
- Likelihood of trauma.
- Lameness or gait abnormality.
- Abnormal stance, e.g. hunched.
- Overt signs of pain:
  - on lifting/handling.
  - on stroking.
  - on jumping.
- Whole body or localised.
- Signs of systemic illness.

2.39.4 Focus of physical examination

- Observe standing and walking.
- Gentle palpation of whole body.
- Palpation of joints – swelling, heat pain, range of movement.
- Muscle mass and tone.
- Abdominal palpation.
- Neurologic examination.

2.39.5 Decision making

- Stiffness associated with pyrexia.
- Musculoskeletal or systemic (metabolic).
- Muscular, spinal or joint associated.
- Traumatic.
- Systemically unwell.

2.39.6 Diagnostic approach

- CPK, AST and electrolytes.
- *Toxoplasma* serology.
- Radiographs of joints, spine ± contrast.
- Arthrocentesis.
- Electromyography.
- Bone, muscle, synovial, fat biopsy.

2.39.7 Management and therapy

Osteoarthritis is a common cause of stiffness in older cats; if initial examination/

investigation is unrewarding consider an NSAID trial. Hypokalaemia can cause muscle stiffness and a stilted gait; it should be excluded early on in the course of any investigation.

2.40 STUPOR AND ALTERED STATES OF CONSCIOUSNESS

2.40.1 Introduction
Altered states of consciousness are associated with interruptions of the structural, metabolic or physiologic function of the brainstem or cerebral cortex. They need to be differentiated from depression, lethargy, disorientation, cognitive dysfunction and other behavioural disorders.
- *Stupor* – partial loss of consciousness with reduced responses to external stimuli.
- *Disorientation* – cat is responsive but the response is inappropriate.
- *Cognitive dysfunction* – behavioural changes including anxiety, fears, phobias, aggression, stereotypic behaviour, night waking and house soiling.

2.40.2 Causes
- CNS disease:
  - Hydrocephalus.
  - Cranial trauma.
  - Space-occupying lesion:
    - Neoplasia – primary or metastatic.
    - Haemorrhage.
    - Inflammation.
    - Cerebral oedema.
    - Parasitic cyst.
  - Feline ischaemic encephalopathy.
  - Post seizure.
- Metabolic:
  - Hepatic encephalopathy.
  - DM.
  - Hypoglycaemia.
  - Uraemia.
  - Hypoxia.
  - Acid–base disturbance.
  - Marked dehydration.
  - Hyperlipidaemia.
  - (Hypothyroidism, hypoadrenocorticism).
- Cardiovascular:
  - Hyperviscosity.
  - Hypotension.
  - Hypertension.
  - Anaemia.
  - Cardiomyopathy.
- Hyperthermia.
- Hypothermia.
- Toxic:
  - Ethylene glycol.
  - Lead.
  - Alcohol.
  - Cannabis.
  - Other hallucinogenic drugs.
  - Sedative drugs.
- Infectious:
  - FIP.
  - Sepsis.

2.40.3 Key history
- Age.
- Onset – acute or chronic.
- Duration and progression.
- History of trauma.
- Lifestyle – access to toxins, likelihood of trauma.
- Drug, herbal or nutritional supplements.
- History of seizures.
- Other signs of systemic disease.

2.40.4 Focus of physical examination
- Evidence of trauma.
- State of circulation:
  - Mucosal colour.
  - Capillary refill time.
  - Pulse quality.
  - Level of dehydration.
- Blood pressure.
- Rectal temperature.
- Thoracic auscultation.
- Evidence of bleeding disorder.

CLINICAL SIGNS

- Neurological examination:
  - Posture and muscle tone.
  - Pupillary light response.
  - Ocular examination – papilloedema, ocular movement.
  - Respiratory pattern.
  - Neck pain.
  - Reflexes and skeletal motor responses.
  - Modified Glasgow coma scale.

2.40.5 Decision making

- Is it an intra- or extracranial disease?
  - Is there likely to be increased ICP?
- Is there history or evidence of trauma?
- Is intoxication likely?
- Hypo- or hyperthermia?
- Hypo- or hypertension?

2.40.6 Diagnostic approach

- Exclude metabolic, cardiovascular and musculoskeletal disease.
- If negative then central causes:
  - coagulation profile.
  - CSF analysis.
  - electroencephalogram and brainstem auditory-evoked potentials.
  - cranial MRI or CT.

2.40.7 Management and therapy

Most cats showing stupor or coma have life-threatening disease requiring immediate diagnostics and treatment. Venous access and a patent airway should be established and ventilation ensured. Blood pressure supported whilst checking that ICP is not raised excessively. Elevating the head reduces excessive cerebral blood flow. Confirmed or suspected cerebral oedema should be treated with furosemide, mannitol, corticosteroids and hyperventilation instituted once BP stabilised. Seizures controlled with diazepam or phenobarbital. Drugs should be given intravenously.

2.41 TREMOR

2.41.1 Introduction

Tremor results from simultaneous or alternating contractions of opposing muscle groups. When tremor is observed effort should be made to describe the type of tremor and distinguish it from other processes involving muscle contraction such as seizure or myoclonus.

Tremor is pathologic when it impairs the cat's normal function.

- *Shiver* – involuntary increase in high-frequency skeletal muscle activity primarily of the torso.
- *Tremble, quiver* – involuntary, moderate-frequency, coarse muscle contraction and relaxation.
- *Tremor* – involuntary contraction and relaxation of antagonistic muscle groups:
  - *Intention tremor* – exacerbated when cat attempts to coordinate movement, e.g. jumping, eating suggest cerebellar disease.
  - *Postural or continual* – more pronounced at rest.
- *Fasciculation* – rapid alternate contraction/relaxation of adjacent muscle groups producing wave-like or writhing sensation on palpation, often associated with nerve root irritation (*root signature*).
- *Myoclonus* – episodic jerking of one or more muscle groups, may continue in sleep.
- *Myotonus* – sustained contraction of a muscle group.

2.41.2 Causes

- Generalised tremor:
  - Temperature regulation.
  - Fatigue.
  - Post-anaesthetic.
  - Exposure to toxins:
    - Organophosphates.
    - Metaldehyde.

○ Metabolic disease:
  ▪ Hypocalcaemia.
  ▪ Hyperkalaemia.
  ▪ Hypoglycaemia.
  ▪ Uraemia.
  ▪ Hepatopathy.
  ▪ Hypothyroidism.
  ▪ Hyperadrenocorticism.
○ Lysosomal storage disease.
○ Spongy degeneration.
• Head tremor:
  ○ Cerebellar disease:
    ▪ Abiotrophy.
    ▪ Hypoplasia (FPV infection *in utero*).
    ▪ Trauma.
    ▪ Neoplasia.
    ▪ Ischaemia.
    ▪ Inflammatory/necrotizing disease.
• Hind limb tremor:
  ○ Nerve root disease:
    ▪ Entrapment.
    ▪ Neoplasia.
  ○ Disc extrusion/discospondylitis.
  ○ Myasthenia gravis.
  ○ Polymyopathy.
  ○ Polyneuropathy.

2.41.3 Key history
• Age and breed.
• Vaccinal status of queen.
• Health of littermates.
• Diet (nutritional secondary hyperparathyroidism).
• Likely exposure to trauma or toxins.
• Speed of onset.
• Duration and progression.
• Description of tremors:
  ○ Type and distribution.
  ○ Present continuously.
  ○ What happens in sleep?
  ○ What happens when eating or jumping?
• Alertness.
• Recent surgery (thyroidectomy).
• Other clinical signs.

2.41.4 Focus of physical examination
• Temperature.
• Palpation of muscles.
• Response to stimuli.
• Evidence of pain.
• Abdominal palpation.
• Neurological examination.
• Observe walking or jumping.

2.41.5 Decision making
• Whole body, head or hindlimbs.
• Congenital or acquired.
• Intra- or extracranial cause.
• Is there intention tremor?
• Evidence of other neurological signs ⇒ cerebellar.
• Evidence of systemic signs ⇒ metabolic/toxic.

2.41.6 Diagnostic approach (see Table 14 page 40–41)
• Muscle enzymes (AST and CPK).
• Fibroblast culture and urinalysis for lysosomal storage disease.
• Acetylcholine esterase activity.
• Acetylcholine receptor antibodies.
• Spinal radiography ± myelogram.
• CSF analysis.
• Electromyography.
• Electroencephalography.
• Cranial MRI or CT.

2.41.7 Management and therapy
Options and need for intervention depend on the severity of the tremor, likelihood of progression, location and type of disease process that is occurring. Apart from metabolic causes, corticosteroids (± other immunosuppressive drugs) and surgery are likely to be the two main therapeutic modalities.

2.42 VOMITING

2.42.1 Introduction
Vomiting is an active process that occurs in three phases – nausea, retching and

CLINICAL SIGNS

CLINICAL SIGNS

vomition. It needs to be distinguished from regurgitation (see section 2.36), expectoration and retching associated with swallowing difficulties (see section 2.14).

- *Nausea* – first phase of vomiting characterised by depression, ptyalism, licking lips and repeated swallowing.
- *Expectoration* – at the end of a bout of coughing, cat expectorates and may produce white, frothy phlegm or can be seen to swallow.

2.42.2 Causes

- Vestibular:
  - Motion sickness.
- Higher CNS centres:
  - Fear.
  - Stress.
  - Excitement.
  - Inflammatory lesions.
  - Increased ICP.
- Chemoreceptor trigger zone:
  - Uraemia.
  - Bacterial toxins.
  - Hyperthyroidism.
  - Acid–base disturbance, e.g. diabetic ketoacidosis.
  - Radiation.
  - Histamine release.
  - Drugs – morphine, salicylates, chemotherapeutic agents.
  - Toxins.
- Visceral:
  - Anatomical areas:
    - Conditions of intestinal tract from stomach to colon – especially duodenum.
    - Pancreas.
    - Liver and gall bladder.
    - Peritoneum.
    - Mesenteric vasculature.
    - Cardiomyopathy.
  - Pathology:
    - Dietary.
    - Obstructive.
    - Foreign body.

- Neoplasia.
- Hypertrophic.
- Functional.
- Intussusception.
- Dysautonomia.
- Ulceration.
- Inflammatory/infiltrative.
- Parasitic.

2.42.3 Key history

- Age and breed.
- Diet.
- Likelihood of access to toxins.
- Drug, herbal or nutritional supplement use.
- Exposure to infections.
- Worming history.
- Onset.
- Duration and progression.
- Weight loss.
- Appetite.
- Health of other cats in household.
- Pattern of vomiting:
  - Relationship to feeding.
  - Frequency.
  - Pain or discomfort.
  - Improved demeanour after vomiting.
  - Nature of vomit:
    - Froth.
    - Bile.
    - Food (state of digestion).
    - Blood – frank vs. coffee grounds.
    - Projectile.
    - Foetid smell.
- Faecal colour and consistency.
- Systemically unwell.
- Excessive grooming.
- Excessive plant eating or pica.

2.42.4 Focus of physical examination

- Temperature.
- Evidence of hypovolaemia or dehydration:
  - Blood pressure.
- Mucosal colour.
- Halitosis – CKD, pneumonia, gastritis.

Table 21 Appropriate symptomatic therapy for vomiting

Therapy that is unlikely to worsen or prolong clinical signs or interfere with further investigation	Therapy that may worsen or prolong the clinical signs, interfere with further investigation or mask worsening of clinical status	Therapy that will interfere with further investigation
Starvation	Antimicrobials	Corticosteroids
Bland diet	Atropine	
Mucosal protectants, e.g. sucralfate, kaolin	Non-steroidal anti-inflammatory drugs	
Antacids, e.g. magnesium hydroxide, H_2-blockers	Anti-emetics and prokinetics, e.g. maropitant, metoclopramide, cisapride	
Vitamin supplementation		
Pro-/prebiotics		

- Abdominal palpation:
  - Distension, pain, organ displacement, dilation of stomach/bowel, amount of faeces.
- Nasal discharge.
- Food/saliva staining around mouth.
- Neurological signs.

2.42.5 Decision making
- Is it true vomiting?
- Is the vomiting frequent/severe enough to justify further investigation?
  - Is it likely to be self-limiting with symptomatic and supportive treatment?
  - Systemically unwell – depression, malaise, pallor, dehydration.
- GI or systemic cause.
- Obstructive.
- Drug related.
- Intoxication.

2.42.6 Diagnostic approach
- Cease all medicaments possible.
- Observe eating.
- Faecal parasitology:
  - Trial therapy with fenbendazole.
- Additional blood tests:
  - Pancreatic lipase, vitamin B_{12}, folate, thyroxin.
- Imaging:
  - Plain radiographs.
  - Barium meal.
  - Barium-impregnated polyspheres.
  - Ultrasound of liver, kidney, pancreas and intestine.
- Stomach and intestinal biopsies:
  - Endoscopy.
  - Laparoscopic.
  - Laparotomy.
- Cranial CT/MRI.

2.42.7 Management and therapy (Table 21)
In many cases, symptomatic and supportive treatment is sufficient. More aggressive management is likely to be required in recurrent cases and those that are systemically unwell.

2.43 WEIGHT LOSS

2.43.1 Introduction
Weight loss is a common clinical sign in cats and is associated with a very wide variety of disease processes. In the majority of cases, the primary presenting signs should be investigated. Less commonly, weight loss is the major/only presenting sign and requires investigation of itself.

2.43.2 Causes
- Inadequate caloric intake:
  - Anorexia/inappetence.
  - Lack of food availability.

- ○ Deliberate starvation.
- ○ Inappropriate diet.
- ○ Failure to meet increased demand – pregnancy, lactation.
- Failure to absorb nutrients – maldigestion/malassimilation:
  - ○ Severe vomiting/diarrhoea.
  - ○ Inflammatory bowel disease.
  - ○ EPI.
  - ○ Intestinal neoplasia.
- Hypermetabolism:
  - ○ Cachexic states, e.g. neoplasia, chronic inflammatory disease.
  - ○ Hyperthyroidism.
- Excessive caloric loss:
  - ○ Protein-losing nephropathy.
  - ○ Protein-losing enteropathy.
  - ○ DM.
  - ○ Renal tubular disease.
  - ○ Severe exfoliating skin disease, e.g. burns.
- Iatrogenic:
  - ○ Repeated drainage of effusions.
  - ○ Drugs e.g. corticosteroids.

2.43.3 Key history

- Age.
- Appetite and attitude to food.
- Diet.
- Approximate amount eaten – caloric intake.
- Duration and severity of weight loss.
- Is the loss becoming more rapid?
- Other signs of disease:
  - ○ Did weight loss precede or follow other signs?

2.43.4 Focus of physical examination

A full physical is required with special attention to the oral cavity and palpation of the thyroid area and intestinal tract.

2.43.5 Decision making

- How accurately has the weight loss been documented?
- Is there an organ disease process to target?
- Can the weight loss be explained by a lack of calorie intake?
  - ○ Caloric requirements in cats 60–75 kcal/kg/day.
  - ○ Maximum weight loss with total starvation is 2–3% bodyweight/week.
  - ○ Weight loss >3%/week $\Rightarrow$ hypermetabolism or caloric loss.

2.43.6 Diagnostic approach

- Investigate primary clinical signs.
- Additional blood tests:
  - ○ Thyroxin level, TLI, pancreatic lipase, FeLV/FIV.
- Oral examination.
- Survey imaging:
  - ○ Dental radiographs.
- Endoscopic or surgical intestinal biopsies.

2.43.7 Management and therapy

Management depends heavily on the primary disease process that is occurring. In the short term, whilst investigation is being conducted a highly palatable, highly digestible, calorie-dense diet can be fed. Food intake can be maximised by ensuring that the environment is conducive; appetite stimulants may be appropriate. Force feeding is not advised as rarely can clients give sufficient and it risks increasing food aversion.

SECTION 3

COMMON ABNORMALITIES OF HAEMATOLOGY, BIOCHEMISTRY AND URINALYSIS

COMMON LAB. ABNORMALITIES

Notes on Feline Internal Medicine, Second Edition. Edited by Kit Sturgess. ©2013 John Wiley & Sons, Ltd.
Published 2013 by Blackwell Publishing Ltd.

INTRODUCTION

- Where lists of differentials are given, conditions more commonly encountered in cats are given first.
- Ranges given by diagnostic laboratories cover 95% of normal animals, so minor changes outside the range may be a normal variant.
- If large numbers of parameters are measured then the chances that one or two of these parameters will lie outside of the reference range are high, without them being necessarily of any significance with respect to the disease process that is causing the clinical signs.
- Laboratory tests are at their most valuable and powerful when used to confirm or deny a clinical hypothesis; e.g. this cat's halitosis is caused by renal disease. When a 'scatter gun' approach is used in the hope of illuminating the cause of a cat's presentation, the risks of being taken down the wrong diagnostic pathway are higher.
- Single abnormal values that are unexpected should be considered to be artefacts until supported by other findings.
- Inter-assay variation is around 10–15% so changes of this magnitude on serial testing cannot be interpreted as evidence of a change in disease status; i.e. a day 3 creatinine of 256 μmol/l when compared to a day 1 creatinine of 290 μmol/l is not necessarily evidence of a fall in creatinine as it could be inter-assay variation.
- Whilst most laboratories quote an upper and lower limit for enzymes, levels below the reference range are very rarely of clinical significance.
- In-house machines tend to produce less accurate and consistent results than those used at external laboratories and can be more affected by lipaemia, haemolysis and jaundice:
  - Total calcium and albumin are difficult to measure accurately on most in-house machines.

3.1 LOW HAEMATOCRIT

HCT is a derived cell parameter (red blood cell count [RBCC] × MCV) and is often used interchangeably with PCV (% volume occupied by the red cells) that is measured by centrifugation of a blood sample in a capillary tube. At the extremes of measurement, HCT and PCV can differ significantly.

Anaemia (see also section 2.30) describes a fall in the red cell mass usually identified as a low HCT. HCT can be affected by cell swelling, e.g. in transport (artificial increase) or haemolysis (artificial lowering); the most reliable and stable parameter to describe anaemia is the Hb level. Levels of various red cell parameters that indicate the severity of the anaemia are given in table 22.

Table 22 Benchmarking reductions in red cell parameters

Parameter	Marked	Moderate	Mild
PCV (%)	12	18	22
RBCC (× 10^{12}/l)	1.7	3.4	5.2
Hb (g/dl)	3	5.5	7
MCV (fl)	32	37	39
MCH[a] (pg)	22	27	30

[a]Mean cell Hb.

COMMON LAB. ABNORMALITIES

COMMON LAB. ABNORMALITIES

3.1.1 Notes

- Derived cell parameters are less reliable in cats as their red cells tend to be more spherical and susceptible to artefacts associated with handling.
- Two types of reticulocyte are identified in cats: aggregate and punctate. Evidence of regeneration is indicated by an increased aggregate reticulocyte count.

3.1.2 Is it regenerative?

Regeneration is indicated by
- Increased MCV.
- Red cell morphology – anisocytosis, polychromasia, macrocytosis.
- Increased reticulocyte count.
- Absolute count >65 000/µl (50 × 10⁹/l) in mild–moderate anaemia and >175 000/µl in severe anaemia.
- Corrected reticulocyte count >1%.
- Reticulocyte production index >1.

3.1.3 Is it haemorrhagic or haemolytic?

Unless the haemorrhage is acute (i.e. within the last 2–4 hours, when the PCV may still be normal as plasma volume has yet to have expanded), haemorrhage is characterised by a loss of whole blood, hence protein levels will also be low.

3.1.4 Why is the cat haemorrhaging?

- Traumatic – internal (3rd space) or external.
- Coagulopathy.
- Thrombocytopenia.
- Occult disease – neoplasia, ulceration, amyloidosis.
- Check urine, faeces and body cavities for evidence of bleeding.

NB – *Chronic external loss can lead to iron deficiency and eventually a non-regenerative anaemia.*

3.1.5 Causes of haemolytic anaemia

- Feline infectious anaemia (haemoplasma).
- Microangiopathy – DIC, vascular tumours (uncommon).
- Oxidative damage – paracetamol, onions.
- Immune-mediated:
  ○ Primary (uncommon).
  ○ Secondary, e.g. drug reaction, retrovirus related, paraneoplastic.

3.1.6 Non-regenerative anaemia

- Extra-marrow disease:
  ○ CKD.
  ○ Most chronic diseases (anaemia usually mild).
  ○ FeLV.
  ○ Iron deficiency.
  ○ Vitamin B₁₂/folate deficiency.
- Intra-marrow disease:
  ○ FeLV, lymphoma, leukaemias, myelophthisis, myelodysplasia, immune-mediated destruction of red cell precursors (red cell aplasia), other neoplasia, drugs, chemotherapy.

3.2 HIGH HAEMATOCRIT

When HCT is high, the disparity with PCV can be marked at 5% or greater.

Absolute polycythaemia describes an increased red cell mass usually identified as a high HCT. A relative increase in HCT can occur in response to dehydration but resolves with fluid therapy. Haematologic changes indicating the severity of the polycythaemia are shown in Table 23

Polycythaemic cases are usually divided into primary or secondary causes (Figure 11).

Table 23 Benchmarking increases in red cell parameters

Parameter	Marked	Moderate	Mild
PCV (%)	70	60	55
RBCC (× 10¹²/l)	15	13	11
Hb (g/dl)	23.5	20	18.5
MCV (fl)	62	59	56

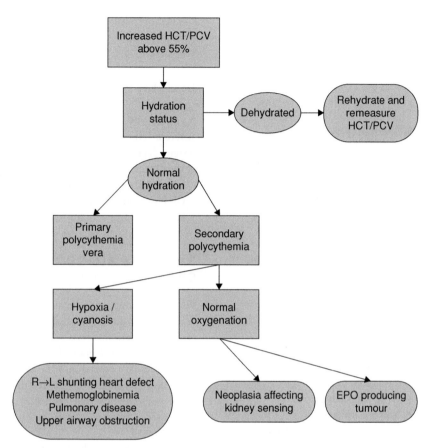

Figure 11 Differential diagnosis of elevated HCT

3.3 PLATELET ABNORMALITIES AND CLOTTING SYSTEM

- Machine artefacts are common, particularly in cats, where platelet clumping occurs very easily.
- A manual smear should be made in all cases before a diagnosis of thrombocytopenia is made.
- Bleeding associated with platelet abnormalities can occur in the face of normal counts (thrombocytopathy).

3.3.1 Laboratory investigation

- Platelet count.
- Buccal mucosal bleeding time.
- Anti-platelet antibodies.
- Thromboelastometry.
- Dynamic clot formation (platelet aggregation factor [PAF] 100).
- Flow cytometry.

3.3.2 Assessment

- Decrease:
  - Mild $< 120 \times 10^9/l$.
  - Moderate $< 50 \times 10^9/l$.
  - Marked $< 10 \times 10^9/l$.

- Increase:
  - Mild > 700×10^9/l.
  - Moderate > 1000×10^9/l.
  - Marked > 1500×10^9/l.
  - Values over 1000×10^9/l strongly suggest primary bone marrow disease.

3.3.3 Thrombocytopenia
- Bleeding rarely occur unless the platelet count drops below 40×10^9/l.
- Typically causes petechiae or ecchymoses, mucosal bleeding or prolonged postsurgical haemorrhage
- Decreased production:
  - FeLV, FIV, *Ehrlichia*, FPV.
  - Drugs – chemotherapeutic agents, chemicals, toxins.
  - Myelophthisis.
  - Marrow aplasia/pancytopenia.
  - Anti-megakaryocyte antibodies.
- Increased destruction:
  - Immune-mediated:
    - Primary.
    - Paraneoplastic.
    - Drug-associated.
    - Vaccine-induced.
  - Microangiopathic neoplasia.
- Increased consumption:
  - Haemorrhage.
  - DIC.
  - Neoplasia.

3.3.4 Thrombocytosis
- Rebound/reactive thrombocytosis.
- Generalised marrow stimulation.
- Polycythaemia vera.
- Primary thrombocyte neoplasia.

3.3.5 Thrombocytopathy
- Inherited – very rare.
- Acquired:
  - Infectious disease, e.g. FIV.
  - Coating of platelets by proteins preventing them from functioning normally – myeloma, dextrans (usually more than 40ml/kg over 24 hours).
  - Drugs – NSAIDs, heparin.

- Platelet dysplasia – common in myeloproliferative disease and other neoplasia.

3.3.6 Clotting system
See Section 2.7.6.
- A variety of tests are available to assess different components of the clotting system depending on the potential site of the defect:
  - Clotting cascade (intrinsic/extrinsic).
  - Global clotting function – includes vascular component and clot stability.

3.4 WHITE BLOOD CELL CHANGES

- White cell changes can be as a result of changes in production, distribution or rate of destruction.
- A large marginated pool of neutrophils can be rapidly released into the circulation, causing a sudden rise in neutrophil count without increased production or the presence of immature forms in the circulation.
- Cats do not readily show a stress leucogram.
- White cell numbers can appear normal but function can be abnormal. Very rarely this is a primary hereditary defect, e.g. Chédiak–Higashi syndrome in Blue-smoke Persians or more commonly secondary to corticosteroids or disease, e.g. DM, FeLV.

3.4.1 Leucocytosis
- Infection – bacterial, fungal.
- Inflammation – immune-mediated, trauma, tissue necrosis, neoplasia.
- Marrow stimulation:
  - Stress.
  - Glucocorticoids.
  - Response to anaemia.
- Leukaemia.

3.4.2 Leucopenia

- Decreased production.
- Increased consumption exceeding marrow response.
- Redistribution, e.g. peritonitis.
- Sample taken during sedation or anaesthesia.

3.4.3 Neutrophilia

- Left shift (band forms present) indicates increased marrow production.
- Mature neutrophilia associated with demarginalisation or a chronic inflammatory or infectious process:
  - Infection – bacterial, *Toxoplasma*, (mycotic).
  - Inflammatory – immune-mediated, trauma, tissue necrosis, neoplasia.
  - Marrow stimulation.
  - Chronic granulocytic leukaemia.

3.4.4 Neutropenia

- Decreased production:
  - Myelophthisis – myeloproliferative disease, lymphoproliferative disease, metastatic neoplasia.
  - Myelofibrosis.
  - Drug induced – methimazole, carbimazole, azathioprine, griseofulvin, oestrogens, chloramphenicol, phenobarbital.
  - Infection – retroviruses, parvovirus, *Ehrlichia*.
- Increased consumption:
  - Bacteraemia.
  - Septicaemia.
  - Hypoadrenocorticism.
- Margination or redistribution.

3.4.5 Lymphopenia

- FIP.
- Retroviruses.
- Lymphangiectasia.
- Drugs – chemotherapy.

3.4.6 Lymphocytosis

- Chronic antigen stimulation – IBD, cholangiohepatitis.
- Post-vaccination.
- Lymphocytic leukaemia.

3.4.7 Monocytosis

- Chronic inflammation.
- Chronic infection.
- Granulomatous disease.
- Myelomonocytic leukaemia.
- Monocytic leukaemia.

3.4.8 Eosinophilia

- Allergic disease – atopy, food allergy, airway disease.
- Parasitic – fleas, *Aelurostrongylus*, *Dirofilaria*, gastrointestinal.
- Eosinophilic granuloma complex.
- Eosinophilic enteritis.
- Sinusitis/rhinitis.
- Pregnancy.
- Neoplasia – mast cell tumour, lymphoma, solid tumours.
- Hypereosinophilic syndrome.
- Eosinophilic leukaemia.
- Fungal infection.

3.5 ACID–BASE DISTURBANCES

Acid–base disturbances are common in cats that are clinically unwell but the level of abnormality is not always predictable. Renal and respiratory compensation will occur with time.

3.5.1 Assessment (Table 24)

3.5.2 TCO$_2$

Total CO_2 – estimates the dissolved CO_2 and the bicarbonate and therefore exceeds bicarbonate by 1–2 units.

COMMON LAB. ABNORMALITIES

Table 24 Interpretation of acid–base changes

| | | Primary | |
	pH	H+ change	Compensation
Metabolic acidosis	↓	↑	↓ HCO_3^- ↓ pCO_2
Metabolic alkalosis	↑	↓	↑ HCO_3^- ↑ pCO_2
Respiratory acidosis	↓	↑	↑ pCO_2 ↑ HCO_3^-
Respiratory alkalosis	↑	↓	↓ pCO_2 ↓ HCO_3^-

3.5.3 Anion gap

This is the difference between the commonly measured cations which exceed the concentrations of the commonly measured anions:

- Reference range – 13–27 mmol/l.
- Tries to give an estimate of the unmeasured anions (phosphate, sulphate, lactate, other organic acids and proteins).
- Used to help identify mixed acid–base disturbances.

3.5.4 Base excess

- Definition – the amount of strong acid required to titrate 1 l of blood to pH 7.4 at 37°C while pCO_2 (partial pressure of carbon dioxide) is held constant at 40 mmHg.
- Derived from pCO_2, pH and HCT.
- Base excess (BE) is changed by non-volatile acids hence reflects metabolic acid–base disturbances.
- A more negative BE reflects acidosis.

3.5.5 Metabolic acidosis

- Normal anion gap:
  - diarrhoea, renal tubular acidosis, drugs (acetazolamide, NH_4Cl).
- Increased anion gap:
  - azotaemia, diabetic ketoacidosis (DKA), lactic acidosis (cardiac, shock, hypoxia), toxins (metaldehyde, ethylene glycol).

- Azotaemia due to reduced tubular ability to produce ammonia and therefore excrete H^+.

3.5.6 Metabolic alkalosis

- Vomiting (pyloric outflow obstruction).
- Loop diuretics.
- Excess alkali.

3.5.7 Respiratory acidosis

Decreased alveolar ventilation.

- Neuromuscular:
  - Organophosphate poisoning, myasthenia gravis, drugs, polyradiculoneuritis.
- Respiratory:
  - Airway obstruction, pneumothorax, pleural disease, severe pneumonia/pulmonary oedema, diffuse metastatic disease, massive pulmonary embolus, cardiac arrest.

3.5.8 Respiratory alkalosis

Caused by hyperventilation blowing of CO_2.

- Central stimulation – anxiety, stress, fever, pain, CNS disease.
- Peripheral stimulation – pneumonia, interstitial lung disease.
- Gram-negative septicaemia.
- Over-ventilation.

3.6 AMYLASE AND LIPASE

- Changes in amylase and lipase are of little diagnostic value. Pancreatitis, both acute and chronic, does not cause a reliable increase in enzyme levels
  - Increased amylase tends to be associated with a decreased GFR.
- Feline pancreatic-specific lipase is a more sensitive and specific test for pancreatitis.
- Increased feline trypsin-like immunoreactivity (fTLI) may be associated with pancreatitis, but lacks sensitivity and specificity.

3.7 AZOTAEMIA

3.7.1 Definitions
- Azotaemia – describes an increase in urea and creatinine outside of the reference interval. It may or may not be associated with clinical signs.
- Uraemia – describes the clinical signs (halitosis, weight loss, etc.) associated with a clinically significant azotaemia.
- Urea and creatinine – used to reflect changes in GFR, but is a non-linear relationship – doubling of urea is not equivalent to a halving of GFR. Severity of clinical signs depends not only on the absolute value but also on the rate of rise.
- Urea and creatinine will only start rising once >75% of renal mass is lost.

3.7.2 Assessment
See page 240–241 for IRIS classification
Urea – reference range 4–12 mmol/l.
Creatinine – reference range 80–140 µmol/l.
- Decreased urea:
  - Mild – 3.5 mmol/l.
  - Moderate – 2.5 mmol/l.
  - Marked – 1.5 mmol/l.
- Increased urea:
  - Mild – 15 mmol/l.
  - Moderate – 23 mmol/l.
  - Marked – 40 mmol/l.
- Increased creatinine:
  - Mild – 200 µmol/l.
  - Moderate – 350 µmol/l.
  - Marked – 500 µmol/l.

3.7.3 Causes of azotaemia
- Pre-renal.
- Renal.
- Post-renal.

Pre-renal disease
- Can be caused by any condition that results in a fall in renal blood flow, e.g. dehydration, hypovolaemia, shock, heart failure, excessive use of diuretics. Urea and creatinine will tend to normalise with fluid therapy. Urine volume is low and urine specific gravity (USG) is usually high unless drug use or disease is affecting concentration ability, e.g. diuretics.

Intrinsic renal disease
- Acute renal failure (acute kidney injury) oligoanuria, hyperkalaemia, phosphate normal:
  - Polyuric, acute renal failure is reported.
- Chronic renal (kidney) disease – normal to increased urine output, isosthenuria (1.007–1.015), potassium normal to low, phosphate often increased.

Post-renal disease
- Secondary to urinary tract obstruction – uroliths, plugs, reflex dyssynergia, UMN bladder (post-trauma), neoplasia.

Other causes of changes in urea and creatinine
See Table 25.

Table 25 Non-renal conditions causing changes in urea and creatinine

Increased urea	Decreased urea	Increased creatinine	Decreased creatinine
Recent feeding	Diuresis	None	Decreased muscle mass
GIT haemorrhage	Liver failure		Neonate
Fever	Low-protein diet		
Drugs, e.g. tetracyclines	Malnutrition		
High-protein diet	Neonate		

COMMON LAB. ABNORMALITIES

3.8 CALCIUM IMBALANCE

- Calcium levels are tightly regulated.
- Calcium exists in three forms in the blood:
  - 40–50% protein bound.
  - 10% complexed.
  - 40–50% ionised biologically active form.
- Most assays measure total calcium and hence can be affected by the blood protein levels.
- No correction factor is available to estimate calcium levels in hypoalbuminaemia in cats (cf. dogs).
- Total calcium can be difficult to assay, hence spurious results are not uncommon.

3.8.1 Assessment
Calcium (total) – reference range 2–3 mmol/l.
Calcium (ionised) – reference range 1.2–1.3 mmol/l.
- Decreased calcium:
  - Mild – 1.8 (T); 1.1 (I) mmol/l.
  - Moderate – 1.5 (T); 0.8 (I) mmol/l.
  - Marked – 1.0 (T); 0.5(I) mmol/l.
- Increased calcium:
  - Mild – 3.5 (T); 1.5 (I) mmol/l.
  - Moderate – 4.0 (T); 1.8 (I) mmol/l.
  - Marked – 5.0 (T); 2.5(I) mmol/l.
    T – total; I – ionised

3.8.2 Hypocalcaemia
- Renal secondary hyperparathyroidism.
- Parathyroidectomy (post-thyroidectomy).
- Pancreatitis.
- Malabsorption.
- Measurement on EDTA or oxalate anticoagulated blood.
- Diabetic ketoacidosis.
- Alkalosis.
- Eclampsia.
- Ethylene glycol poisoning.
- Rhabdomyolysis.
- Excess phosphate – diet, enema.
- Hypoparathyroidism.
- Hypercalcitoninism.

- (Haemodilution and hypoalbuminaemia [total]).

3.8.3 Hypercalcaemia
- Idiopathic (most common cause in cats).
- Hypervitaminosis D – calciferol rodenticides, vitamin D ointments, jasmine ingestion.
- Iatrogenic – use of vitamin D analogues in CKD, dietary formulation error.
- Paraneoplastic syndrome – lymphoma, carcinoma, bone metastasis.
- CKD (usually low).
- Primary hyperparathyroidism.
- Acidosis.
- Osteolysis.
- Granulomatous disease.
- (Haemoconcentration and hyperalbuminaemia [total]).

Management of ionised hypercalcaemia
- Address underlying cause if identified.
- Diuresis – fluids (0.9% NaCl), furosemide.
- Corticosteroids.
- Bisphosphonates.

3.9 CHOLESTEROL AND TRIGLYCERIDE CHANGES

- Useful indicators of systemic disease.
- Marked increases may cause primary pathology.

3.9.1 Assessment
Cholesterol – reference range 1.5–6 mmol/l.
Triglyceride – reference range 0.5–1.5 mmol/l.
- Decreased Cholesterol:
  - Mild – 1.4 mmol/l.
  - Moderate – 1.1 mmol/l.
  - Marked – 0.8 mmol/l.
- Increased cholesterol:
  - Mild – 9 mmol/l.
  - Moderate – 18 mmol/l.
  - Marked – 25 mmol/l.

- Increased triglyceride:
  - Mild – 2 mmol/l.
  - Moderate – 3.5 mmol/l.
  - Marked – 5 mmol/l.

3.9.2 Hypercholesterolaemia
- Renal failure.
- Endocrine disease – DM (HAC, hypothyroidism).
- Nephrotic syndrome.
- Obstructive hepatic disease.
- Hepatopathy.
- Acute pancreatitis.
- Recent meal/high-fat diet.
- Hepatic lipidosis.
- Primary hyperchylomicronaemia in cats.
- Lipoprotein lipase deficiency.
- Idiopathic.

3.9.3 Hypocholesterolaemia
- Maldigestion/malabsorption.
- Hepatic failure.
- Starvation.
- Portosystemic shunt.
- Protein-losing enteropathy.
- Lymphangiectasia.
- (EPI, hypoadrenocorticism).

3.9.4 Hypertriglyceridaemia
- Biliary obstruction.
- Pancreatitis.
- Nephrotic syndrome.
- Endocrinopathy – DM, (hypothyroidism).
- High-fat diet.
- Obesity.

3.9.5 Hypotriglyceridaemia
- Acute liver disease.

3.10 ELECTROLYTE DISTURBANCES

- Electrolyte levels are generally fairly tightly regulated so even quite modest changes are likely to be of clinical significance.

3.10.1 Assessment (see Table 26)

3.10.2 Hypokalaemia
Hypokalaemia can be the result of a whole body deficiency or redistribution to the intracellular space. Serum potassium levels can change very fast if the hypokalaemia is due to redistribution, and high levels of i/v supplementation are given.
- The most common electrolyte disturbance in cats associated with inadequate dietary intake and chronic kidney disease.
- Alkalosis.
- Potassium-free fluids.
- Vomiting.
- Post-obstructive diuresis.
- Hypokalaemia of Burmese cats.
- Drugs – loop diuretics, penicillins.
- HAC (rare).
- Hyperaldosteronism (rare).
- Insulin therapy.

3.10.3 Hyperkalaemia
- Post-renal disease and acidosis.
- Bladder rupture.
- Acute kidney injury.
- Spurious (due to poor sample handling/separation especially if associated with leucocytosis or thrombocytosis).

COMMON LAB. ABNORMALITIES

Table 26 Benchmarking changes in electrolytes

Electrolyte	Low			Reference range	High		
	Marked	Moderate	Mild		Mild	Moderate	Marked
Sodium (mmol/l)	115	125	130	135–160	164	168	172
Potassium (mmol/l)	2	2.5	3.5	3.5–5.5	6.5	7.5	8.5
Chloride (mmol/l)	90	97	105	110–130	135	140	145

- Diffuse tissue damage following ischaemia or trauma.
- Dehydration.
- Acidosis especially diabetic ketoacidosis.
- Hypoadrenocorticism (rare).
- Drugs, e.g. ACE inhibitors, potassium-sparing diuretics, propranolol.

3.10.4 Hyponatraemia
- Vomiting and diarrhoea (including intestinal sequestration e.g. obstructive disease).
- DM.
- Chronic effusions.
- Polyuric renal failure.
- Hypotonic fluids.
- Severely sodium-restricted diets.
- Burns.
- Hypoadrenocorticism (rare).
- DI (rare).

3.10.5 Hypernatraemia
- Dehydration or adipsia.
- Decreased water (food) intake.
- Excess sodium-containing food or fluids.
- Vomiting and diarrhoea.
- Renal failure.
- Fever.
- Hyperaldosteronism (rare).
- DI (rare).

3.10.6 Hypochloraemia
- Gastric vomiting.
- Metabolic alkalosis.

3.10.7 Hyperchloraemia
- Dehydration.
- Metabolic acidosis.

3.10.8 Magnesium
Hypomagnesaemia
- Decreased intake – nutritional, prolonged i/v fluid without magnesium.
- Diabetic ketoacidosis.
- Increased loss – GIT or renal.
- Altered handling – diuretics, hyperthyroidism, primary hyperparathyroidism.

- Alteration in distribution – acute administration of glucose, insulin, surgery, sepsis, trauma, hypothermia, pancreatitis.

3.11 GLUCOSE ABNORMALITIES

- Cats are more prone than dogs to stress-related hyperglycaemia. Stress factors can include hospitalisation, handling, transport and underlying disease process. In some cases, blood glucose can exceed the renal threshold and lead to glycosuria.
- Blood glucose as high as 30 mmol/l can occur in non-diabetic cats.
- Fructosamine (primarily glycosylated albumin) reflects glycaemic control over the past 2–3 weeks. It will not reliably detect episodes of hypoglycaemia.
- PU/PD is associated with glycosuria not hyperglycaemia.
- The most common cause of low glucose is measuring blood samples that have not been separated or stored in oxalate fluoride resulting in WBC metabolism of glucose.
- Hand-held glucometers tend to underestimate blood glucose.

3.11.1 Assessment
Glucose – reference range 3.5–6.5 mmol/l.
- Decreased glucose:
  ○ Mild – 3 mmol/l.
  ○ Moderate – 2.2 mmol/l.
  ○ Marked – 1.5 mmol/l.
- Increased glucose:
  ○ Mild – 10 mmol/l.
  ○ Moderate – 18 mmol/l.
  ○ Marked – 25 mmol/l.

3.11.2 Hyperglycaemia
- Stress.
- DM.
- Glucose-containing fluids.
- Drug therapy – especially glucocorticoids, progestogens, megestrol acetate.

- Renal insufficiency.
- Pancreatitis.
- Acromegaly.
- Laboratory error.
- HAC.
- EPI.

3.11.3 Hypoglycaemia
- Delayed separation of serum.
- Liver failure.
- Excess insulin – insulinoma, iatrogenic.
- Neoplasia.
- Septicaemia.
- Polycythaemia.
- Leukaemia.
- Glycogen storage disease.
- Hypoadrenocorticism.

3.12 LIVER PARAMETERS

- This section covers liver enzymes (alkaline phosphatase [ALKP], ALT, gamma-glutamyl transferase [γ-GT]), bilirubin, ammonia and bile acids.
- See Section 3.13 'Muscle Enzymes' for AST.
- Liver enzyme changes reflect the number of cells involved, not the severity of damage or the level of liver function.
- Normal or even subnormal liver enzymes do not exclude severe liver disease.
- Bile acids must be performed on serum (rather than plasma) to ensure accuracy.

- Bile acids reflect liver function; mild to moderate increases occur with a number of non-hepatic diseases.
- Postprandial bile acid samples are taken 2 hours after feeding.
- Bile acids are difficult to interpret in the face of jaundice (hyperbilirubinaemia).
- Where there is a significant increase in bile acids, there is a poor correlation between magnitude and severity of liver dysfunction in different individuals.
- To be reliable, ammonia needs to be taken into iced tubes in an area where ammoniacal cleaning agents have not been recently used.

3.12.1 Assessment (see Table 27)

3.12.2 ALKP
- Membrane-bound enzyme.
- Half-life in cats 6 hours (in dogs, 24 hours).
- Lower cellular levels in cats vs. dogs.
- Increased ALKP sensitive but non-specific indicator of hepatobiliary disease.
- No steroid-induced isoenzyme in cats.
- Primary sources – liver, kidney, bone, GIT.
- Often mildly exceeds reference range in growing kittens.

Increased ALKP
- Cholestasis.
- Intra-hepatic – cholangitis, cholangiohepatitis, hepatic lipidosis.

Table 27 Benchmarking changes in liver parameters

Liver parameter	Reference range	High		
		Mild	Moderate	Marked
ALKP (iU/l)	<50	200	500	1000
ALT (iU/l)	<50	200	400	600
γ-GT (iU/l)	<10	20	80	150
Total bilirubin (μmol/l)	<10	20	40	100
Bile acids (BA) (μmol/l)	<10	35	60	100
BA – post-feeding (μmol/l)	<25	50	70	100

COMMON LAB. ABNORMALITIES

COMMON LAB. ABNORMALITIES

- Extra-hepatic – cholangitis, cholecystitis, cholelith, inspissated bile, biliary obstruction, biliary carcinoma.
- Hyperthyroidism.
- Pancreatic disease – pancreatitis, pancreatic neoplasia, fibrosis, abscess, cyst.
- Drug induced, e.g. anticonvulsants, glipizide.
- Bone isoenzyme – growth, extensive bone lysis.
- Enteritis.

3.12.3 ALT

- Cytoplasmic and mitochondrial – released following membrane damage.
- Hepatocyte damage:
  ○ Hepatitis.
  ○ Drugs – barbiturates, NSAIDs, glucocorticoids, metronidazole, potentiated sulphonamides, cephalosporins.
- Hepatic lipidosis.
- Endocrinopathy:
  ○ DM, hyperthyroidism, HAC.
- Hypoxia:
  ○ Cardiopulmonary, thromboembolic.
- Infection – FIP.
- Trauma:
  ○ Contusion.
  ○ Diaphragmatic rupture.
  ○ PPDH.
  ○ Liver lobe torsion.
- Hepatocyte regeneration.
- Neoplasia – primary or metastatic.
- Toxins:
  ○ Chemicals.
  ○ Mycotoxins.
  ○ Copper.
- Lysosomal storage diseases.

3.12.4 γ-GT (GGT)

- Membrane-bound, primarily cholestatic.
- Also found in renal medulla and cortex and small intestinal mucosa.
- Cholestasis – intra- or extra-hepatic.

3.12.5 Total bilirubin

- Direct and indirect bilirubin assays rarely of significant value.
- Resolution of tissue jaundice lags behind clearance from serum.
- Pre-hepatic:
  ○ Haemolytic anaemia (see anaemia section 3.1).
- Hepatic:
  ○ Cholangitis/cholangiohepatitis.
  ○ Cirrhosis.
  ○ Hepatic lipidosis.
  ○ Nodular hyperplasia.
  ○ FIP.
- Post-hepatic:
  ○ Cholangitis.
  ○ Biliary obstruction.
  ○ Ruptured gall bladder.
  ○ Duodenal perforation.
- Artefact – haemolysis, lipaemia, oxyhaemoglobin use.
  See also section 2.27

3.12.6 Ammonia

- Upper limit of normal $\approx$ 50 µmol/l.
- Good assay technique important.

Increased
- Hepatic failure – cirrhosis, portosystemic shunt.
- Intestinal haemorrhage.
- Artefact – haemolysis, ammoniacal cleaners.

3.12.7 Bile acids

- Sensitive but non-specific indicator of hepatobiliary dysfunction.
- Significant liver dysfunction can be associated with normal fasting bile acids.
- Postprandial bile acids significantly increase the sensitivity of this test.

Increased
- Decreased liver function – cirrhosis, portosystemic shunt.
- Icterus.
- IBD.

- Hyperthyroidism.
- Pancreatitis.
- HAC.
- Choleretics.
- Corticosteroid use.

3.13 MUSCLE ENZYMES

Creatinine kinase (CK), AST; serum glutamic-oxaloacetic transaminase (SGOT) and LDH are all released following muscle damage. Mild to moderate increases can occur with very low-grade muscular injury, such as prolonged recumbency or i/m injections, and are therefore difficult to interpret. CK has a relatively short half-life (≈6 hours), tending to be the first to increase and then fall following muscle injury. Many muscular diseases are not inflammatory and cause little change in muscle enzymes.

3.13.1 Assessment
Creatinine – reference range <150 iU/l.
- Increased creatinine:
  ○ Mild – 300 iU/l.
  ○ Moderate – 1000 iU/l.
  ○ Marked – 5000 iU/l.
AST – reference range <70 iU/l.
- Increased AST:
  ○ Mild – 250 iU/l.
  ○ Moderate – 700 iU/l.
  ○ Marked – 2000 iU/l.

3.13.2 CK
- Muscle inflammation:
  ○ Immune-mediated, infectious (*Toxoplasma*), eosinophilic, endocarditis.
- Nutritional:
  ○ Hypokalaemic polymyopathy, taurine deficiency.
- Trauma:
  ○ Recumbency, i/m injection, postsurgical, RTA, fall, post-exercise.
- Post infarct ischaemia:
  ○ Aortic thromboembolism, DIC.

- Hypothermia.
- Hyperthermia.
- Post-seizure.

3.13.3 AST
Primarily indicates hepatocyte or muscular damage as it is a mitochondrial enzyme.

3.13.4 LDH
- Rarely assayed in cats, relatively little known about isoenzymes.
- Will also increase in renal and hepatic disease following any organ or tissue damage and haemolysis (*in vivo* or *in vitro*).

3.14 PHOSPHATE

- Phosphate levels are regulated by PTH, dietary intake and renal excretion.
- Closely associated with changes in calcium levels.
- If calcium (mmol/l) × phosphorus (mmol/l) exceeds 6 then the cat is at risk of ectopic calcification occurring.
- Attempt to normalise if phosphate level is below 0.5 mmol/l or chronically over 2.5 mmol/l (see also IRIS recommendations page 240–241).
- Hypophosphataemia is rare but potentially life threatening as it can cause a haemolytic anaemia.

3.14.1 Assessment
Phosphate – reference range 1.2–2.6 mmol/l:
- Decreased phosphate:
  ○ Mild – 1.1 mmol/l.
  ○ Moderate – 0.9 mmol/l.
  ○ Marked – 0.7 mmol/l.
- Increased phosphate:
  ○ Mild – 3 mmol/l.
  ○ Moderate – 3.8 mmol/l.
  ○ Marked – 5 mmol/l.

3.14.2 Hypophosphataemia
- Inadequate dietary intake.
- Primary hyperparathyroidism.

COMMON LAB. ABNORMALITIES

- Secondary to hypercalcaemia.
- Secondary to neoplasms that produce PTH-like hormones (pseudohyperparathyroidism).
- Hyperinsulinaemia.
- Diabetic ketoacidosis (cellular shift), made worse during correction of acidosis.
- Intracellular translocation during glucose administration, alkalosis or correction of acidosis.
- Hypovitaminosis D.
- Eclampsia.
- Hypercalcitonism.

3.14.3 Hyperphosphataemia

- Cats less than 6 months due to bone growth.
- Decreased GFR:
  ○ Acute and chronic renal disease.
  ○ Chronic hypovolaemia.
- Post-renal obstruction.
- Renal secondary hyperparathyroidism.
- Dietary excess – all meat diets leading to renal secondary hyperparathyroidism.
- Artefact due to phosphate release from red cells, haemolysed sample.
- Iatrogenic – phosphate enemas, IV phosphate administration.
- Intoxication – hypervitaminosis D, jasmine.
- Hypoparathyroidism.
- Mild increase in anorexic or vomiting animals.
- Tissue trauma or necrosis.
- Osteolytic bone lesion.

3.15 PROTEIN ABNORMALITIES

- Total protein and albumin are measured; globulin level is obtained by subtraction (protein – albumin = globulin).
- Albumin is a relatively difficult parameter to measure particularly for in-house analysers; error will affect both albumin and globulin results.
- Total solids estimated by refractometry approximates to total protein.

3.15.1 Assessment (see Table 28)

3.15.2 Hypoproteinaemia

- Kittens.
- Hypoalbuminaemia.
- Haemorrhage.
- Protein-losing enteropathy.
- Overhydration.
- Liver failure.
- Repeated drainage of pleural or peritoneal effusion.

3.15.3 Hyperproteinaemia

- Dehydration.
- Hyperglobulinaemia.
- Spurious – haemolysis or lipaemia.

3.15.4 Hypoalbuminaemia

- Decreased intake:
  ○ Malnutrition, malabsorption, maldigestion.
- Decreased production:
  ○ Liver failure, portosystemic shunt, neonate, malnutrition, negative acute phase protein.

Table 28 Benchmarking changes in proteins

Parameter	Low			Reference	High		
	Marked	Moderate	Mild		Mild	Moderate	Marked
Total protein (g/l)	35	42	47	54–80	90	100	110
Albumin (g/l)	15	20	24	26–42	Indicates dehydration		
Globulin (g/l)	15	18	22	24–47	55	60	70

- Excessive loss:
  - Protein-losing nephropathy, protein-losing enteropathy, severe exudative skin disease (e.g. burns), external blood loss, chronic effusions.
- Compensatory decrease as a result of hyperglobulinaemia.

3.15.5 Hyperalbuminaemia
- Dehydration.

3.15.6 Hypoglobulinaemia
- Neonate.
- Protein-losing enteropathy.
- Blood loss.
- Immunodeficiency.

3.15.7 Hyperglobulinaemia
- Dehydration.
- Inflammation.
- Gammopathy – myeloma, *Ehrlichia*.
- Polyclonal activation:
  - FIP, chronic inflammatory disease, e.g. IBD, dental disease, immune-mediated disease, neoplasia.

3.15.8 Fibrinogen
- Increased – inflammation, pregnancy.
- Decreased – liver failure, coagulopathies, primary hypofibrinogenaemia.

3.15.9 C-reactive protein (CRP)
- Cytokine (primarily IL-6)-mediated acute phase protein.
- Synthesised in the liver.
- Increases within 4 hours and normalises 36–48 hours after inflammation subsides.
- Used as a marker for a wide range of acute and chronic inflammatory
  - Bacterial, viral or fungal infections.
  - Diseases.
  - Malignancy.
  - Tissue injury or necrosis.

3.15.10 α_1-Acid glycoprotein
- Acute phase protein.
- Increases in response to acute and chronic inflammation.
- Increased in FIP cases BUT it is not disease specific.

3.15.11 Serum protein electrophoresis (Figure 12)
- Separates globulins into sub-fractions:
  - Alpha-1, alpha-2, beta and gamma globulin fractions.
  - Alpha and beta globulins are mostly synthesised by the liver.
  - Alpha-2 region also contains acute phase reactant proteins and lipoproteins.
- Immunoglobulins can migrate in the alpha-2, beta and gamma fractions.
- Gammopathies can be monoclonal (single spike) or polyclonal.
- Haemolysis can result in a broad alpha-2 band.
- In iron-deficient, anaemic patients transferrin migrates as a band in the beta region.

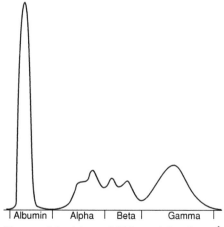

Figure 12 Normal SPE result (total protein 72 g/L)

COMMON LAB. ABNORMALITIES

3.15.12 Monoclonal gammopathy

- FIP.[a]
- Inflammatory bowel disease.[a]
- Lymphoma.
- Amyloidosis.[a]
- Multiple myeloma.[b]
- Plasma cell leukaemia.
- Plasmacytoma.
- Chronic lymphocytic leukaemia.[b]
- Ehrlichiosis.[a]

[a] Gammopathy usually polyclonal.
[b] Monoclonal gammopathy common.

3.16 URINALYSIS

- False-positive proteinuria result if urine is very alkaline.
- Time of urine collection – sample analysis influenced by time stored in bladder:
  - *Morning* – most concentrated, highest yield of cells, glycosuria may be masked, cytology altered by pH and osmolality exposure.
  - *Recently formed* – better for culture, cells (unless dilution causes lysis) and glucose.

3.16.1 Volume

- Increased – causes of PU/PD see section 2.33

NB – *Polyuric acute renal failure does occur.*

- Decreased (oligoanuria) – associated with acute kidney injury, dehydration, hypovolaemia.

3.16.2 Physical characteristics

- Colour – usually straw to yellow:
  - Colourless ⇒ dilute.
  - Amber ⇒ bilirubinaemia.
  - Red ⇒ haematuria, haemoglobinuria, myoglobinuria.
  - Brown ⇒ pyuria with haematuria.

- Clarity – clear:
  - Turbid ⇒ increased cells, crystals or mucus.

3.16.3 Urine solute concentration

- *Osmolality* – solutes lower the freezing point/vapour pressure regardless of molecular weight. Most accurate results are obtained by simultaneously testing the osmolality of urine and serum.
- *SG* (density relative to water) ≡ *refractive index* (bending of light) – depends on the number, nature and temperature of particles as they bend light. Artificially raised by glycosuria, heavy proteinuria and radiographic contrast media.

Assessment of SG

- Dipstick assessment is unreliable, refractometer should be used.
- Normal cats usually >1.035 (can be up to 1.090).
- Hyposthenuria – SG <1.007:
  - Active renal dilution – DI, other causes PU/PD.
- Isosthenuria – SG 1.007 → 1.015:
  - Osmolality similar to plasma – renal disease, fluid therapy, diuretics, PU/PD.
- Hypersthenuria – SG >1.015:
  - Active renal concentration of solutes.

3.16.4 Urine pH

- Normally – 5.5 → 7.5.
- Range – 4.5 → 8.5.

Alkaline

- Urinary tract infection.
- Postprandial.
- Renal tubular acidosis.
- Diet – high vegetable-based protein content.
- Drugs/chemicals – detergents/disinfectants, carbonic anhydrase inhibitors,

thiazides, sodium bicarbonate, lactate and acetate, potassium citrate.

Acidic

- Normal (mildly acidic).
- Acidifying diets.
- Systemic acidosis.
- Drugs – phosphate salts, DL-methionine, ammonium chloride, ascorbic acid, furosemide.

3.16.5 Protein

- Small amounts of mucoprotein (Tamm–Horsfall) are normally secreted by urothelium.
- *Dipstick test* – amino groups bind and alter indicator dye:
  - Dependent on the number of free amino groups.
  - Albumin 2–3 × > globulins or haemoglobin.
  - Increased binding; in strongly alkaline urine or if stick is immersed too long.
- *Biochemical analysis* – normal <65 mg% with SG in normal range.
- *Proteinuria* – protein:creatinine ratio >0.4 (equivocal UPC 0.2–0.4).
- Must always combine with urine sediment analysis.
- Pre-renal – low molecular weight:
  - Myeloma.
  - Paraproteinaemias.
  - Haemolytic anaemia.
  - Rhabdomyolysis.
- *Renal* – sediment must be inactive:
  - Glomerular damage – amyloid, glomerulonephritis.
  - Tubular defect – acute tubular necrosis, renal failure, PKD, Fanconi's syndrome.
- *Post-renal* – active sediment (cannot exclude renal component):
  - Inflammation of ureters or lower urinary tract – FLUTD, UTI, uroliths, trauma, prostatitis, vaginitis.

3.16.6 Glucose

- *Glucose oxidase method*:
  - false positive with hypochlorite or chlorine, formaldehyde generated from methenamine.
  - false negative with high doses of ascorbic acid.
- *Glycosuria:*
  - DM.
  - Stress.
  - Proximal tubular disease – Fanconi's syndrome, primary renal glycosuria, aminoglycosides.
  - Glucose-containing IV fluids.

3.16.7 Ketones

- Does NOT detect beta-hydroxybutyrate which tends to rise first.
- Level reduced by bacteria.
- Ketonaemia resolves before ketonuria:
  - Ketonaemia can be measured using patient-side ketone meters.
- Ketonuria occurs very rarely in non-diabetic animals.

3.16.8 Urobilinogen, nitrite and bacteria

- Dipstick results are of no diagnostic value in cats:
  - Urobilinogen positive result ⇒ sticks have expired.

3.16.9 Bilirubin

- Always abnormal in cats.

Bilirubinuria

- Haemolytic anaemia.
- Hepatic disease.
- Mild increase in starvation and fever.
- False positive with phenothiazines.

3.16.10 Blood

- See Figure 8 (Section 2.21) for differentiation of haematuria, haemoglobinuria and myoglobinuria.

COMMON LAB. ABNORMALITIES

Haemoglobin/myoglobin
- Pseudoperoxidase activity is also mimicked by white cells, epithelial cells and sperm.
- Normally the haemoglobin from red cells is bound to haptoglobin and is not filtered. Myoglobin is not bound and is readily filtered.

Haematuria
- See Section 2.21.

Haemoglobinuria
- Typically port wine urine.
- Red cells lysed.
- Severe haemolysis.
- Babesiosis.

Myoglobinuria
- Severe muscle necrosis.
- Trauma – crush injuries.
- Rhabdomyolysis.

Table 29 Types of urinary crystals, their appearance, significance and favoured pH for formation

Crystal	Appearance	pH	Significance
Ammonium urate	Thorn-apple, yellow/ brown	Any	Rarely in normal animals
Amorphous urate	Amorphous/spheroid yellow/brown	Acidic	Common in cats, PSS
Calcium oxalate – dihydrate monohydrate	Small colourless envelopes Small spindles, dumbbells or ring forms	Any, favoured by acid pH	Associated with haematuria as irritant Normal and with uroliths As dihydrate but more likely in ethylene glycol poisoning
Calcium phosphate	Amorphous or long thin prisms	Alkaline	Large numbers in normal animals and with calcium phosphate uroliths
Cystine	Flat, colourless, hexagonal plates	Inhibited by very alkaline	Rare in cats
Struvite	6–8 sided colourless prism in cats. Occasionally fern-like	Favoured by alkaline	Normal, infection induced (urease producing organisms), with uroliths that may be non-struvite or mixed. LUTD without uroliths
Sulphonamide	Sheaves of needles, fan shaped	Acidic	Drug associated, can obstruct renal tubule
Xanthine	Circular, yellow brown in colour	Any	Very rare in cats
Uric acid	Diamond or rhombic rosettes, oval plates or pointed ends	Acidic	As for urates

3.16.11 Bacteria

- Ideally from a cystocentesis sample into a plain tube.
- Use a boric acid tube only for a free-catch sample.
- Quantitative culture using standard volume loop >10 000 colonies/ml significant.

3.16.12 Urine microscopy

- Easily altered by storage:
  - Prepare direct and centrifuged sediment samples (casts may breakdown if spun too fast).
  - Staining; e.g. Sedistain can be helpful.

Cells

- *Red cells* – differentiate from fat droplets which are more refractile:
  - Normally <5/hpf (hpf refers to high power field) in centrifuged urine.
  - Grossly seen >50/hpf.
  - Swell and lyse in urine SG <1.008.
- *White cells*:
  - <5/hpf normal.
  - 5–50/hpf equivocal.
  - >50/hpf ⇒ pyuria due to infection or inflammation.
- *Epithelial cells* – normally <2/hpf:
  - Increased – inflammation, infection, neoplasia, iatrogenic (catheterisation).

Bacteria

- There is a poor correlation between bacteria 'identified' on sediment microscopy and positive culture.

Crystals (see Table 29)

- Commonly precipitated in urine as it cools, especially in cats fed some dry food. Crystalluria in stored urine has a positive predictive value of 40% for the presence of crystals in fresh urine in cats fed on dry food or mixed diets.

Casts

- Significant numbers indicate tubular involvement (absence does not rule out active renal tubular disease).
- *Hyaline* – serum proteins tend to facilitate aggregation of Tamm–Horsfall proteins ⇒ pre-renal and glomerular causes of proteinuria. BUT also occur in physiologic transient proteinuria.
- *Cellular* – always of pathological significance:
  - Red cells – renal haematuria.
  - White cells – tubulointerstitial inflammation but will degenerate forming granular casts.
  - Epithelial will degenerate into fatty or granular (first coarse, then fine) and are affected by duration of disease. Associated with ischaemia or toxic tubular insults.
- *Granular* – can result from hyaline, epithelial or white cell casts.
- *Waxy/fatty* – degenerating tubular epithelial cells or lipid relatively common in cat urine.

COMMON LAB. ABNORMALITIES

SECTION 4

ORGAN SYSTEMS

ORGAN SYSTEMS

Notes on Feline Internal Medicine, Second Edition. Edited by Kit Sturgess. ©2013 John Wiley & Sons, Ltd.
Published 2013 by Blackwell Publishing Ltd.

4.1 RESPIRATORY DISEASE

4.1.1 General examination of the respiratory system

- Observe the general demeanour and body stance and look for evidence of mouth breathing.
- Observe the rate, pattern and character of breathing.
- Listen to the breathing for stridor (laryngeal disease), stertor (snoring), snuffles (nasal or nasopharyngeal disease) or rattles (tracheal FB).
- Check mucosal colour and lymph nodes of the head and neck.
- Examine nasal area for symmetry, hair discoloration and nasal discharge.
- Check air flow from both nares using a small piece of cotton wool or a glass slide.
- Palpate the URT and thorax (for integrity, compressibility and position of the apex beat).
  - Cranial mediastinal mass reduces thoracic compressibility; differentiate from reduced compliance due to increased respiratory effort especially if there is air trapping.
- Gently squeeze larynx to assess cough response.
- Auscult the thorax and trachea for the location, intensity, normality of breathing and cardiac sounds.
  - Moist crackles:
    - Parenchymal disease, e.g. bronchopneumonia, oedema.
  - Expiratory wheeze:
    - Small airway disease, e.g. asthma.
  - Loud inspiratory noise audible throughout lung field:
    - Upper airway obstruction referred noise.
  - Harsh respiratory sounds:
    - Airway disease, e.g. chronic bronchitis.

- Muffled heart or lung sounds:
  - Various possibilities, e.g. pleural effusion, diaphragmatic hernia, pericardial effusion, pneumothorax (reduced lung sounds), consolidation of lungs (usually more focal muffling).
- Altered position of apex beat:
  - Mass lesions displacing the heart, e.g. thymic lymphoma.
  - Consolidation or collapse of lung tissue.
  - Diaphragmatic rupture.
- Abnormal heart sounds, e.g. murmur, gallop, arrhythmia:
  - Various possibilities, e.g. primary cardiac disease, hyperthyroidism, anaemia.
  - Murmurs may be 'created' in old thin cats with firm pressure of the stethoscope causing a shift in the heart position.
  - Murmurs are variable and often rate dependent in cats. They are often more sternally located than in dogs.
- Percuss the thorax for increased (air) and decreased (fluid, soft tissue) resonance.
- Look for evidence of non-respiratory disease causing respiratory signs:
  - Stress, pain, trauma, hyperthermia, cardiovascular disease, anaemia, acid–base disturbances, abdominal enlargement, hyperthyroidism, muscle weakness.

Patterns of respiration

- Normal:
  - Ribs move craniolateral, diaphragm contracts, and abdomen moves outwards.
- Increased work:
  - Secondary respiratory muscles recruited to elevate the first and second ribs, pull sternum cranially, flare the nostrils.

- ○ There is greater abdominal movement.
- ○ Open mouth (generally a sign of severe respiratory distress in cats).
- ○ Expiration becomes active using abdominal and internal intercostal muscles.
- ○ Postural adaptations by standing, sitting or sternal recumbency.
- ○ Extend head and neck and abduct elbows.
- Marked inspiratory effort with deep, laboured chest movements:
  - ○ Major airway, nasal or nasopharyngeal obstruction – inspiratory noise usually present.
  - ○ Sometimes seen in pulmonary parenchymal or pleural disease – inspiratory noise absent.
- Restrictive breathing:
  - ○ Rapid and shallow breathing $\Rightarrow$ pulmonary parenchymal or pleural disease.
- Prolonged expiration with increased end effort using abdominal muscles:
  - ○ Indicates small airway obstruction, e.g. asthma or chronic bronchitis.
- CNS damage:
  - ○ Cheyne–Stokes – progressively deeper and sometimes faster breathing, followed by a gradual decrease that results in a temporary apnoea.
  - ○ Cushing breathing – irregular breathing caused by increased ICP.
- Respiratory fatigue:
  - ○ Paradoxical movement is a sign of severe respiratory fatigue and requires urgent intervention to reduce respiratory work:
    - ▪ Intercostal muscles collapse on inspiration as they fatigue and are no longer able to counteract the pull of the diaphragm reducing the inspiratory volume. On expiration the abdominal muscles push abdominal contents cranially to aid expiration, but in obstructive conditions, e.g. feline asthma, this may

lead to outward movement of the ribs rather than increased air flow.

4.1.2 Disease of the upper respiratory tract

Nares and nasal planum (Anatomy – Figure 13)

Congenital
- Brachycephalic cats may have collapsed alar cartilages obstructing the nares causing increased inspiratory effort. This is made worse by cats' reluctance to mouth breathe. If obstruction is significant surgical correction is necessary.

Ulceration/erosion
- Eosinophilic granuloma complex (see Section 4.3.2) and squamous cell carcinoma (SCC):
  - ○ Differentiation may require biopsy.
  - ○ SCC tends to be more extensive and destructive and is particularly common in older cats with lightly pigmented noses.
  - ○ Superficial SCC can be managed with surgery, cryosurgery, intralesional carboplatin, radiation and photodynamic therapy.
  - ○ Deep and invasive SCC requires radical surgery or radiation therapy.
  - ○ Further lesions may occur as UV light exposure is the trigger.

Nasal cavity disorders

Clinical signs
- Obstructed or noisy breathing that resolves when the cat open mouth breathes:
  - ○ Stridor occurs on inspiration; vibrating noise common with nasopharyngeal polyps.
- Sneezing (Section 1.38).
- Nasal discharge (Section 1.38).
- Pain on palpation.
- Distortion of the nasal/frontal bones or soft tissue.

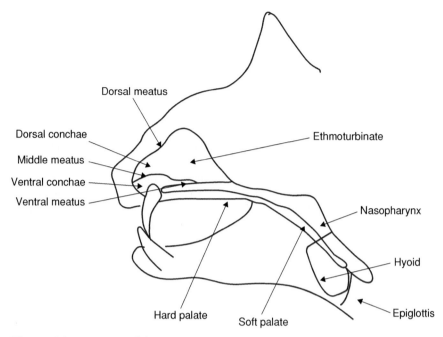

Figure 13 Anatomy of the upper respiratory tract

- Changes in coat colour in 'pointed' breeds.
- Rubbing face.
- Ocular discharge.
- Infectious and neoplastic processes may extend into the brain giving signs of CNS disease.

Diagnostic approach
- Examination of the nasal discharge:
  - Cytology looking for infectious agents particularly Cryptococcus or neoplastic cells.
  - Fungal culture.
  - Bacterial culture is usually unhelpful as primary bacterial infection is extremely rare.
- Radiography using intraoral films or open-mouth views together with lateral and oblique skull:
  - Distortion.
  - Soft tissue or bony lesions.
  - Destruction of turbinates.
  - Uni- or bilateral.

- Advanced imaging (CT or MRI) produces more detailed images than radiography and allows the extent of any mass lesions to be better evaluated; in particular, whether the cribriform plate is intact or whether there is invasion into the CNS as this will affect the choice of further diagnostic procedures
- Rhinoscopy:
  - The oral cavity should always be carefully inspected prior to rhinoscopy.
  - Antegrade using an auriscope (limited) or rigid arthroscope preferably with a flushing sheath:
    - Use an appropriate sized, cuffed endotracheal tube and pack the pharynx.
  - Retrograde using a flexible endoscope; the caudal nasopharynx can be examined using a dental mirror and spey hook to move the soft palate rostrally.

- Anaesthesia required, but the cat may still react (reduce using topical local anaesthetics):
  - Anaesthetic complication rates seem higher in cats with nasal disease.
  - Pre-oxygenate and induce with the minimum agent necessary.
  - Post-operative observation is essential as some cats will suffer respiratory arrest post extubation as they are reluctant to mouth breath but their meati are temporarily obstructed following the rhinoscopy procedure
- Biopsy/nasal flush:
  - Aspirates or saline flush – the pharynx is packed and warm saline is flushed forcibly through the meati. Samples are collected on the packing or in a suitable collection device but may fail to identify underlying disease.
  - Brush cytology – diagnostically useful where disease is superficial; relatively atraumatic.
  - Traumatic flush – urinary catheter cut to length (medial canthus) with the edge roughened by small nicks in the surface. Catheter moved up and down the DORSAL surface whilst flushing with saline. The ventral, vascular floor, of the nasal chambers should be avoided.
  - Pinch biopsies – obtained using small cup biopsy forceps. Guided biopsies are usually diagnostically the most valuable but if facilities for rhinoscopy are not available, blind biopsies can be obtained. The biopsy forceps should not be introduced further caudally than the medial canthus of the eye.
  - Core biopsy – where a mass lesion is identified, a catheter can be cut and pushed into the mass to obtain a core biopsy.
  - Exploratory surgery is sometimes required particularly when biopsies cannot be obtained or are non-diagnostic.

NB – *Ulceration of the surface of nasal tumours is common; hence superficial biopsies may be diagnosed as chronic inflammatory disease.*

- Serology for Aspergilla and Cryptococcus.

Congenital disease
- Deviation of the septum and malformed turbinates occasionally occur, associated with a chronic mucopurulent nasal discharge.

Viral URTD – see section 5.2.
Bordetellosis – see section 5.1.

Chronic rhinitis/sinusitis
- Usually sequelae to viral URTD.
- Consider fungal, neoplastic or foreign body causes.
- Permanent damage and metaplasia of the mucosa results in an inability to prevent recurrent bacterial colonisation.
- Clinical signs variable, usually periodic sneezing, mucopurulent nasal discharge and noisy breathing.
- Rarely systemically unwell but may become inappetent.
- Diagnosis based on rule out of other diseases.
- May be an immune-mediated/allergic component as some cats improve significantly if kept outside.

NB – *Bacterial culture is a waste of time and money.*

Management
- Humidification.
- Antimicrobial treatment:
  - Broad spectrum – tetracyclines, cephalosporin, penicillins.

○ Difficult to medicate patients – consider azithromycin (q48h) or long acting cephalosporin e.g. cefovecin (q14 days)

○ Pulse or continuous therapy.

○ Same antibacterial should be used until it becomes ineffective (may take years).

- Anti-inflammatories – glucocorticoids or NSAIDs.
- Antihistamines.
- Therapeutic lavage.
- Topical nasal decongestants marketed for children may be helpful (e.g. oxymethazoline – one drop in each nostril q24hr for a maximum of 3 days).
- Surgical turbinectomy is described but should be reserved for severe cases that are non-responsive to medical management
- Acupuncture.
- Antiviral – interferon, L-lysine.
- Immunotherapy.

Fungal rhinitis

Fungal elements can be present in the nasal cavity (particularly saprophytic) as incidental or commensal organisms, so positive fungal cultures or fungal elements in nasal discharge need to be interpreted with care.

- Uncommon:
  ○ Can be seen secondary to underlying neoplasia.
- *Cryptococcus neoformans* most common cause (see Section 5.14.4).
- *Aspergillus, Penicillium, Sporothrix* and saprophytic fungi are responsible in some cases.
- Often begins unilaterally.
- Mucopurulent discharge.
- Bony involvement and facial distortion may occur in chronic cases.
- Diagnosis of stained smears of nasal discharge is suggestive.
- Biopsy evidence of invasion important as treatment is expensive, and side effects are common.
- Serology for cryptococcal antigen.

Management

- Long-term anti-fungal treatment is required.
- Surgical excision, if there are large aggregates of fungal-infected tissue, may be necessary.
- May not be curative.
- Ideally based on culture and sensitivity results especially for unusual fungi.

Cryptococcosis

- Itraconazole – given with food to maximise bioavailability, relatively few side effects. Suspension has greater bioavailability than capsules. Dose at 10–20 mg/kg PO q24h for 6–18 months.
- Fluconazole – expensive but fewer side effects, and may be more effective at 5–10 mg/kg PO q12h for 6–18 months.
- Amphotericin B – for unresponsive cases, very nephrotoxic in cats. Administration of micro-encapsulated drug with aggressive diuresis significantly reduces toxicity but is very expensive.

Polyps

- Non-neoplastic inflammatory masses.
- Result of chronic inflammatory disease likely associated with FHV-1 or FCV infection.

Nasopharyngeal polyps

- Originates in the middle ear, traverses the eustachian tube and emerges in the nasopharynx.
- Young cats <6 years; no sex or breed predilection.
- Clinical signs:
  ○ Obstruction, stertor, gagging, sneezing and nasal discharge.
  ○ Less common – dysphagia and dysphonia.
- Diagnosis on examination of nasopharynx (usually requires general anaesthesia):
  ○ Frequently by digital palpation of the soft palate.

ORGAN SYSTEMS

- Radiographs of the skull, including tympanic bulla will show the extent of the lesion.
- Polyps can often be twisted free as they have narrow stalks.
- Bulla osteotomy is required if the polyp involves the middle ear or there is regrowth (about 1/3rd of cases).

Nasonasal polyps (nasopharyngeal stenosis)

- Inflammatory membrane rather than polyp across the caudal nares in response to injury (infectious, traumatic).
- Can cause almost complete bilateral obstruction of air flow.
- Diagnosis on retrograde rhinoscopy.
- Membrane can be torn away with forceps but may regrow:
  ○ Consider ballooning, surgery or stenting.

Neoplasia

- Relatively uncommon.
- Lymphoma, adenocarcinoma, SCC.
- Usually present as obstructive disease.
- Mucopurulent nasal discharge ± blood usually unilateral.

Diagnosis

- Radiography may also show destruction of overlying bone due to pressure or invasion.
- Advanced imaging if CNS invasion suspected.
- Biopsy is important to distinguish from inflammation and to elucidate tumour type.
- Lymphoma may not be localised, CNS involvement is relatively common.

Management

- SCC – may be responsive to surgical debulking and radiation therapy
- Adenocarcinoma – radiation therapy is the treatment of choice with median survival times of around 1 year; the value of piroxicam/meloxicam for palliation is unknown
- Nasal lymphoma usually middle-aged to older cats, there is a relatively high incidence of involvement of other sites (20%)
  ○ Chemotherapy (see 4.12)
  ○ Radiotherapy
  ○ Combined therapy seems to give the best median survival time (2.5 years)

Trauma

- Usually following RTA.
- Splitting of hard palate.
- Fracture of nasal/frontal bones with sequestrum formation resulting in chronic nasal discharge.
- Extension of dental disease (particularly canines) causing oronasal fistula, may present as chronic unilateral nasal discharge.

Foreign bodies

- Grass seeds tend to cause acute signs but can be difficult to locate resulting in a misdiagnosis of idiopathic rhinosinusitis.
- Aggressive retrograde flushing may be helpful.
- Blades of grass can become lodged in the caudal nasopharynx and irritate the larynx causing coughing or reverse sneezing without nasal discharge being present.

Laryngeal disease

Laryngeal disease is relatively uncommon in cats but can present as acute dyspnoea.

Laryngeal paralysis

- Male predisposition suggested.
- Usually progressive history though occasionally acute onset, often bilateral.

Clinical signs

- Dyspnoea.
- Inspiratory noise.
- Dysphagia.
- Dysphonia.
- Gagging.
- Vestibular signs.

Diagnosis
- Observation of movement under a light anaesthetic plane (do not use diazepam in the induction protocol).
- Ultrasound.

Cause
- Trauma.
- Myasthenia gravis.
- Hypothyroidism.
- Generalised neuromuscular disease.
- Neoplasia.
- Idiopathic cases are rare.
- Post thyroidectomy

Treatment
- Surgical tie-back.

Prognosis
- Guarded as many of the underlying causes are progressive.

Laryngeal neoplasia
- Clinical signs are of progressive obstruction; can present acutely.
- Older cats.
- Treatment depends on type – lymphoma (most common), SCC, adenocarcinoma, carcinoma.

Laryngitis
- Commonly associated with infection (FHV-1, FCV).
- Presentation usually fever, anorexia, dehydration, ptyalism, lethargy:
  - Less commonly causes change in meow, dyspnoea, gagging, stridor.
- Diagnosis based on presenting history and clinical signs:
  - Examination of the larynx may show poor function, inflammation and thickening of the vocal folds and mucosa.
- Usually self-limiting and treatment is symptomatic and supportive:
  - Rarely temporary tracheotomy is required.

Laryngospasm/oedema
- Typically acute onset lasting from a few seconds to 1 minute.
- Can be unprovoked.
- Cat crouches with head extended and low.
- Inspiratory wheeze and cough.
- Larynx appears normal on examination.
- Diagnosis – presumptive on history.
- Can occur following intubation usually when this has been difficult or intubation repeated during an anaesthetic.

Treatment
- To induce swallowing, owners should use 1–2 ml of water in a syringe to dislodge mucus/saliva.
- If accompanying pharyngitis, then short-term anti-inflammatories – NSAIDs or prednisolone.
- Post-anaesthetic laryngeal oedema may require glucocorticoids or even short term tracheotomy.

Upper airway disease

Tracheal/bronchial foreign bodies
- Variety – often plant material.
- Usually acute onset then chronic history – often partially antibacterial responsive.
- Often initial response to antibacterials and anti-inflammatories.
- Coughing is usually the primary presenting sign.

Diagnosis
- Halitosis.
- Localised radiographic density.
- Purulent ± eosinophilic bronchial wash.
- FB seen on bronchoscopy.
- Chronic cases may be difficult to locate – CT can be very helpful in this respect.

NB – *If a foreign body is present but not seen leading to a bronchoalveolar lavage (BAL) being performed, there is a risk of disseminating the infection.*

ORGAN SYSTEMS

Treatment
- Bronchoscopic removal.
- Thoracotomy and bronchotomy.
- Occasionally lobectomy.
- If a foreign body is suspected, but pattern is diffuse, then 4–6 weeks of antibacterial treatment followed by repeat radiographs may define the affected area more clearly.

Tracheal collapse/stenosis
- Very rare, usually secondary to granuloma, polyp or trauma.
- Dyspnoea.
- Gagging.
- Coughing that is exacerbated by tracheal palpation.

Diagnosis
- Inspiratory and expiratory radiographs of intra- and extrathoracic trachea.
- Bronchoscopy.
- Fluoroscopy.

Treatment
- Inflammatory masses often respond to corticosteroids.
- Surgical removal.
- Tracheal resection.
- Tracheal stent.

Tracheal rupture
- Overinflation of endotracheal tube:
  ○ Most commonly occurs associated with dental procedures.
- High-rise syndrome – cats falling from height can avulse the trachea from the carina.
- Bite wounds.

Clinical signs
- Acute dyspnoea.
- Pneumomediastinum and pneumothorax.
- Subcutaneous emphysema.
- Some cats do not present with dyspnoea immediately post trauma.

Diagnosis
- Clinical signs and history of trauma or recent anaesthesia.
- Radiography.
- Bronchoscopy.

Treatment
- Conservative management of small defects may be appropriate.
- Surgical repair.
- Risk of post-surgical stricture.

Neoplasia
- Rare.
- Usually progressive dyspnoea but coughing, gagging, sonorous respiration, stridor, sneezing and dysphagia can also be a feature.
- Treatment – tracheal resection, chemo- or radiotherapy depending on type.

4.1.3 Mediastinal disease
Mass lesions are the most common cause of localised mediastinal disease but fluid and air (pneumomediastinum) as part of pleural disease or inflammation (mediastinitis) usually associated with infection (e.g. penetrating oesophageal injury) occur. Rarely mediastinal haemorrhage.

Clinical signs of mediastinal disease
- Dysphagia.
- Regurgitation.
- Dyspnoea.
- Coughing.
- Horner's syndrome.
- Head and neck oedema.

Mediastinal mass
- Coughing primarily due to large airway compression.
- Regurgitation associated with oesophageal compression.
- Dyspnoea due to size ± pleural effusion.
- Lymphoma most common (see section 5.11).

Diagnosis
- Non-compliant cranial thorax.
- Widened mediastinum on radiographs.
- The trachea cranial to the heart is displaced dorsally.
- Lung fields displaced caudally.
- ± free pleural fluid.

Other mediastinal masses
- Benign thymomas, which respond well to surgery, are seen in older cats (4–18 years).
- Thymic cysts.
- Tracheobronchial lymph node enlargement.
- Mediastinal granuloma (usually fungal) are reported.

4.1.4 Lower airway disease – feline bronchopulmonary disease

Feline inflammatory airway disease
- Group of conditions which include asthma, bronchitis, bronchopneumonia, chronic obstructive pulmonary disease, etc.
- Feline asthma more specifically refers to eosinophilic inflammation and reversible airflow limitation but standardised tests are lacking.
- Coughing is a major presenting clinical sign due to
  - Airway inflammation – allergic, irritant.
  - Airway irritation – mechanical, chemical.
  - Excessive airway secretion.
  - Severe bronchoconstriction.

Signalment
- Young to middle-aged (2–8-year-old) cats.
- Female.
- Siamese over-represented.

Clinical presentation
- Chronic coughing.
- Acute-onset severe dyspnoea.
- Paroxysmal gagging.

- Expiratory wheeze.
- Persistent tachypnoea.

Physical examination
- Can be unremarkable particularly in cats with episodic signs.
- Majority have persistently increased lung sounds (wheezes and crackles) on auscultation.

Diagnosis
- Haematology – changes are variable (many normal), most frequent changes eosinophilia and neutrophilia.
- Biochemistry – unremarkable unless other concurrent disease.
- Serology – FeLV/FIV status whilst not directly relevant can affect longer term prognosis.

Radiology
- Good-quality plain radiographs (lateral and DV or VD) are required.
- Easy to create/obliterate lung changes with exposure, positioning and phase of the respiratory cycle.
- General anaesthesia with the cat intubated allowing consistent inspiratory films is desirable.
- Radiographic changes are not always seen despite severe disease.
- Usually, some degree of bronchial or bronchointerstitial pattern is seen caused by thickening of the bronchial walls and peribronchial infiltration.
- Air trapping is also sometimes seen as a flattening of the diaphragm, an increase in thoracic size, hyperlucent lung fields.
- Occasionally emphysematous change.

Cytology
- Produces the most useful information.

Tracheal wash
- Safe, simple and inexpensive.
- Disease needs to be in the major airways to produce diagnostic samples.

ORGAN SYSTEMS

Transthoracic lung aspiration

- Inexpensive and simple.
- Associated with significant risks.
  - Primarily pneumothorax.
  - Haemothorax and haemorrhage into airways can occur.
- Most useful where lesion appears mass-like and non-aerated.

Bronchoalveolar lavage

- Technique of choice.
- Blind lavage via endotracheal tube produces more limited and less diagnostically useful samples as penetration of the wash fluid to the small airways and alveoli is poor.
- Need bronchoscope for specific lobe lavage, also allows cytology brushing and biopsy.
- Complications are relatively rare.
- Technique:
  - Advance the endoscope until airway is being plugged.
  - Flush with isotonic sterile saline (5–10 ml per flushing).
  - Flush a little air through to clear any dead space in the tubing.
  - Coupage.
  - Aspirate – should contain froth and alveolar macrophages indicating a truly alveolar wash.
  - Divide sample for cytology (EDTA) and culture:
    - For cytology, make direct preparations as well as sending fluid.

Normal parameters

- Variable – may be dependent on technique and depth of wash.
- Columnar epithelial cells.
- 60–90% macrophages.
- 2–30% eosinophils.
- Few neutrophils and lymphocytes.
- Bacteria only significant if some are intracellular or seen on direct preparations as overgrowth of contaminants can occur in transport.

NB – *Pseudomonas is not infrequently cultured from BAL samples; it usually represents contamination from growth within the bronchoscope.*

Management of inflammatory airway disease

Aims

- Remove primary cause (where possible).
- Reduce exacerbating factors – smoke, dust, cat litter, aerosol use, etc.
- Weight reduction can be of great value in obese cats (Pickwickian syndrome).
- Decrease inflammation.
- Increase removal of secretion.
- Bronchodilators – beta-2 adrenergic agonists, theophylline.
- Humidification.
- Mucolytics.

Corticosteroids

- Inflammation is a major component of disease associated with airway hyper-responsiveness, i.e. an exaggerated response to minor stimuli.
- Bronchodilators alone will relieve clinical signs, but can be associated with a poor long-term prognosis.
- Oral prednisolone initially 1–2 mg/kg PO q12h and reducing.
- For long-term management, the use of inhaled corticosteroid reduces the total dose received:
  - Inhaled corticosteroids – beclometasone, fluticasone propionate (more expensive but no systemic absorption 125–250 mg/cat q12–24h).

Bronchodilators

- Beta-2 adrenergic agonists:
  - Not licensed for use in cats.
  - Clenbuterol has been widely used with few reported problems at a dose of 1–2 µg/kg initially twice daily.
  - Terbutaline is easier to dose than clenbuterol at 1.25 mg q12h available as a syrup.

- Inhaled salbutamol (100 μg/cat q4–6h) and is particularly useful if acute bronchospasm occurs.
- Potential side effects – tachycardia, cardiomegaly, hypotension (especially with concurrent steroid use), GIT upset, depression and lethargy.
- Theophylline:
  - Weak bronchodilator.
  - Improves mucociliary transport, decreasing respiratory muscle fatigue.
  - Reduces late phase of allergic response.
  - Narrow therapeutic window.
  - Sustained-release products preferable at 20–25 mg/kg PO q24h.
  - Side effects include GIT irritation, hyperactivity, tachycardia (potentially arrhythmogenic), muscle tremors and seizures.
- Anticholinergic drugs:
  - Inhibit vagally mediated broncho-constriction; tachycardia and dry oral mucosa are unacceptable side effects prohibiting long term use.

Other treatments
- Ciclosporin:
  - Has shown some benefits for poorly responsive cats and as a steroid-sparing medication.
  - 3–5 mg/kg (of microemulsion-based products) PO q12h.
- Leukotriene inhibitors:
  - Leukotrienes are part of the inflammatory cascade.
  - Used in a few cases in cats (Zafirlukast 10 mg/cat PO q12h).
  - Value not determined.
- Antitussives:
  - Limited use/value in cats.
- Omega-3 polyunsaturated fatty acids:
  - Studies have shown decrease in airway hyper-responsiveness.
- Mucolytics:
  - Bromhexine is a bronchial secretolytic acting to improve removal of mucus from the airways.

- Efficacy in the management of respiratory disease is unproven.
- Demulcents:
  - Soothing action and are used for dry, irritating cough.
  - Flavours rarely acceptable to cats.
- Antihistamines:
  - Benefit has not been shown.
- Expectorants:
  - Increase the volume but reduce the viscosity of bronchial secretions, improving removal.
  - Not used in cats.
- Humidification:
  - May be helpful.
  - Room humidifiers are relatively inexpensive.

Management of chronic disease
- Owner compliance is a key factor in successful long-term management.
- Must understand that cure is very unlikely.
- Each cat requires an individual regime based upon the lowest drug use over a long term, i.e. low-dose continual treatment may be more effective with fewer side effects than intermittent high-dose therapy.
- Must suit the cat and owner.
- Depot corticosteroids should be avoided if possible.

Acute decompensation
- Crisis:
  - IV adrenaline – 0.5–1 ml of 1:10,000 solution.
  - Atropine – 0.02–0.04 mg/kg IM.
- Keep restraint to a minimum.
- Check that history and clinical signs fit, i.e. not some other cause, e.g. RTA, cardiomyopathy.
- Cage rest with increased oxygen.
- Inhaled salbutamol absorbed and may be the least stressful method of drug administration.
- Corticosteroids.

ORGAN SYSTEMS

Infectious bronchitis/ bronchopneumonia

Bacterial

- Rarely primary bacterial invasion – *Bordetella*, mycoplasma, mycobacterium, *Streptococcus equi* subsp. *zooepidemicus*.
- Important to search for underlying cause:
  - Extension of URT viral infection or cow pox.
  - Secondary to aspiration pneumonia (megaoesophagus).
  - Immune deficiency – congenital or acquired.
  - Ciliary dysfunction.
  - Inflammatory airway disease.
  - Laryngeal dysfunction.
  - Foreign body.
- Antibacterial use:
  - Based on culture and sensitivity.
  - 3–6 weeks treatment.
  - Initially IV in severe cases.
  - Empirical choices – cephalosporin, potentiated amoxicillin, fluoroquinolone ± metronidazole.

Fungal

- Very rare in UK:
  - Non-UK – sporotrichosis, aspergillosis, histoplasmosis, blastomycosis, coccidioidomycosis, Cryptococcosis reported.
- Pneumocystis carinii been reported in immunosuppressed cats.

Lungworm

- Primarily *Aelurostrongylus abstrusus*:
  - Non-UK – *Eucoleus aerophilus*, paragonimiasis, *Troglostrongylus* sp., cuterebrosis, *Capillaria*.
- Small airways and pulmonary arterioles.

Life cycle of Aelurostrongylus

- Eggs deposited in airways expectorated and swallowed.
- Intermediate host slugs or snails.
- Reinfect cats eating transport hosts – birds or rodents.
- Reinfect lungs via blood or lymphatics.

Clinical signs

- Low worm burdens are asymptomatic.
- Coughing is the major sign of symptomatic disease.

Diagnosis

- Larvae in faeces on flotation.

Management

- Fenbendazole – 50 mg/kg for 3 days repeated in 3 weeks:
  - Other parasiticides such as moxidectin, ivermectin and selamectin may also be effective.
- Prevent access to transport host.

Feline idiopathic pulmonary fibrosis

- Uncommon/rare condition of middle-aged to older cats.
- No apparent sex or breed predisposition.
- Causes chronic history of progressive dyspnoea and coughing.
- Physical examination – tachypnoea, inspiratory or mixed inspiratory and expiratory effort, and adventitial lung sounds.
- Radiographic changes – dense patchy or diffuse interstitial, bronchiolar, and alveolar infiltrates.
- BAL showed mild neutrophilic inflammation.
- Response to therapy (corticosteroids, antibiotics, bronchodilators, and diuretics) poor.
- Most cats died within days to months.

Acute respiratory distress syndrome, acute lung injury

- Acute respiratory distress syndrome (ARDS) and acute lung injury (ALI) are syndromes of pulmonary oedema and inflammation.

- Common causes include pneumonia, smoke inhalation, non-cardiogenic oedema, trauma.
- ARDS is also associated with systemic inflammatory conditions:
  - Pancreatitis, shock, sepsis, DIC.
  - ARDS forms part of systemic inflammatory response syndrome (SIRS) and multiple organ dysfunction syndrome (MODS):
    - Caused by inflammation that has spiralled outside the normal control of natural anti-inflammatory mechanisms.
- ARDS and ALI are best managed by addressing the underlying cause but prognosis is poor:
  - Oxygenation and ventilation are crucial.
  - Conservative fluid management, furosemide and albumin may be helpful.

Lung neoplasia

Primary tumours

- Rare.
- Nearly all are adenocarcinomas.
- Clinical signs are slowly progressive.
- Initially non-specific signs – weight loss, anorexia.
- Pleural effusion is common.
- Present as space-occupying lesions causing dyspnoea, coughing.
- Multiple primaries have been reported.
- Diagnosis on radiography, CT, bronchoscopy and biopsy.
- Surgical removal of solitary lesions may be successful but, despite radiographic appearance, many will have spread by the time of presentation.
- Little evidence that adjunctive chemotherapy is helpful.

Secondary tumours

- Lungs are a common site for metastases.
- Look for primary tumour.

- Clinical presentation as for primary lung masses ± signs that are attributable to the primary site.
- Treatment is palliative.

4.1.5 Pleural disease

- Common emergencies in veterinary practice frequently requiring a rapid diagnosis and treatment.
- Cat is often physiologically unstable and even a moderate increase in oxygen demand (e.g. stresses associated with handling) can lead to death.
- Prognosis tends to be either good (e.g. pyothorax, ruptured diaphragm) or very poor (e.g. FIP, lung adenocarcinoma).
- Presents as restrictive breathing associated with a space-occupying lesion of the thoracic cavity.
- Pleural space can be filled with air, fluid, viscera or soft tissue.
- Dyspnoea is the major clinical sign.

Anatomy

- Mediastinal barrier between the left and right hemithorax is incomplete in the cat.
- Most effusions are bilateral.
- Pyothorax and chylothorax most frequently lead to unilateral effusions, presumably due to inflammation causing loculation.
- Capillary vasculature supplying the visceral pleura originates from the right side of the heart, and those supplying the parietal pleura from the left, hence pleural effusions can arise from both left and right-sided heart failure.

Clinical presentation

- Pathogenesis often chronic.
- Present acutely, since cats are able to compensate well to a decreased oxygen reserve.
- Pleural disease is the most common cause of respiratory distress in cats.

ORGAN SYSTEMS

- Typically causes a restrictive breathing pattern with decreased depth, increased rate and open-mouth breathing.
- Lung sounds are reduced and percussion is abnormal.
- History of trauma is usual in cases of pneumothorax, haemothorax and diaphragmatic rupture:
  - BUT haemothorax and pneumothorax can be caused by other disease processes, such as a coagulopathy or bulla rupture.

Differential diagnosis of clinical signs
- See dyspnoea in Section 2.15.

Differential diagnosis of pleural disease
Primary diseases of the pleura
- Suppurative exudation – pyothorax.
- Exudative vasculitis – FIP.
- Primary neoplasia – mesothelioma.
- Pleuritis (rare).
- Pleuropericardial diaphragmatic hernia.

Secondary diseases of the pleura
- Pleural effusion secondary to neoplasia, chylothorax, heart disease.
- Haemothorax.
- Diaphragmatic rupture.
- Pneumothorax.
- Rarely – lung lobe torsion, pancreatitis, pulmonary infarction, thymic branchial cysts, lungworm, *Dirofilaria*, pacemaker implantation.

Diagnosis
- Clinical signs.
- Thoracic imaging:
  - Ultrasound, radiography or CT.
- Thoracocentesis.

Ultrasound
- Rapid assessment for the presence of fluid, air or intestines within the pleural space:
  - Facilitates sampling or draining of fluid.

- Diagnosis of lung masses.
- Investigation of diaphragmatic integrity.
- Cardiac assessment.

Thoracic radiography
- Challenge with regard to handling.
- Should the cat be sedated or anaesthetised?
- Sedation – various protocols (see Section 1.6).
- Two views should be taken wherever possible – a lateral and DV (severely dyspnoeic cats should never be placed in dorsal recumbency for a VD view).
- Standing lateral may be appropriate.

Interpretation
- Assessment of diaphragmatic integrity, especially ventrally, can be difficult when the line is obscured by fluid.
- Inclusion of the caudal abdomen in the films can be helpful as it allows the position of the liver and stomach axis to be assessed.
- Heart size and position can be obscured by the presence of an effusion.
- Pericardial fluid can appear to increase the cardiac dimensions, as well as causing a raised trachea.
- Compression of the lung field by a space-occupying lesion and the difficulty of achieving inspiratory films in the dyspnoeic cat can make the assessment of lung patterns, especially diffuse increases in density, impossible.
- Pleural fluid generally (Figure 14)
  - Pushes the lungs centrally in the thorax.
  - Causes scalloping of the ventral lung lobes especially if chronic.
  - Increases the separation of the lungs from the vertebral column at the diaphragmaticolumbar recess.
  - Elevates the heart.
  - Obscures the diaphragmatic line.
  - Separates the lung shadow from the chest wall on the DV view.

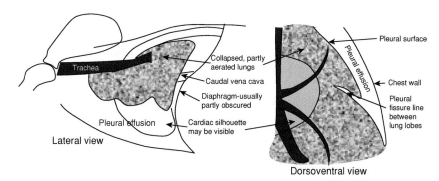

Figure 14 Diagram of radiographic appearance of free pleural fluid

- Masses tend to push the lung field radially away from themselves.
- The differentiation of soft tissue masses from loculated fluid and the fact that some thoracic masses also cause effusions, does not always allow for easy interpretation.
- Where the possibility of diaphragmatic rupture remains, a small quantity of barium (5–10 ml) can be given orally to better demarcate the stomach and small intestines.

Thoracocentesis and analysis of fluid
- Thoracocentesis prior to radiography may be required.
- Removal of 10 ml/kg of fluid can produce a major improvement in the cat's condition as well as providing valuable diagnostic material.
- Normally performed at the 7th–8th intercostal space at the level of the costochondral junction.
- 19g butterfly needle attached to a three-way tap and a 50 ml syringe.

Aspirate types and their causes
- Air – pneumothorax (trauma, pneumonia, neoplasia, spontaneous).
- Chylous – idiopathic, CHF, neoplasia, constrictive pleuritis, diaphragmatic rupture, pericardioperitoneal diaphragmatic hernia, *Dirofilaria*, obstruction of the thoracic duct, lung lobe torsion, post-pacemaker implantation.

- Haemorrhage – trauma, coagulopathy (especially coumarin poisoning), neoplasia.
- Transudate/modified transudate – neoplasia, CHF, diaphragmatic rupture, pericardioperitoneal diaphragmatic hernia, hypoproteinaemia.
- Pure transudates – rarely encountered associated with hypoproteinaemia.

Transudates
- Moderate total proteins (20–30 g/l).
- SG (1.010–1.030).
- Cell counts (<5 × 10^9/l).
- LDH (<200 iU).
- Caused by increased hydrostatic pressure.
- Clear to cloudy and yellow to amber.
- Predominant cell type tends to be macrophages.

Exudates
- Higher protein levels, SG, cell counts and LDH than transudates.
- Some overlap.
- Caused by increased capillary permeability.
- Variable appearance.
- Septic (pyothorax) or sterile (FIP, neoplasia, immune-mediated).

Management
- Initially oxygen, cage rest, pain relief.
- Treatment of underlying disease.

ORGAN SYSTEMS

Placement of chest drains

- Placed where repeat drainage over a short period of time is necessary.
- Normally performed under local anaesthetic ± sedation.
- Flexible but not collapsible, sterile tube 50–70% of the space between the ribs (12FG; 4.0 mm for adult cat).
- Cat should be placed in sternal or lateral recumbency.
- Local anaesthetic infiltrated between the 10th and 11th rib about halfway up the chest wall.
- Small skin incision is made and the tip of the catheter inserted to create a tunnel to the 8th intercostal space.
- Tube is then raised perpendicular to the chest wall and passed through the chest wall.
- Catheter is then advanced to lie in the cranioventral thorax.
- Trocar is removed, a gate clamp applied, and a Chinese finger trap suture used to secure the tube to the body wall; fittings can be glued together for increased security.
- Bandaged in place and monitored carefully.
- Cats tolerate drains relatively poorly, so they should be maintained for the minimum time necessary and monitored 24/7.
- Bilateral drains are rarely necessary unless there is a loculated effusion, e.g. chronic pyothorax.
- Drainage:
  - Continuous suction (low pressure) rarely necessary except if severe pneumothorax.
  - Heimlich valve – inappropriate for cats even the mini-Heimlich are unreliable in cats.
  - Intermittent suction via a three-way tap is most suitable for cats – maximum of 5 ml of negative pressure.

Chylothorax

- Relatively common in cats.
- Usually truly chylous:
  - Triglyceride >plasma.
  - Cholesterol ≤plasma.
- Most commonly associated with CHF, although a significant number appear to be idiopathic.
- Occurs secondary to a production/drainage mismatch, usually due to poor lymph return to the brachycephalic vein following obstruction or raised intrathoracic pressure. This causes lymphangiectasia and the development of collateral lymph vessels that drain into the thoracic cavity.
- Management should be directed towards identification and treatment of the underlying cause.
- Spontaneous resolution of idiopathic chylothorax can occur.

Medical management

- Recommended for initial management.
- Long-standing chylothorax can lead to the development of fibrosing pleuritis.
- Where medical management over 5–10 days is proving unsuccessful, surgical intervention should be considered.

Drainage

- Palliative drainage to relieve respiratory distress, and to enable potential underlying causes to be investigated.
- Repeat drainage can have a variety of negative consequences; physical and biochemical parameters should be monitored at regular intervals:
  - Dehydration.
  - Weight loss.
  - Hypoproteinaemia.
  - Hyponatraemia.
  - Hyperkalaemia.
  - Immune compromise.
  - Restrictive pleuritis.

Dietary management

- Traditionally managed with low fat diet on the basis that this will reduce the flow of chyle.
- Medium-chain triglycerides, as a fat and energy source.
- Recent evidence does not support either approach.
- Trying to maintain body weight and muscle mass is however crucial.

Diuretics

- Valuable treatment in chylothorax of cardiogenic origin.
- Contraindicated in the treatment of idiopathic chylothorax as they do not result in a significant reduction in the rate of fluid accumulation and may serve to worsen dehydration.

Corticosteroids

- Have been used in the therapy of idiopathic cases, as inflammation may be an underlying aetiology.
- Value in management is anecdotal.

Pleurodesis

- Not recommended.
- Painful and ineffective.

Rutin

- Rutin is a flavone benzo-[γ]-pyrone plant extract (bioflavonoid).
- Mode of action is unknown, but proteolysis and macrophage enhancement appear to be the most likely mechanisms.
- Dose rate – 250 mg three times daily.
- Side effects not reported.
- Efficacy has not been well documented.

Surgical management

- Various surgical techniques have been described for the management of idiopathic chylothorax.
- None have proved universally effective.

Thoracic duct ligation ± removal of pericardium

- Most widely used and reported surgical intervention for the management of idiopathic chylothorax.
- Resolution of the effusion occurs in around 50% of cases.

Other

- Cisterna chyli ligation.
- Thoracic duct embolisation.
- Passive and active shunts moving the chyle into the peritoneal cavity.

Prognosis

- Where the underlying cause is not treatable – prognosis is guarded to poor.

Neoplasia

- Relatively common cause of pleural effusion.
- Thymic lymphosarcoma accounts for nearly 80% of cases, with a strong bias towards young cats:
  - Lymphoblastic cells identified on thoracocentesis.
  - Response rates to treatment (chemotherapy or radiation) are around 45% with a median survival time of 2.6 months.
  - Survival unaffected by FeLV status.
- Pulmonary carcinoma account for vast majority of remaining cases, prognosis very poor.

Exudative effusions

FIP (see Section 5.6)

- Pleural effusion occurs in approximately 50% of cases of wet FIP and will, infrequently, occur without evidence of an abdominal effusion.
- Fluid is always a sterile exudate, having a high protein content and variable cell count (which can be low).

Pyothorax

- Effusion characterised by a high cell count with a predominance of neutrophils, many of which are degenerate.

ORGAN SYSTEMS

- Phagocytosis of bacteria by macrophages is often seen together with free bacteria in the fluid.
- Various causes of pyothorax have been reported but in many cases haematogenous spread is assumed.
- There is no evidence of an association between pyothorax and immunosuppressive conditions such as retrovirus infection, or the use of glucocorticoids or cytotoxic drugs:
  - FeLV/FIV status can affect the prognosis.
- A variety of organisms have been identified, with obligate and facultative anaerobes occurring most commonly – some are potentially zoonotic.

Treatment
- Best approach remains controversial.
- Main aim of therapy should be to prevent loculation of the infection.
- Recent cases:
  - Drainage.
  - Followed by prolonged antibacterial therapy.
  - Initially antibacterials should be given intravenously:
    - Metronidazole (10 mg/kg q12h).
    - Ampicillin (10–20 mg/kg q6–8h) or potentiated amoxicillin (12.5–25 mg/kg q12h).
    - Fluoroquinolones if Gram-positive rods identified.
  - Followed by a 4–6 week course of oral medication.
- Chronic cases:
  - Implantation of a chest drain.
  - Lavage with warm saline:
    - Addition of antibacterials or proteolytic enzymes to the lavage fluid has not been shown to be of any benefit.
  - Some cases require thoracotomy to break down adhesions and facilitate lavage.

Pneumothorax
Cause
- Usually follows trauma.
- Post-anaesthetic.
- Lung bulla are rare in cats.
- Erosive tumours.
- Tracking foreign body.

Presentation
- Dyspnoea with reduced lung sounds.
- Hyperresonance on percussion.
- Diagnosis on radiography – lungs retracted centrally.

Management
- Needle/catheter drainage to achieve a seal.
- If unable to achieve a seal, or rapid reaccumulation, then place chest drains.
- If it fails to resolve over 2–3 days, thoracotomy indicated.

4.1.6 Diaphragmatic disease
- Usually presents as space-occupying pleural lesion.
- Pleuroperitoneal diaphragmatic hernia – see cardiology section.

Diaphragmatic rupture
- Usually present as an emergency following trauma especially RTA:
  - Some cases may have bilateral involvement associated with an earlier rupture that can have occurred years previously – always check previous history of RTA/trauma.
- Can be chronic; these cats tend to present with lethargy, inappetence and weight loss with vague GI signs.
- Rarely an incidental finding.
- Dyspnoea, major presenting sign.

Diagnosis
- Challenging, particularly in cats that are haemodynamically and unstable with respiratory compromise:
  - Thoracic ultrasound is often the least stressful and most definitive confirmatory test.

- Mass-like lesion or effusion.
- Physical examination:
  - Empty abdomen.
  - Borborygmi in thorax.
  - Dull thoracic percussion.

Radiography
- Loss of diaphragmatic line.
- Pleural fluid.
- Free gas in thorax.
- Loss of abdominal liver shadow.
- Cranial rotation of stomach.
- Bowel displacement can be highlighted with barium swallow.

Management
- Prior patient stabilisation crucial before anaesthesia.
- Surgical repair.

4.1.7 Pulmonary vascular disease

Pulmonary thromboembolism
- Usually presents as sudden onset of severe dyspnoea ± cyanosis, coughing, collapse.
- Result of a combination of hypercoagulability, vascular endothelial damage and abnormal blood flow/stasis.
- Major emboli produce profound respiratory distress.
- Hypercoagulability (balance of coagulation and fibrinolysis):
  - Sepsis – coagulation activated (± fibrinolysis depressed), e.g. DIC.
  - High endogenous/exogenous steroids.
  - Specific loss of ATIII – renal failure, decreased production in liver disease.
- Vascular endothelial damage – directly activates coagulation cascade:
  - Following sepsis.
  - Inflammatory disorders – pancreatitis.
  - Immune-mediated diseases.
  - Specific infections – FIP, *Dirofilaria*.
- Vascular stasis:
  - Poor perfusion.
  - Shock.
  - Vascular obstructive disorders.
  - Cardiomyopathy.

Diagnosis
- Hypoxia – blood gas analysis.
- Variable radiographic change:
  - Normal to hyperlucent lung fields.
  - Areas of alveolar disease.
  - Pleural effusion.
- Sudden decrease in platelet count.
- Definitive diagnosis requires selective angiography or scintigraphic ventilation/perfusion scanning.

Management
- Thrombolytic therapy is controversial.
- Support – ensure tissue perfusion and oxygenation.
- Heparin – value is unclear.
- Treat underlying disease.
- Autolysis takes a few days to 2–3 weeks.

Prophylaxis
- Identify cats at risk and try and reduce that risk.
- Anticoagulants have not been shown to be efficacious – heparin, aspirin, clopidogrel:
  - Heparin acts via ATIII, ineffective if serum ATIII low.
  - Rebound hypercoagulability occurs, so withdraw heparin slowly.

Pulmonary hypertension
- Rarely reported in cats.
- Results from increased impedance to pulmonary venous drainage, pulmonary over-circulation or increased pulmonary vascular resistance.
- Secondary to underlying cardiac or lung disease.
- Signs usually relate to underlying disease process.
- Diagnosis is most usually made by demonstrating high-velocity tricuspid regurgitation (>2.8 m/s) in the absence of pulmonic stenosis.
- No therapeutic studies have been conducted – vasodilators and bronchodilators would be logical.

ORGAN SYSTEMS

ORGAN SYSTEMS

4.2 CARDIOLOGY

4.2.1 Introduction

- Clinical signs attributable to heart disease can result from primary intrinsic dysfunction or can occur as a result of another non-cardiac disease process, e.g. hyperthyroidism, CKD.
- Heart disease initially involves one of the five main parts of the heart:
  - Gross cardiac anatomy.
  - Cardiac muscle.
  - Heart valves:
    - Acquired valvular disease is uncommon.
  - Electrical conducting system.
  - Pericardium:
    - Significant pericardial is rare in cats.
- Most commonly seen in middle-aged to older cats as a result of degenerative conditions.

4.2.2 History and presentation

Congenital heart disease

- Majority of cases of congenital disease have a genetic basis (usually polygenic and not elucidated).
- Consider other factors including environmental, infectious, toxic, nutritional and drug-related causes that have affected cardiac development *in utero* or in the neonatal period.
- Congenital heart disease is relatively common accounting for 0.2–1% of Feline University Hospital admissions in the USA.
- The majority of congenital cardiac disease will result in a murmur; such murmurs need to be distinguished from 'innocent' or 'flow' murmurs.
- Flow murmurs can also be associated with significant extracardiac pathology, such as anaemia or a PSS.

Innocent murmurs

- Usually I–III/VI, craniodorsal, ejection type.
- Variable with heart rate and body position.
- Often musical.
- Typically diminishing with age and resolving by 16 weeks.

Congenital murmur

- Usually loud unless
  - Large defect.
  - Tricuspid valve (TV) dysplasia.
  - Mild semilunar valve stenosis.
  - R → L shunting.
- May be associated with clinical signs:
  - Failure to grow and poor appetite.
  - Cyanosis.
  - Exhaustion after brief periods of play.
  - Weakness.
  - Collapse.
- Source of congenital murmurs can be difficult to identify in some cats.
- Complex and multiple defects seem more common in cats than dogs.

Presenting clinical signs

- Cardiovascular assessment is a mandatory part of any physical examination of a sick cat, as part of a health or pre-vaccination check, or prior to anaesthesia.
- Due to the cardiac reserve, and the cat's ability to modify its behaviour, significant disease can be present without the owner reporting obvious clinical signs.
  - This means that a chronic, progressive disease will often present as an apparent acute condition.

Clinical signs

- Commonly
  - Dyspnoea.
  - Weight loss.
  - Anorexia/inappetence.
  - Pallor.
  - Exercise intolerance.

- Posterior paralysis.
- Ascites.
- Syncope/collapse.
- Less commonly → rarely
  - Sudden onset blindness.
  - Coughing.
  - Cyanosis.
  - Peripheral oedema.
  - Pyrexia.
  - CNS signs.
  - Sudden death.

Differential diagnosis of clinical signs
- See Sections 2.1 Abdominal enlargement, 2.3 Arrhythmia, 2.9 Collapse/syncope, 2.10 Cardiac murmurs, 2.15 Dyspnoea, 2.17 Failure to grow, 2.29 Ocular changes associated with systemic disease, 2.30 Pallor, 2.43 Weight loss.

Physical examination
- Indicators of primary cardiovascular disease:
  - Grade III–IV/VI systolic murmur.
  - Any diastolic murmur.
  - Gallop heart sounds.
  - Palpable precordial thrill.
  - Peripheral cutaneous thrill.
  - Generalised venous engorgement.
  - Localised absence of arterial pulse.
  - Radiographic evidence of cardiac enlargement.
  - Bundle-branch block on ECG.
  - Cardiac arrhythmias.
  - AF.
  - Paroxysmal tachycardia.
  - Frequent/persistent APC or VPC.
  - Frequent second-degree Mobitz type II and third-degree AV block.
- Examination focus in cases of suspected cardiac abnormalities:
  - Breathing – rate, depth, cat's posture.
  - Mucosal colour – cranial and caudal mucous membranes.
  - Abdominal shape – fluid thrill.
  - Examination of jugular vein.
- Pulse quality and rate, synchrony with heart.
- Thoracic auscultation and percussion.
  - Auscultation of heart sounds, in particular murmurs, is often better achieved by listening sternally in cats (see Figure 15).
  - Palpation of neck – evidence of hyperthyroidism.
  - Ocular examination – evidence of hypertension.
- Classification of murmurs:
  - Classification of heart murmurs in cats tends to be more difficult as their heart rates are faster and the murmur is frequently not valve associated.
  - As the murmur is often dynamic in nature, intensity is more affected by rate (how stressed the cat is in the consulting room) making serial recording of murmur intensity an unreliable indicator of progression or lack thereof.
- *NB* – More than one murmur may be present, e.g. VSD.
- *NB* – Murmurs can be created in old, thin cats merely by the pressure with which the stethoscope is applied to the body wall.
- Intensity:
  - Grade I–VI (Table 30).
  - Pitch (quality or frequency) – stenotic murmurs are a higher frequency than regurgitant.
  - Shape (modulation) – often difficult to appreciate in cats.
- Location (point of maximum intensity) and radiation.
- Timing and duration:
  - Systolic – is it holosystolic (pansystolic) or only early/late in systole?
  - Diastolic – rare; aortic insufficiency, AV stenosis, dirofilariasis.
  - Continuous – usually PDA, sometimes aortic stenosis with diastolic regurgitation.

ORGAN SYSTEMS

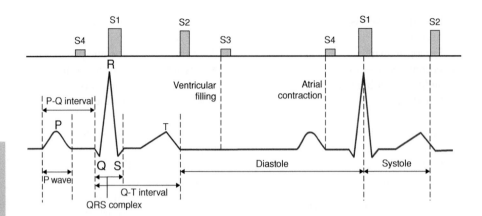

Figure 15 Parts of the ECG complex and the temporal relationship of the heart sounds with the cardiac cycle and ECG. S1 – closure of atrioventricular valves; S2 – closure of aortic and pulmonary valves; S3 (rapid ventricular filling) and S4 (ventricular filling associated with atrial contraction) – not normally heard in cats

- Gallop rhythms:
  - Usually S4 associated with poor ventricular compliance (e.g. HCM); the sounds are enhanced by the increased LAP associated with heart failure.
  - Especially in older cats, gallop rhythms may be a more reliable indicator of significant myocardial disease in cats than a murmur.
- Jugular examination – persistent jugular distension when the cat is standing with its jaw parallel to the floor and/or

Table 30 Heart murmur intensity grading

Grade I	Quiet – need good listening conditions to hear
Grade II	Soft but easily heard
Grade III	Moderate – similar to intensity of normal heart sounds
Grade IV	Loud – louder than intensity of normal heart sounds
Grade V	As IV but with precordial thrill
Grade VI	Very loud, precordial thrill, can be heard with stethoscope away from body wall

pulse extending more than one-third way up the neck implies an elevation of systemic venous pressure:
  - Right-sided CHF.
  - Pericardial disease.
  - Hypervolaemia.
  - Obstruction of the cranial vena cava.
  - Contraction of right atrium against a closed TV:
    - AF.
    - Third-degree AV block.
- Pulmonary evaluation:
  - Observation of the rate and rhythm of breathing.
  - Posture – dyspnoeic cats frequently crouch with their elbows abducted and the head and neck stretched forward.
  - Thoracic and tracheal auscultation.
  - Percussion – needs practice and knowledge of normal resonance:
    - Helps to differentiate between cardiac and respiratory disease as well as differentiating pulmonary oedema (increased respiratory noise, dyspnoea, normal percussion) from pleural effusion

ORGAN SYSTEMS

(decreased respiratory noise, dullness on percussion, restricted breathing pattern) in cats with significant LV disease.

4.2.3 Diagnostic aids

Summation of history, clinical examination and diagnostic tests

- Cardiac-specific biomarkers – cardiac troponin I (cTnI) and N-terminal pro-brain natriuretic peptide (NT-proBNP):
  - If both markers are elevated this tends to suggest a more guarded prognosis.
- ECG – primarily evaluates rate and rhythm.
- Radiography – heart size and shape, pulmonary evaluation.
- Ultrasound – dynamic function, evaluation of valves, heart size (chamber size and myocardial thickness).
- Blood pressure (BP) – primary or secondary disease, therapeutic decisions.

General laboratory evaluation

- Will provide little information in many cases of heart disease.
- Useful in
  - Deciding whether the heart disease is primary or secondary to another systemic problem, e.g. hyperthyroidism.
  - Older cats to evaluate other major organ function, particularly when therapeutic options are being considered:
    - Renal function will be affected by heart disease due to reduced renal perfusion but pre-existing renal dysfunction leads to worsening of heart disease and complicates management especially the use of diuretics and agents causing significant reductions in BP.
  - Monitoring of drug levels and side effects as part of long-term case management.

- Laboratory changes in heart disease:
  - Polycythaemia in right-to-left shunting diseases, e.g. tetralogy of Fallot.
  - Normoblasts seen in CHF without anaemia (probably associated with EPO stimulation due to mild hypoxia).
  - Hypoproteinaemia – effusions.
  - Pre-renal azotaemia due to reduced renal perfusion.
  - Raised liver enzymes associated with hypoxia.
  - Neutrophilia ± left shift, monocytosis, increased fibrinogen – endocarditis.

Cardiac-specific biomarkers

cTnI

- Evaluates cardiac myocyte damage.
- Relatively stable in serum and starts to rise 5–7 hours after injury peaking 1–2 days post injury and persisting for 1–2 weeks.
- Can be elevated in non-cardiac disease.
- Predictive value for mortality in cats with cardiac and non-cardiac disease.
- Highest values are seen with ischemic injury or arrhythmias.
- Can be used to monitor success of therapy, e.g. management of cats with hyperthyroid myopathy; values should return to normal with successful management of their hyperthyroidism.
- More sensitive assays now available may allow subtle cardiac muscle damage in early myocardial disease to be detected but not potential non-cardiac disease leading to mild elevations in cTnI.

NT-proBNP

- Produced primarily in response to LV stretch.
- Requires to be either sent frozen or in special tubes containing proteases for analysis.

ORGAN SYSTEMS

ORGAN SYSTEMS

Table 31 Recommendations for the interpretation of NT-proBNP results in cats

	NT-proBNP level (pmol/l)
Normal – low probability of significant heart disease	<50
Elevated – possible heart disease as a cause	50–100
Heart disease is likely to be present with volume overload	100–270
Suggests CHF	>270

- Limited clinical utility in the diagnosis of subclinical or occult disease.
- Value in distinguishing dyspnoea associated with cardiac disease from dyspnoea associated with respiratory disease (Table 31).
- Value in acute medicine is limited by the need for external assay.

Genetic testing

- Genetic screening tests are available for HCM in Maine Coons and Ragdolls:
  - Heterozygous or homozygous results are reported associated with mutations in the *MYBPC3* gene.
  - Cats that are homozygous for the genetic mutation are thought likely to develop HCM.
  - A negative result does not mean that HCM associated with other mutations/causes will not occur.

Electrocardiography

Use of ECGs

- Evaluation of arrhythmias.
- Limited evaluation of anatomic change.
- Evaluation of anti-arrhythmic therapy.
- Prognostication.
- Serially for evaluation of progression.
- Non-specific disease.

- Monitoring anaesthesia:
  - Most valuable for monitoring trends and changes in the shape of the complexes.
  - Atropine causes an initial, centrally mediated *bradycardia* before vagolytic effects increase the heart rate.
  - Bigeminal rhythm following short-acting barbiturates.
  - Rare persistent supraventricular tachycardia with thiopentone.
- Holter monitoring of cats has become significantly easier with lighter (150–200 g) solid-state devices that also have the advantage of easy, rapid download via the internet for interpretation.

Electrode systems

See Figure 16.

Practical points

- Standard positioning is right lateral recumbency but for rhythm analysis let the cat adopt a comfortable, minimally stressed position.
- Electrodes can be attached to the fur rather than the skin if plenty of coupling gel is used.
  - Some cats tolerate small, paediatric sticky electrodes applied to the metacarpal/tarsal pad better.

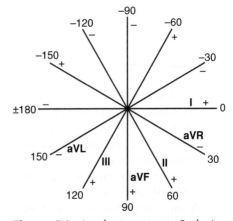

Figure 16 Lead orientation in Bailey's hexaxial system

- Electrodes: red – right fore; yellow – left fore; green – left hind; black – right hind.
  - Chest (V) leads very rarely used in cats.
- Complexes often small – use 20 mm/mV sensitivity at 50 mm/second.
- T wave can be difficult to see – use multiple leads.

ECG interpretation
- Diagnostic quality:
  - Can the complexes be distinguished from artefact?
- Rate:
  - Measure the overall rate over 15 cm that gives a minute rate by multiplying by 10 (paper speed 25 mm/second) or 20 (paper speed 50 mm/second).
  - Measure individual R-R rates using an ECG ruler.
- Rhythm:
  - Sinus rhythm – P for every QRS and a QRS for every P wave.
  - Unlike dog, cats do not normally have a sinus arrhythmia so variations in R-R interval are usually indicative of disease.
- Mean electrical axis (MEA) (Box 2 for example):
  - Calculation:
    - MEA is orientation (direction is sum of positive and negative deviation) of the lead at 90° to the isoelectric lead (see Figure 15).
    - The isoelectric lead is the lead in which the sum of the positive and negative deviation of the QRS approximates to zero.
    - If no isoelectric lead exists, choose the one closest to it; if the sum is overall positive, MEA is towards the positive terminal of the isoelectric lead.
- Abnormal beats or artefact.
- Measure and multiply to determine size and duration of parts of each complex (see Table 32 for reference ranges).
- Miscellaneous.

Box 2 Approximating the mean electrical axis

1. Lead I was the most isoelectric of this ECG but the sum is overall positive
2. Lead at 90° is aVF (+90 → ⁻90°) that is this case had a positive summation
3. Lead I has a positive overall sum; the MEA is towards the positive pole of lead I (0°)
4. MEA in this cat is therefore approximately 80°, i.e. normal

Criteria for evaluating feline ECG
P wave
- Right atrium depolarizes before left, so left atrial enlargement accentuates asynchrony and widens P, except in some cats where LA enlargement causes increased height of P.

Table 32 Reference ranges for lead II complex measurements in adult cats with normal heart rates

	Adult cat
Heart rate	120–240 bpm
P wave	<0.04 seconds × 0.2 mV
PQ interval	0.05–0.09 seconds
QRS complex	<0.04 seconds
R wave	<0.9 mV
QRS deviation	<1.2 mV
ST segment – elevation or depression	<0.1 mV
T wave	<0.3 mV
QT interval	0.12–0.18 seconds
MEA	0–160°°

QT, the section of the ECG between the Q and the T wave; ST, the section of the ECG between the S and the T wave

ORGAN SYSTEMS

- P pulmonale (tall P wave):
  - TV disease.
  - Atrial septal defect.
  - Dilated cardiomyopathy (DCM).
  - Pulmonic stenosis.
  - Pulmonary hypertension.
  - Rapid heart rates.
- P mitrale (wide P wave):
  - LA enlargement.
  - Ischaemia.
  - Anoxia.
  - Myocarditis.
- Biatrial (wide and tall):
  - Cardiomyopathy.
  - AV valve disease.
  - Severe pulmonary venous congestion.

PR interval
- Should be constant beat to beat, if variable suggests ectopic rhythm.
- If PR interval is variable then check association of P with QRS as there could be two independent rhythms (i.e. idioventricular rhythm).
  - Often if the P and QRS complexes are disassociated variation in QRS morphology will be noted as P and QRS complexes are superimposed.

  PR interval consistent but increased:
- First degree AV block:
  - Increased vagal tone – usually marked by a wandering pacemaker.
  - Bradycardia.
  - Atrial myocardial disease.
  - AV nodal disease.
  - Drugs slowing atrial conduction – digitalis, β-blockers, calcium antagonists.
  - Metabolic disease (hyperkalaemia).
  - Toxaemia, endotoxaemia.
  PR interval consistent but shortened:
  - Accessory pathway.
  - Rapid rate.
  - Increased sympathetic tone.
  - Drugs: beta-agonists – terbutaline, salbutamol, dobutamine, dopamine, vagolytic drugs.

QRS complex
- Increases in height and width with ventricular enlargement, hypertrophy or dilation, bundle-branch block.
- Small complexes associated with poor electrode contact, obesity, pleural or pericardial effusion, intrathoracic masses, hypovolaemia.

ST segment
- Early phase of repolarisation occurring.

  ST segment slurring:
- LV enlargement.
- Myocardial hypoxia.

  ST segment elevation/depression:
- Ventricular hypertrophy.
- Pericarditis.
- Myocarditis.
- Myocardial ischaemia.
- Electrolyte disturbances (hypo- and hyperkalaemia).
- Trauma.

T wave
- Few restrictions – affected by ventricular hypertrophy, myocardial hypoxia, electrolyte disturbance.
- Most useful in sequential observations – T wave reversal of polarity is significant (e.g. during anaesthesia) as this indicates myocardial hypoxia.
- Tall T wave – hypoxia, ventricular enlargement.
- Tall peaked T wave – hyperkalaemia.
- Small biphasic T wave – hypokalaemia.

QT interval
- Varies inversely with heart rate.
- Prolonged QT – hypocalcaemia, hypokalaemia, ethylene glycol poisoning, hypothermia, CNS disease.
- Shortened QT – hypercalcaemia, hyperkalaemia, digoxin.

Table 33 ECG changes classically associated with chamber enlargement

RA	Tall, peaked P wave
LA	Wide P wave
RV	MEA >180°
LV	Wide QRS; tall R wave
Biventricular	MEA <0°
	Wide QRS; tall R wave
	MEA – normal
	Wide QRS; tall R wave

Criteria for chamber enlargement
ECG is an unreliable method of determining chamber enlargement when results are compared to echocardiographic findings. Expected changes in the ECG are outlined in Table 33

Effect of electrolyte disturbances on ECG
See Table 34.

ECG and myocardial hypoxia
- ECG sensitive to small changes in oxygenation.
- Severe pulmonary disease can also cause hypoxic ECG change.
- Evidence of developing hypoxia:
  - Change in heart rate – initial fall, then rise.
  - ST segment elevation/depression.
  - ST segment slurring.
  - T wave change from previous.
  - Development of arrhythmias – most commonly VPC but can be anything.

Radiographic assessment of the heart and pulmonary vasculature
Changes in heart size
- Less marked changes occur in cats compared to dogs.
- Cardiomegaly tends to cause elongation of the heart on lateral thoracic radiographs.
- Changes associated with LA enlargement – straight caudal border, splitting of main stem bronchi are rarely seen even where there is a marked dilation.
- DV view illustrates atrial enlargement more readily.
- Valentine heart shape on DV view is associated with biatrial enlargement.
- Microcardia:
  - Dehydration/hypovolaemia.
  - Over-inflation of lungs.
  - Shock.
  - Pneumothorax.
  - Obstruction to venous flow.
- Normal heart size and shape, but heart disease present:
  - Mild–to-moderate HCM.
  - Small VSD.
  - Mild congenital or acquired valvular disease.
  - Conduction disturbance.
  - Neoplasia.
  - Congestive failure over-treated with diuretics.

ORGAN SYSTEMS

Table 34 ECG changes associated with abnormalities in electrolyte levels

Electrolyte	ECG change
Hyperkalaemia	Tall peaked T waves, flattened P wave, bradycardia, prolonged PR and QT intervals, widened QRS, atrial standstill, sinoventricular rhythm, 3° AV block, cardiac arrest
Hypokalaemia	Prolonged QT, small biphasic T wave, bradycardia
Hypercalcaemia	Elevated ST, bradycardia, altered T wave shape, ? shortened ST segment
Hypocalcaemia	Prolonged QT, tachycardia
Hypomagnesaemia	Prolonged PR, widened QRS, depressed ST, peaked T

Criteria to assess presence of cardiomegaly
- Buchanan heart score (vertebral heart score) >6.5–8.5 (Figure 17).
- Craniocaudal width of heart – cranial to 5th and/or caudal to 7th rib.
- Craniocaudal width of heart on lateral up to two intercostal spaces and <70% of height of thorax.
- <50% of width of thorax on DV/VD view.

Causes of cardiac enlargement
- Generalised enlargement:
  ○ Volume overload.
  ○ Myocardial failure.
  ○ Pericardial effusion.
  ○ Pericardioperitoneal diaphragmatic hernia.
- LA enlargement results from volume overload – usually associated with LV enlargement:
  ○ Left-sided CHF.
  ○ High output states, e.g. hyperthyroidism.
  ○ Chronic severe anaemia.
  ○ Congenital or acquired MV disease.
  ○ Left-to-right shunts.
- LV enlargement alone results from pressure overload, or myocardial thickening:
  ○ Cardiomyopathy.
  ○ Systemic hypertension.
  ○ Aortic stenosis.

- Right atrial enlargement results from volume or pressure overload – usually associated with right ventricular enlargement:
  ○ Cardiomyopathy and right CHF.
  ○ TV disease (uncommon).
  ○ Right atrial haemangiosarcoma (rare).
- Right ventricular enlargement results primarily from pressure overload:
  ○ Cardiomyopathy.
  ○ Secondary to LV failure.
  ○ Pulmonary hypertension – heart worm, pulmonary thromboembolism, idiopathic.
  ○ Large ventricular septal defects.
  ○ Eisenmenger's complex and right-to-left shunting defects.

Pulmonary vasculature and lung fields
NB – *Although VD projections tend to give more information about the lung fields than DV views, it is inadvisable to turn a dyspnoeic cat on its back.*

- Veins are ventral and central.
- Lateral view:
  ○ Arteries lie dorsal and are of a similar size to the veins.
  ○ Vessels lie on either side of the bronchus.
  ○ Cranial pulmonary vessels are less than the diameter of the proximal third of the 4th/5th rib.

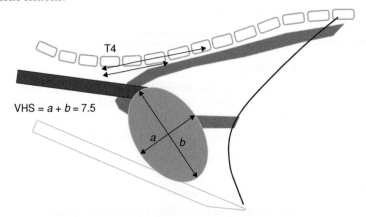

$$VHS = a + b = 7.5$$

Figure 17 Calculation of the Buchanan vertebral heart score

- DV view:
  - Arteries are lateral to veins.
  - Caudal pulmonary vessels are less than the diameter of the 10th rib as they cross it.

Normal pulmonary vessels but cardiac disease present:
- Cardiomegaly may or may not be evident.
- Mild valvular disease.
- Small VSD.
- Multiple defects.
- Pericardioperitoneal diaphragmatic hernia.

Under-perfused lungs – pulmonary vessels are narrowed and lung lucency appears increased.
- Usually associated with right atrial enlargement.
- Severe pulmonic stenosis.
- Tricuspid dysplasia.
- Tetralogy of Fallot.
- Pulmonic stenosis and right-to-left shunting ASD.
- Pulmonary thromboembolism.
- Hypovolaemia, shock.

Prominent pulmonary veins:
- Usually associated with left-sided enlargement.
- Aortic stenosis and LV failure.
- MV malformation/stenosis.
  Over-perfused:
- Prominent arteries and veins:
  - CHF.
  - Left–to-right shunts.
  - Fluid overload.
- Look for evidence of pulmonary oedema:
  - Early stages will appear as an interstitial pattern (loss of clarity of blood vessels).
  - More advanced alveolar oedema is seen as fluffy, cotton wool density within the lung fields.
  - Poorly defined edges.
  - Can occur anywhere (unlike dog where it usually begins in perihilar area).

Tortuous and truncated:
- Heartworm (not UK).
  Pleural fluid:
- For the appearance of free pleural fluid on radiographs see page 148–149.

Investigating 'asymptomatic' heart murmurs

- It is not possible to assess the severity of heart disease in a cat with a newly acquired murmur on history and physical examination
- 10–20% of older 'healthy' cats had heart murmurs
- 3 common causes – dynamic subaortic stenosis, dynamic right ventricular outflow tract obstruction, positional and iatrogenic murmurs.
- Generally routine blood tests, ECG and radiography have low sensitivity for establishing diagnosis and assessing severity
- Cardiac troponin and pro-BNP have low to moderate sensitivity
- Echocardiography is required in most cases
  - Echocardiographic changes present in 50% of these cats
- Clear treatment benefits only evident if CHF present
  - May be some value in using beta-blockers in non-CHF cases with moderate-severe dynamic subaortic stenosis.

Echocardiography
- Particularly important in feline heart disease as obvious chamber enlargement is not common.
- Mild-to-moderate cardiomyopathy is frequently associated with no radiographic or ECG changes.
- It should be performed on a conscious, unsedated, cat where possible.
- It is often preferable to shave the cat sometime prior to the procedure.
- Concurrent ECG recording improves interpretation.

ORGAN SYSTEMS

Right parasternal views

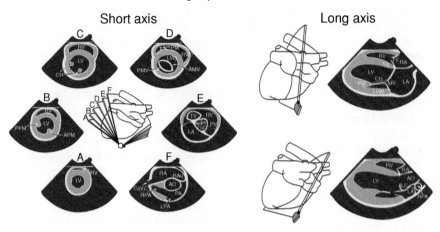

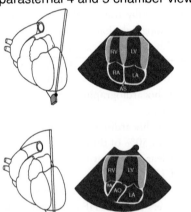

Left parasternal 4 and 5 chamber views

AMV – anterior mitral valve leaflet, Ao – aorta, APM – anterior papillary muscle, AS – atrial septum, CaVC – caudal vena cava, CH – chorda, LA – left atrium, LC – left coronary cusp of the aortic valve, LPA – left pulmonary artery, LV – left ventricle, LVO – left ventricular outflow, LVW – left ventricular wall, NC – non-coronary cusp of the aortic valve, PA – pulmonary artery, PM – papillary muscle, PMV – posterior mitral valve leaflet, PPM – posterior papillary muscle, PV – pulmonary valve, RA – right atrium, Rau – right auricle, RC – right coronary cusp of the aortic valve, RPA – right pulmonary artery, RV – right ventricle, RVO – right ventricular outflow, TV – tricuspid valve, VS – interventricular septum
From Thomas et al. (1993)

Figure 18 Standard echocardiographic views of the heart. From Thomas WP, Gaber CE et al *J Vet Intern Med* 1993; *7* :247–252. Reproduced with permission from John Wiley & Sons.

- 7.5 MHz phased array probe improves detail.
- A diagnosis can be obtained in many cases with 2D/M-mode (motion mode).
- Doppler and colour flow is necessary to accurately assess diastolic disease and the presence/degree of LV outflow obstruction, as well as many congenital defects.
- Standard right and left lateral parasternal views (Figure 18).

Right parasternal long axis
- Beam perpendicular to long axis of body and parallel to left atrium of heart, 4 chamber view.
- LV outflow view by cranial angulation or clockwise rotation.

Right parasternal short axis
- Rotate transducer by 90° clockwise.
- Left ventricle with circular symmetry.

ORGAN SYSTEMS

- Progressive dorsal angulation – with slight clockwise rotation to obtain cross section of aorta.

Left parasternal 4 chamber
- Left caudal to right cranial orientation, relatively flat to the body wall directed dorsally towards the heart base.
- 4 and 5 chamber views allowing measurement of trans-atrioventricular and aortic valve velocities.

M-mode
See Table 35.

Table 35 Comparison of M-mode and 2D echocardiography in the diagnosis of heart disease

M-mode more suitable for	2D more suitable for
Precise axial dimensions	Examining spatial orientations and
Accurate measurement of axial motion	global myocardial function
Timing of cardiac events associated with ECG trace – systolic time interval, relaxation time index	Assessing defects in cardiac structures, e.g. VSD
	Determining lateral dimensions
	Assessing lateral motion

- Provides a commonly used index of LV systolic function, the fractional shortening (FS), and is obtained by determining the percent decrease in the minor (transverse) axis of the left ventricle.
- Positioning is important to ensure an accurate cross section.

Normal values for M-mode indices
See Table 36.

Basic ultrasound examination
The following information is valuable in further management:

- Does the heart wall motion assessed from the long- and short-axis view look normal?
- What is the thickness of the IVS and LV free wall – is the thickening global or focal?
- Is there evidence of
  - Left atrial enlargement?
  - Thromboembolism?
  - Diastolic dysfunction?
  - Systolic dysfunction?
  - Right heart disease?

Table 36 Reference ranges for M-mode measurements in adult cats

Diastole	LV diameter	11–19 mm
	LV free wall	2.5–5.5 mm
	IVS	2.5–5.5 mm
	Left atrial – aortic ratio	0.8–1.6
Systole	LV diameter	4–11 mm
	LV free wall	4–9 mm
	IVS	5–9 mm
FS		35–60%

Interpreting the results
- Wall thickness is increased if M-mode measurements in diastole are >6 mm. In some cats it can be difficult to obtain an accurate M-mode measurement of the LVFW as the papillary muscles get in the way, in which case measurements can be obtained from a short-axis, 2D diastolic frame.
- CHF is suggested if there is significant left atrial enlargement:
  - Normal aortic diameter is 8–10 mm.
  - Normal LA:Ao ratio <1.4, values over 1.6 or a LA greater than 17 mm indicates congestion.
- Diastolic failure is indicated by
  - Changes in transmitral flow and therefore requires Doppler.

ORGAN SYSTEMS

Table 37 Arrhythmias associated with changes in impulse formation or conduction

Location of arrhythmia	Impulse formation		Impulse conduction	
	Excitation	Depression	Excitation	Depression
Sinus node	Tachycardia	Bradycardia, pause, arrest or block		Sinoatrial block or standstill
Atrium	Prematurity, tachycardia, flutter or fibrillation			
AV junction	Prematurity or tachycardia	Escape	Pre-excitation	
AV node				Blockade
Ventricle	Prematurity, tachycardia, flutter or fibrillation	Escape or arrest		Bundle-branch block

- ○ Is suggested when the wall of the heart is globally thickened with a small ventricular volume in systole (lumen tends to disappear) and diastole often accompanied by a high FS; these are the typical changes seen in HCM.
- Systolic failure is indicated by
  - ○ FS of <35% especially when accompanied by increased LV diameter in systole (>11 mm).

4.2.4 Arrhythmias
- Also see Section 2.3.

Clinical effect
- Reduces CO.
- Depends on severity of arrhythmia – cerebral blood flow reduced 10% by VPC/APC, 40–75% by ventricular tachycardia, slightly smaller reduction in coronary and renal circulation occurs.
- Mild arrhythmia leads to weakness, fatigue, lethargy, decreased activity.
- Severe arrhythmia leads to profound weakness, ataxia, disorientation, collapse, seizure, coma, sudden death.

Causes (see Table 37)
- Primary or secondary.
- Ectopic rhythms generated outside sinoatrial (SA) node – cardiac cell irritated through metabolic, inflammatory, ischaemic, hypoxic, toxic or physical injury may develop abnormal membrane potential.

Management of supraventricular arrhythmias
Arrhythmia is characterised by normal-looking QRS complexes, P waves may or may not be seen and, if present, may not be associated with the QRS complexes.
- Atrial tachycardia – can be physiologic; usually associated with atrial myocardial disease/enlargement.
- AF/flutter – rare in cats compared to dogs, indicates severe atrial enlargement.
- Junctional tachycardia.

Drugs
Acute therapy of sustained/paroxysmal arrhythmias requires i/v drug administration. The following injectables should be considered as part of an 'emergency box'. 2% lidocaine without adrenalin, propranolol and verapamil.

Acute therapy

- Vagal manoeuvre – massage carotid sinus by gentle continuous pressure to the area just caudodorsal to the larynx or with 15–20 seconds of bilateral ocular pressure over closed eyelids:
  - If rate slows ⇒ sinus tachycardia rather than a re-entrant tachycardia involving AV node.
- Vagal manoeuvre ineffective – give i/v verapamil (0.025 mg/kg slowly repeat every 5 minutes to maximum dose of 0.15–0.2 mg/kg) and try vagal manoeuvre after each dose.
- Verapamil ineffective – propranolol (0.02 mg/kg slowly repeat every 5–10 minutes to maximum five times).
- Propranolol ineffective – try lidocaine.
- BP and ECG should be monitored if i/v drugs are given.

Chronic therapy

- Manage underlying cause.
- Atenolol or diltiazem, if episodes of tachycardia still occurring in cats with normal BP and any CHF is controlled.

Management of ventricular arrhythmias

- Isolated VPCs or ectopic beats do not need to be treated although investigation of their cause should be considered.
- Treat if
  - Significant effect on CO (clinical assessment).
  - Likely to degenerate (R on T, multifocal).

Acute therapy for sustained or paroxysmal ventricular tachycardia

- If the cat is not in CHF and has reasonable systolic function
  - Propranolol as above.
- Propranolol ineffective or in CHF
  - Lidocaine – 0.25–0.5 mg/kg i/v over 5 minutes can repeat boluses of 0.15–0.25 mg/kg up to a total of 4 mg/kg.

- Effective rhythm control – 10–40 µg/kg/minute as continuous rate infusion (CRI).

Chronic therapy

- Manage underlying heart disease, if present.
- Little information is available but sotalol (0.5–2.0 mg/kg q12h) is the most widely used drug.

Management of bradyarrhythmias

- Atrial standstill or arrest secondary to fibrosis associated with muscular dystrophy, or long-standing atrial enlargement.
- AV block in cats is relatively common and is usually pathologic though often relatively asymptomatic, as ventricular escape rate is rapid.
- Treatment
  - Only if symptomatic.
  - Sympathomimetics – terbutaline, theophylline.
  - Pacemaker.

Bundle-branch block

- Common rhythm abnormality but not haemodynamically important.
- Reflects underlying cardiac disease.
- Common in HCM.

4.2.5 Congenital heart disease

Cause

- Genetic.
- Environmental.
- Infectious.
- Toxic.
- Nutritional.
- Drug related.

Common congenital defects

- Approximate order of prevalence:
  - MV dysplasia.
  - TV dysplasia.
  - VSD.
  - Atrial septal defects.

ORGAN SYSTEMS

○ PPDH.

○ AV canal and AV septal defects.

• Defects can often be complex involving several structures in cats.

Approach

• Physical examination and breed – what is the likely defect?
• Why does the owner want to know?
• Should the kitten be returned?
• Estimation of life expectancy.
• Costs of investigation and treatment.
• Is knowing the precise defect likely to change my management?
• Is it surgical?
• How often should I monitor?
• What signs are likely to be seen by the owner?
• Could sudden death occur?
• What treatments can I offer?

Diagnosis

• Occurrence and severity of clinical signs, ECG, radiographic and echocardiographic changes will depend on the exact nature and degree of the congenital defect.
• Ultrasound is usually necessary.
• Point of origin of some cardiac murmurs can be difficult to define in kittens.

Treatment

• Dependent on clinical signs.
• Only PDA and PPDH are likely to be amenable to surgical intervention.
• Balloon valvuloplasty is limited due to patient size.
• Therapy should be based on improving CO and reducing cardiac work.

Aortic stenosis

• Rare in cats.
• Dynamic, valvular and supravalvular forms described:
  ○ Dynamic disease occurs secondary to a variety of other conditions, e.g.

fixed stenosis, mitral dysplasia and HCM.
  ○ Concurrent MV anomalies not uncommon.

Pulmonic stenosis

• Rarely seen in cats.
• Leads to right-sided CHF.
• 2° tricuspid insufficiency.

Clinical signs

• Reduced playing (exercise intolerance).
• Stunted.
• Syncopal.

ECG

• Often normal.

Radiography

• Post-stenotic dilation may be seen on DV.
• Reverse D shape on DV.
• Hypovascular lung pattern.

Echocardiography

• Right ventricular concentric hypertrophy.
• 2D changes can be valvular, sub- or supravalvular.
• Flattened IVS ± paradoxical motion, i.e. IVS bows into LV in diastole.
• Increased transvalvular velocity.

Treatment

Beta blockade to reduce dynamic component.

Balloon valvuloplasty reported with favourable outcome.

Atrial septal defects

• Common in cats – account for 10% of abnormalities.
• Failure of fusion of endocardial cushion to form the septum *in utero*.
• Several forms exist, depending on the location of the defect.

Clinical signs
- May be none.
- Pulmonary over-circulation and syncope.
- Soft murmur over pulmonic valve.
- Split S$_2$.

Radiography
- Right-sided volume overload.
- Dilation of pulmonary artery (PA).
- Pulmonary vascular prominent.

ECG
- Often normal.
- Intraventricular conduction disturbance.

Echocardiography
- Need to view septum in several planes.
- Bubble study for reverse shunt.

NB – *Echo dropout over the membranous portions of the atrial septum can mimic a defect.*

Prognosis
- Overall prognosis for cats with endocardial cushion defects is guarded to poor as they tend to develop severe cardiomegaly and CHF.

Ventricular septal defects
- Common in cats – accounts for 15% of abnormalities.
- Ventricular septum is formed from two principal parts – a membranous dorsal part developed from fibrous skeleton and an extensive muscular septum forming the ventricular outflow tract.

Pathophysiology
- Depends on the amount of blood being shunted, i.e. size/pressure difference between left/right ventricles.
- Initially right over-circulation and LV volume overload.
- If the defect is high, the large volume of blood pumped into pulmonic trunk causes increased LV but not right ven-

tricular work, and increased preload to the left atrium.
- Eventually results in pulmonary hypertension and right ventricular hypertrophy, causing reversal of shunt (Eisenmenger's syndrome).
- Usually associated with TV dysplasia in cats, but can be other defects (ASD, PDA, aortic or pulmonic stenosis, tetralogy).

Clinical findings
- Diagonal, holosystolic murmur 2nd to 4th intercostal space on the right, 5th to 6th intercostal space on the left.
- Thrill.
- Split S$_2$.
- Reversal of shunt – attenuated murmur and cyanosis.

ECG
- Biventricular enlargement.
- Arrhythmia.
- Bundle-branch block.
- Early ventricular septal activation characterised by a wide Q wave.

Radiographic
- Right enlargement.
- Pulmonary over-circulation.
- Progressing to generalised cardiomegaly and CHF.

Echocardiography
- Demonstrate defect in several planes.
- Flow across defect ± aortic regurgitation.
- Left ventricle hyperkinetic.
- LV and left atrial dilation.
- Right ventricular hypertrophy.
- High velocity (pressure) across the shunt implies the shunt is restrictive and is likely to have less haemodynamic consequences as pressure difference between the left and right ventricle is maintained.

ORGAN SYSTEMS

Prognosis
- Small defects can be asymptomatic and well tolerated.
- Large defects progress to CHF.

Patent ductus arteriosus
- Accounts for 10% of the defects in cats in the USA, appears to be rarer in the UK.

Pathophysiology
- Pulmonary over-circulation.
- LV overload.
- Pulmonary venous and arterial hypertension.
- Chronic mitral incompetence and LA enlargement.
- Large defect – pulmonary vascular pressure increases markedly with reversal of shunt in the first few months – Eisenmenger's physiology.

Clinical findings
- Left-sided heart failure.
- Continuous 'machinery' murmur classically heard in dogs may be less obvious in cats as the diastolic component can be difficult to hear.
- Murmur can be quite localised.
- Palpable thrill over cranial thorax.
- Water hammer pulse.
- Murmur is often more caudoventral in cats.

ECG
- Wide P.
- Tall R.
- Prolonged QRS.
- AF and ventricular premature complexes – if decompensation occurs.

Radiography
- Three-knuckled bulge is less obvious in cats.
- Pulmonary over-circulation.
- Left-sided enlargement.
- Left apex displaced to right.

Echocardiography
- Left atrial and LV enlargement.
- Decreased contractility with chronic overload.
- Septal motion exaggerated.
- Continuous flow/disturbance/turbulence and high retrograde pulmonic flow towards the pulmonic valve in the main pulmonary artery (requires Doppler).

Prognosis
- Good if treated before heart failure develops – surgical or by coil embolisation.

Atrioventricular valve dysplasia
- 15–20% of lesions in cats.
- Insufficiency is more common than stenosis – but can co-exist.
- Regurgitation with volume overload of ipsilateral chamber and poor CO.
- Ipsilateral atrial dilation with eccentric ventricular hypertrophy.
- Predisposition to arrhythmia especially AF.
- Obstructed filling when stenotic.
- Often tolerated for years; onset of clinical signs variable, reported from 6 months to 8 years.
- Cats with MV dysplasia may develop CHF early.
- Significant cardiomegaly is a poor prognostic indicator.

Mitral valve dysplasia
- Most common defect in cats.
- ± Chorda (fused, thickened or elongated) and papillary muscles involvement.
- Thickened cusps and incomplete closure.
- SAM causing dynamic left ventricular outflow tract (LVOT) obstruction.
- Aortic stenosis may also co-exist.

Clinical signs
- Usually evident at 6 months of age but can be older.
- Holosystolic murmur, rarely diastolic rumble of stenosis, loud gallop.

Radiography
- Left-sided cardiomegaly.
- CHF.

Echocardiography
- Wide excursion of valves during systole and diastole.
- Initial increase in FS followed by a progressive fall and LV dilation due to myocardial failure.
- LV hypertrophy due to SAM making the condition difficult to distinguish from HCM.

Treatment
- Beta blockade may reduce LVOT obstructive element and minimise LV hypertrophy

Mitral stenosis
- Infrequent, often associated with sub-aortic stenosis.
- Thickening and fusion of leaflets obstructing flow, increasing diastolic pressure gradient and mean LA pressure causing pulmonary oedema.
- Supraventricular arrhythmias and left CHF.
- Decreased diastolic excursion of valve leaflets that are thickened.
- Left atrial enlargement more severe than LV changes.

TV dysplasia
- Second most common defect in cats.
- Lesions similar to MV dysplasia.

Clinical signs
- Holosystolic right apical murmur.
- Poor correlation between intensity of murmur and severity.
- Palpable precordial thrill.
- Harsh regurgitant murmur; careful listening required to detect murmur in some cases.
- Jugular pulse.

ECG
- Usually abnormal with intraventricular conduction disturbances.
- Wide P.
- AF.
- Right bundle-branch block.

Echocardiography
- Abnormal valve motion – stenosis is rare.
- Right-sided enlargement.
- Flattened IVS and paradoxical motion.

Prognosis
- Poor once signs of right CHF develop.
- Treatment difficult.

Endocardial fibroelastosis
- Familial Burmese and Siamese.
- LV and left atrial dilatation with severe endocardial thickening.
- Diffuse hypocellular, fibroelastic thickening, thin randomly organised layers of collagen/elastic fibres.
- Oedema of endocardium with lymphatics is prominent.
- No evidence of myocardial inflammation or necrosis.

Clinical
- Early development (<6 months old) of left or biventricular failure.
- Failure to thrive.

Radiography
- Left enlargement.

Echocardiography
- Ventricular stiffness.
- Volume overload from mitral regurgitation.

Diagnosis
- Tenuous unless post-mortem histology.
- Chronic LV dilatation may lead to similar changes secondary to mitral dysplasia, aortic stenosis, DCM or myocarditis in man.

ORGAN SYSTEMS

Vascular ring anomalies

- Rare.
- Persistent right aortic arch most commonly reported.

Cyanotic heart disease

- Cyanosis (in heart disease) indicates a right-to-left shunting defect, i.e. deoxygenated blood is entering the systemic circulation.
- Cyanosis is not a reliable sign (interclinician correlation poor).
  - Ease with which cyanosis seen will depend on haemoglobin level.
    - If haemoglobin <5 g/l, cyanosis will not be evident.
- Cyanosis will occur when the PaO_2 falls below 60 mmHg (SaO_2 75% – PCV within the reference range) and is, therefore, an indication of severe hypoxia.
- Tends to suggest that the disease is chronic.
- Physiologic response to low oxygen tension is polycythaemia.

Eisenmenger's physiology

- Eisenmenger's complex – VSD and pulmonary vascular disease/hypertension resulting in secondary right-to-left shunt.
- Occurs due to high flow rates or direct transmission of systemic arterial pressure to pulmonary circulation and the development of pulmonary vascular disease.
- Observed in PDA, VSD, aorticopulmonary communication, atrial septal defect.
- Management:
  - Dependent on whether pulmonary hypertension (see Section 4.1.7) exists (cf. Tetralogy of Fallot when pulmonary resistance is normal).
  - Phlebotomy, hydroxycarbamide (hydroxyurea) or surgical leeches.

Causes of cyanotic heart disease

- Tetralogy of Fallot:
  - Pulmonic stenosis, subaortic VSD, right ventricular hypertrophy, overriding or dextraposed aorta.
- Reverse shunting PDA ($\approx$5% of PDAs).
- Tricuspid dysplasia.
- Double-outlet right ventricle – VSD present to allow LV emptying.
- Transposition of the great arteries – aorta from the RV, and pulmonary artery from the left, i.e. two separate circulations with a shunt (otherwise lethal).
- Truncus arteriosus – large VSD results in both ventricles emptying into a large vessel with mixing of blood. Results in cardiomegaly due to volume overload.

4.2.6 Acquired cardiac disease

Myocardial disease

- Cardiomyopathy – heart muscle disease of unknown aetiology.
  - Most types of cardiomyopathy have been described in cats.
- Whether the aetiopathogenesis of the different forms of cardiomyopathy are distinct is unknown.
  - Anecdotal evidence suggests that the form of cardiomyopathy may change over time.
- Gradual loss of function worsened by conduction/rhythm disturbances and valve incompetence.
  - Damaged myocardial cells are unstable and become ectopic foci.
- If aetiology known, e.g. hyperthyroidism, then the cat has secondary hypertrophy, not HCM.
  - Myocardial changes can occur secondary to
    - Infection.
    - Inflammation.
    - Trauma.
    - Ischaemia.
    - Toxins.
    - Myocardial neoplasia.

- Drugs.
- Thyrotoxicosis.
- Acromegaly.
- Hypertension.
- Inappropriate nutrition (e.g. taurine deficiency).
- Chronic anaemia.

Hypertrophic cardiomyopathy
- Most common form of cardiomyopathy reported.
- Associated with diastolic failure.
- Cardiac filling is dependent on relaxation and compliance of the ventricle which is affected by
  - Wall stiffness.
  - Pericardial constraints.
  - End diastolic volume.
- Relaxation abnormality will initially pseudonormalise by hypertrophy.

Pathophysiology
- Hypertrophied LV free wall and IVS; often symmetrical.
- ± LV outflow tract obstruction.
- Further obstruction of LV outflow tract by forward motion of MV during systole (SAM).
- Reduced wall compliance limiting filling.
- Increased LV end-diastolic pressure.
  - ± worsened by diffuse endocardial fibrosis.
  - ± MV dysfunction and left atrial enlargement.
- Increased intracellular calcium that inhibits relaxation may be a factor.
- Increased circulating growth hormone levels compared to other cardiac diseases.
- Myocardial ischaemia due to
  - Coronary remodelling.
  - Decreased vasodilator capacity.
  - Increased LV wall tension.
  - Tachycardia.
  - Increased myocardial oxygen demand (MVO_2).
- Arrhythmias further decrease LV filling and increase MVO_2.

- MV regurgitation – due to SAM, cranial malposition of valve, papillary muscle.
- Eventually systolic dysfunction occurs.

Presentation
- Young to middle-aged (mean 6.5 years).
- Male.
- Higher prevalence reported in Maine Coon, American short hair, Ragdoll, possibly Persians.
  - Autosomal dominant pattern found in family studies.
  - Rare in oriental.
- Sudden death – uncommon.

Clinical signs
- 60% of cases have an acute history:
  - Signs can be precipitated by a stressful event, e.g. anaesthesia or intercurrent disease.
- Murmur:
  - Variable up to grade IV with PMI over MV/LVOT.
    - 1/3rd cases no murmur
  - Will vary with heart rate.
  - Physical examination can be otherwise normal if CHF not present.
- Gallop sounds (usually S4).
- Anorexia, lethargy (often noticed by owner as increased sleeping), vomiting.
- Dyspnoea and tachypnoea – variable lung sounds/percussion findings depending on whether pleural effusion or pulmonary oedema present.
- Posterior paresis and weak/absent femoral pulses associated with feline arterial (aortic) thromboembolism (FATE).
- Increased capillary refill time.
- Pallor.
- Cyanosis.
- Hypothermia.

ECG
- Highly variable.
- 70% abnormal – increased P and R width and amplitude.

ORGAN SYSTEMS

- Atrial or ventricular premature complexes or AF.
- Occasionally AV conduction disturbances.
- Left anterior fascicular block.
- Left axis deviation.

Radiography
- Valentine heart.
- Pulmonary oedema.
- Pleural effusion.
- Cardiomegaly – often long heart on lateral view.
  - ○ Generalised enlargement/rounding ⇒ pericardial effusion.

Echocardiography
- Symmetric or asymmetric hypertrophy.
- Asymmetric hypertrophy of IVS causing LV outflow obstruction.
- Hypertrophied papillary muscle.
- Decreased LV internal dimensions.
  - ○ In advanced disease as systolic failure develops, dilation may occur.
- FS – normal to increased.
  - ○ FS can fall below the reference range in advanced disease.

- Left atrial enlargement.
  - ○ 'Smoke' or thrombi may be evident.
- SAM of MV.
  - ○ On M-mode the MV moves upwards to the IVS during systole (Figure 19).
- Mild pericardial effusion.
- Mild RV hypertrophy.
- Mitral regurgitation > 90% cases.
- Increased aortic gradient with abnormal Doppler waveform – slow rise.
- Mitral inflow A and E wave changes.

Prognosis
- Progression of HCM is unpredictable with some cats remaining in a stable state for years whilst other cats have a more rapidly progressive course:
  - ○ Median survival time of asymptomatic cats appears good >3years.
  - ○ Median survival time for cats presenting with CHF is 6–12 months.
  - ○ Increased median survival time of cats with SAM is reported.
- Poor prognostic indicators:
  - ○ Age – older cats have poorer prognosis.
  - ○ Marked LV hypertrophy.
  - ○ Significant left atrial enlargement.

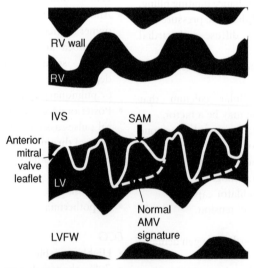

Figure 19 Diagram illustrating SAM on M-mode echocardiography

- ○ Non-obstructive form.
- ○ Thromboembolism.
- ○ Heart rate >200 bpm.
- ○ Attenuated diuretic response.
- ○ CHF.

Therapy

- According to clinical presentation (see Section 4.2.7).
- Hyperechoic blood flow in the left atrium 'smoke' indicates an increased risk of thrombosis due to blood stasis, platelet activation secondary to mitral regurgitation, endothelial damage. Anticoagulant therapy should be considered.

HCM in Maine Coon

- Equal male and female incidence.
- Autosomal dominant – genetic test available.
- Usually evident by 2 years, except in some females.
- Severe by 2–4 years.
- Sudden death and heart failure.
- Consistent papillary muscle hypertrophy.
- 60–70% patients have dynamic obstruction of outflow tract.

HCM in American Shorthairs

- Benign course.
- Few develop severe HCM and die.

HCM in Ragdoll cats

- Ragdolls over-represented in UK studies.
- Survival time post diagnosis poor.
- Genetic test available

Restrictive cardiomyopathies

- Endocardial and myocardial forms.
- Associated with extensive fibrosis.

Endocardial form

- Younger cats.
- Associated endocarditis.
- Parvovirus genomic DNA found.
- Secondary fibrosis.

- Severe fibrosis of endocardium causing mid-ventricular stenosis or fusing and distortion of MV apparatus.
- Myocardial infarction.
- Mural thrombi.
- Coronary artery atherosclerosis.
- Endocardial infiltrate.

Myocardial (non-infiltrative) form

- Middle-aged older cats; no breed predisposition.
- Neither amyloid nor deposition of abnormal metabolic material reported.
- Mild-to-moderate increase in heart weight.
- Patchy endocardial and interstitial fibrosis.
- Myocyte necrosis.

Clinical findings

- Weight loss.
- Effusions.
- Soft systolic murmur.
- Gallop.
- Thromboembolism common.
- Arrhythmias common.

Radiography and ECG

- LA → biatrial enlargement.
- LV → generalised cardiomegaly.
- ECG often abnormal:
  - ○ Wide QRS with tall R.
  - ○ Disturbed interventricular conduction.
  - ○ Wide P with atrial tachycardia/fibrillation.

Echocardiography

- Impaired diastolic filling.
- Normal or decreased ventricular diastolic volume.
- Normal to increased wall thickness.

Endocardial

- Pronounced scarring and constriction in the mid-ventricular area.
- Severe left atrial enlargement.

ORGAN SYSTEMS

- Mild LV hypertrophy.
- Non-homogeneous LV wall.
- MV insufficiency.
- Contractility usually normal.

Myocardial
- Marked left atrial or biatrial enlargement.
- Relatively normal left ventricle.
  - Regional wall dysfunction present in some cats.
- Normal to mildly increased wall thickness.
- Lack of severe LV volume overload.
- Relatively normal LV internal cavity size.
- Mild reduction in FS (usually >25%).

Therapy
- According to clinical presentation.

Prognosis
- Generally worse than HCM.
  - Refractory pleural effusion or thromboembolism common.

Dilated cardiomyopathy
- Rare in cats (since the discovery of taurine-associated dilation).
- Approximately 5% of cardiomyopathies.
- May be a terminal phase of HCM/restrictive cardiomyopathy (RCM) in some cats.

Potential underlying cause
- Should be ruled out before treatment:
  - Nutritional.
  - Tachycardia induced – AF, supraventricular tachycardia, anaemia.
  - Viral.
  - Immune-mediated.

Clinical findings
- Older cats.
- Usually present in heart failure.
- Initially signs are vague – anorexia, lethargy.
- Vomiting a few days prior to presentation.
- Dyspnoea – pleural effusion very common.
- Ascites.

- Weak and rapid pulse, pulsus alternans.
- Hypothermia.
- Gallop rhythm.
- Jugular distension.

Biochemistry
- Often pre-renal azotaemia, raised liver enzymes and stressed leucogram.
- Taurine – contact laboratory for sampling protocol:
  - Plasma <20–30 µmol/l indicates deficiency.
    - Supplement if plasma taurine <60 µmol/l.
  - Whole blood <140 µmol/l indicates deficiency.

ECG
- Wide P wave.
- Tall and wide QRS.
- Ventricular extrasystole and ventricular tachycardia.
- First-degree heart block.

Radiography
- Generalised cardiomegaly.
- Pleural effusion common.
- Pulmonary oedema.
- Ascites.
- Hepatomegaly.

Echocardiography
- Increased chamber size.
- Decreased contractility.
- Wall thickness is normal to focally hypertrophied.
- Hypokinesis is usually global and symmetric.
- Decreased FS.
- Pericardial effusion.

Therapy
- According to clinical presentation
  - Over-aggressive diuretics can worsen hypotension.
  - Venodilation.

○ Pimobendan.

○ Anti-thrombotic medication.

• Taurine 500 mg/cat/day.

○ Expect clinical improvement in 1–2 weeks in truly deficient cases.

Prognosis

• Many cats die/are euthanised within days of presentation.

• Those that survive 1 month have 50% survival at 1 year.

Unclassified cardiomyopathy

• 10–15% of cardiomyopathies have features that are inconsistent with the described forms.

• May represent intermediate phases.

• Prognosis seems relatively good.

Increased left ventricular moderator bands

• Rare form of cardiomyopathy.

• Moderator bands carry conducting fibres across the ventricle.

• Become thickened and hypertrophied restricting LV relaxation.

• Usually other cardiac changes.

• Two groups – young (possibly congenital) and older (acquired).

Arrhythmogenic right ventricular cardiomyopathy

• Rare.

• Progressive fibrofatty infiltrate of myocardium.

Clinical presentation

• Vague history.

• Dyspnoea.

• Syncope.

• Right-sided congestive failure.

• Holosystolic murmur.

ECG

• Variable.

• Supraventricular tachycardia.

• Ventricular ectopia or tachycardia.

• Right bundle-branch block.

Radiography

• Marked right-sided enlargement.

• Effusions – pleural, pericardial, peritoneal.

Echocardiography

• Right ventricular dilation and non-homogeneous wall kinetics.

○ Paradoxical IVS motion.

• Severe right atrial enlargement.

• Mild-to-moderate left atrial change.

Treatment and prognosis

• Guarded once CHF.

• Diuretics, positive inotropes and ACEi.

Corticosteroid-induced CHF

• Increased rates of CHF noted in cats given corticosteroids.

• Acute onset lethargy, anorexia, tachypnoea and respiratory distress.

• Radiography:

○ Moderate cardiomegaly.

○ Pulmonary oedema/pleural effusion.

• Variable ECG change.

• Echocardiography – mild wall thickening in diastole and LA enlargement.

• Survivors of acute episode show partial resolution of pathologic changes.

○ Long-term survivors can be withdrawn from medication without recurrence.

Myocarditis

• Viral aetiology suspected in some cases – panleucopenia, coronavirus.

• Other agents that may be involved include Bartonella and Toxoplasma.

• Inflammation commonly (60%) reported in myocardial biopsies from cardiomyopathy cats.

• Endomyocarditis reported in young cats dying suddenly from acute CHF.

ORGAN SYSTEMS

ORGAN SYSTEMS

- Traumatic myocarditis is probably common following RTA but rarely recognised clinically.
- Sporadic occurrences in adult cats associated with marked increases in cTnI.

Endocarditis

- Rarely diagnosed.
- Clinical signs of an infected focus:
  - Depression.
  - Lethargy.
  - Fever.
  - Shifting lameness.
  - Signs of heart failure only occur in late disease.
- Diagnosis:
  - Soft systolic murmur.
  - Leucocytosis.
  - Positive blood culture.
  - Vegetative changes on aortic or MV.
- Therapy:
  - Long-term antimicrobial treatment based on sensitivity.
- Outcome:
  - Sequelae common – myocarditis, thromboembolism, sepsis in other organs.
  - May require permanent antimicrobial treatment.
  - Progress into heart failure.

4.2.7 Management of feline heart failure

Definitions

Heart failure

- Inadequate perfusion in the face of adequate venous return, cf. hypovolaemic shock.

Preload

- Stretching force that determines the pre-contraction length of cardiac muscle fibres – Frank–Starling law.
- Related to LV end-diastolic pressure, when mechanism can no longer cope = backward failure.

Afterload

- Tension that has to develop before contraction occurs, i.e. to overcome resistance to forward flow.
- With an increase in ventricle size or wall thickness, more tension must be generated to produce a given pressure (Laplace's law) – in CHF = forward failure.

Cardiac output

- CO = stroke volume × heart rate.
- CO is regulated in order to maintain BP.
- As the heart fails and stroke volume declines, increases in heart rate maintain CO.
- The maximum effective heart rate in cats is about 240 bpm.
- Chronically tachycardia is an ineffective way of maintaining output.

Pathophysiology

- Regardless of cause, heart disease should be managed on the basis of the major dysfunction(s) causing the low output.
- In cats with heart failure, around one in three develop pulmonary oedema, and two in three develop pleural effusion.
- Oedema occurs when LAP exceeds pulmonary capillary pressure.
  - Initially venous return that cannot be moved forward results in increased left atrial volume and dilation. Dilation serves to normalise the pressure.
  - Eventually venous return exceeds the ability to dilate and LAP increases causing oedema.
- Pleural effusion is thought to occur due to the pleura being supplied by the left and right sides of the heart in cats.
- In HCM, a failure in the diastolic filling of the left ventricle due to increased stiffness results in an increase in left atrial volume at the end of diastole, and increased LAP as pulmonary venous return continues.

- In failure, the heart is working harder and hence myocardial oxygen demand is higher.
- The increased oxygen demand coincides with decreased myocardial oxygen supply, thus compromising myocardial function and increasing the risk of developing rhythm disturbances.
- Oxygenation is further compromised as
  - pulmonary oedema – results in decreased arterial oxygenation.
  - increased heart rate – occurs at the expense of diastolic relaxation time, decreasing coronary circulation time.
  - muscular hypertrophy – compresses the coronary vessels.
- Increased heart rate is not the sole response to decreased CO. A number of other neurohormonal events occur designed to maintain BP. Acutely, such changes are necessary and helpful; chronically, however, they become inappropriate – accelerating the rate of decline in cardiac function.
- Fall in CO associated with fall in BP.
  - Short-term response to decrease vagal and increase α_1-adrenergic stimulation leading to vasoconstriction.
  - Long-term RAAS activation occurs mediated by renin release (Figure 20) and increased levels of angiotensin II causing
    - vascular smooth muscle constriction increasing resistance and reducing capacitance.
    - antidiuretic hormone (ADH) released reducing fluid loss and further stimulating vascular smooth muscle.
    - increased thirst leading to expansion of blood volume and increased pulmonary capillary pressure.
- Decreased noradrenalin uptake increases circulating levels which constrict vascular smooth muscle.
- Downregulation of β_1-adrenergic responses (fight/flight mechanisms).
- Vascular smooth muscle growth leading to arteriolar narrowing and myocardial hypertrophy.
- Free radical production increased damaging cell membranes, leading to cell death and replacement by fibrous tissue.
- Aldosterone production to be increased.

Treatment strategies
- Management of congestive failure can be divided into two main areas:
  - Short-term therapy in patients presenting with acute onset congestion (usually associated with decompensated chronic failure).
  - Long-term strategies aimed at preserving cardiac function.

Aim
- Increased stroke volume.
- Increased CO therefore decreased neurohormonal stimulation and reduced oxygen demand.
- Decrease myocardial oxygen demand.
- Treat inappropriate compensatory response:
  - Heart rate.
  - Atrial/ventricular rhythm.
  - Volume overload.
  - Venous constriction.
  - Diastolic or systolic failure.
- Optimise heart rate, myocardial function, preload and rhythm.

Strategy
Initial management should focus on the area that is causing the most significant reduction in tissue oxygenation.
- Management of underlying disease, e.g. hyperthyroidism.
- Management of volume overload, oedema, effusion.
- Vasodilatation and reduction in cardiac workload.

ORGAN SYSTEMS

- Improving diastolic function.
- Improving systolic function.
- Management of tachycardia.
- Management of thromboembolic risk.

NB – *It is usually inappropriate to attempt to solve all aspects of the heart disease immediately as there is a significant risk of severe hypotension and it is difficult to assess the efficacy of each drug for long-term management.*

General principles
- Where possible, start drugs at a low dose and titrate upwards to effect.
- Regular follow-up until the cat and drug dose rates are stable.
- Home monitoring of respiratory rate is a valuable and sensitive indicator of treatment efficacy in cases with a tendency to develop pulmonary oedema or pleural effusion.
  - Respiratory rate charts can be provided to owners (Apps also available).
  - Relaxed cats at home have a RR <24/minute.
  - Sustained (2–3 days) increases in RR at rest require further investigation/intervention.
- BP monitoring can be used to decide on the safety of increasing dose rate or introducing another therapy.

- In severely compromised cats, always consider rest, increased oxygenation and opiates on arrival or between procedures.

Diet
- Value of dietary modification in cats with heart disease has not been shown.
- Salt is a palatability factor and maintaining food intake is probably more important than severe sodium restriction.
See Table 38

Options for therapy
- Decreasing volume overload → pulmonary oedema/pleural effusion:
  - Diuretics; venodilators.
  - Thoracocentesis.
- Decrease heart rate to below 180 bpm and manage arrhythmias:
  - Class II & IV anti-arrhythmics.
- Increase CO:
  - Reduce rate and arrhythmia.
  - Positive inotropes.
- Increase stroke volume:
  - Arteriodilators.
  - Positive inotropes.
  - Decrease regurgitant volume – arteriodilators.
- Increase force of contraction:
  - Increase preload.
  - Positive inotropes.

Table 38 Dietary recommendations for the management of cats with cardiac disease

Asymptomatic disease	Mild-moderate disease	Severe disease	
n–3 PUFA	Maintain optimal BCS	Enhance palatability to maintain BCS	
Mild sodium restriction?	n–3 PUFA	n–3 PUFA	
	Maintain serum Mg^{2+} and K^+ levels in reference range	Increased Na^+ restriction	
		Taurine	Benefits
	Moderate Na^+ restriction	Carnitine	unproven
		Coenzyme Q	unless specific
		B-vitamins	deficiency
		L-Arginine	demonstrated

PUFA, polyunsaturated fatty acid; BCS, body condition score.

Changing therapy

- Adjustments to therapy are often necessary as heart failure is a progressive condition.
- Increase in dose or the addition of new drugs is relatively straightforward.
- New therapeutic agent has been tried and proven ineffective or has unacceptable side effects and needs to be withdrawn but
  o Replacement drugs may take days, weeks or even months to become fully effective.
  o Sudden withdrawal of existing therapy may cause undesirable rebound effects.
  o The drug may be having significant beneficial effects despite adverse side effects.
  o Where possible gradual withdrawal over several days is advisable.

When to treat

- Obvious when cat is clearly symptomatic and CHF developed.
- Problematic where cardiac abnormality identified (e.g. murmur or mild hypertrophy) and there is no clear evidence of compromised output:
  o Evidence base for therapies beyond diuretics in CHF is lacking.
  o However, truly assessing cardiac compromise in cats can be difficult as a number of asymptomatic cats will improve with therapy!
  o There is no clear evidence to support prophylactic therapy in cardiac disease in cats.

Diuresis

- Overzealous use can reduce force of contraction (by Frank–Starling mechanisms) leading to low output failure.
- Excessive diuretic use is common in cats due to small body size relative to tablet strength.

- Signs of overdose can be similar (lethargy, inappetence, depression) to those of inadequate therapy and the danger is in ever increasing dose rates.

Furosemide

- Most commonly used diuretic.
- Acts on loop of Henlé.
- Acute congestion/pulmonary oedema:
  o Initially 2 mg/kg every 2–6 hours IV or IM.
    - IV furosemide may have venodilatory activity increasing capacitance.
  o CRI – 0.25–1 mg/kg/hour.
  o Subcutaneous absorption may be very poor due to peripheral vasoconstriction.
  o Once clinical signs especially dyspnoea improve, reduce dose to 2 mg/kg q8–12h.
- Maintenance therapy:
  o Aim for 1–2 mg/kg/day.
  o If more than 2–4 mg/kg/day is required, consider a second diuretic.
  o Periodically monitor potassium especially in inappetent cats.
- Side effects:
  o Ototoxicity (clinically apparent disease appears rare).
  o GI disturbances, weakness, leucopenia, anaemia, restlessness.
  o Risk of causing severe dehydration and hypovolaemic shock with low-output heart failure.

Spironolactone

- Aldosterone receptor antagonist.
- Diuretic effect insufficient alone.
- Limited value in acute therapy.
- Benefits:
  o Significant synergistic effect for long-term management.
  o May have additional beneficial effects by inhibition of myocardial fibrosis, vascular remodelling and endothelial dysfunction.
  o Potassium sparing.

- Oral dose – 2 mg/kg q24h.
- Side effects:
  - Severe ulcerative facial dermatitis is reported in USA especially in Maine Coons.
  - Gynaecomastia – rare.
  - Hyponatraemia and hyperkalaemia – rare.

Vasodilation

- Act directly to dilate arterioles and/or veins.
- Venodilators increase capacitance and are useful in the acute management of volume overload.
- Arteriodilators/balance dilators (e.g. ACEi) reduce afterload improving output and are more valuable in chronic therapy.

  ALL are hypotensive.
- Potentially DANGEROUS fall in BP can occur if there is fixed outflow obstruction, e.g. aortic stenosis as the fall in afterload is not balanced with increased CO.

Glyceryl trinitrate

- May have value in the management of severe oedema.
- Active transdermally.
- Direct venodilator activity (also coronary vasodilation).
- Coronary artery dilation.
- 3–6 mm of 2% ointment rubbed well in on hairless area – pinna q4–8h.
- Gloves worn when administering treatment.
- Become refractory to treatment in 2–3 days.
- Can cause significant hypotension and tachycardia.
- Efficacy controversial.

Angiotensin-converting enzyme inhibitors (ACEi) (Figure 20)

- Balanced vasodilation.
- Short-term effects on peripheral resistance and RAAS activation.
- Long-term effects on cardiac and vascular remodelling.
- Shown to improve survival in man and dogs with CHF.
- Inappropriate in hypotensive or dehydrated cats.

Potential beneficial effects
- Reduce angiotensin II levels.
- Arteriolar dilation.
- Decrease aldosterone.
- Decreased noradrenalin.
- Decreased CNS sympathetic activation.
- Improved vascular compliance.

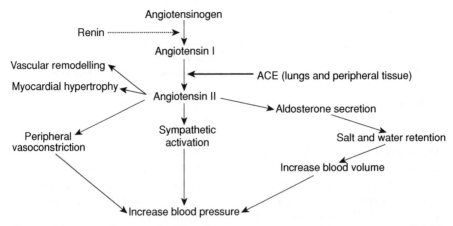

Figure 20   Point of action of ACEi in the renin–angiotensin–aldosterone system (RAAS)

- Decreased maladaptive muscular hypertrophy.
- Increase prostaglandin production causing vasodilation.
- Decrease bradykinin metabolism (vasodilation).
- Decrease vasopressin (ADH).
- Decrease pre- and afterload.
- Reduce risk of arrhythmias (via reduced sympathetic activity).
- Potassium sparing.

Potential side effects:
- Hypotension is the most common side effect particularly in cats with hypertrophic obstructed cardiomyopathy.
- Pre-renal failure – a stable rise in urea is a common occurrence with ACEi therapy presumably due to a fall in GFR secondary to decreased renal perfusion.
  - Urea and creatinine levels should be monitored in high-risk cats (dehydrated, hyponatraemic, pre-existing renal insufficiency) 24–48 hours after beginning therapy.
  - Increases of >50% in urea/creatinine are an indication to reduce the dose or discontinue therapy.
  - Azotaemia does not resolve in all cases.

- Acute kidney injury – avoid high-dose furosemide when initiating therapy.
- Hyperkalaemia (very rare).

Improving diastolic function

Consequences of poor diastolic function
- Reduced ventricular compliance reducing passive filling of ventricle.
- Decreased compliance resulting in increased end-diastolic pressure for a given volume.
- Excessive HR.
- Atrial dysfunction.

β-Blockers and calcium channel antagonists (Box 3)
- Reduce contractility and heart rate.
- Lower contractility may reduce dynamic outflow obstruction.
- Have anti-arrhythmic activity (β-blockers class II; diltiazem class IV).
- Dose rate:
  - Atenolol – 6.25–12.5 mg/cat q12–24h.
  - Propranolol – 0.2.5–1.0 mg/kg q8h.
  - Diltiazem – 0.5–1.25 mg/kg q8h.

Box 3 Comparison of β-adrenergic blockers and calcium channel antagonists in the management of cardiomyopathy in cats

β-Blockers	Calcium channel antagonists – diltiazem
Negative inotrope	Negative inotrope
Reduce outflow gradient	Reduce outflow gradient
Negative chronotrope	Negative chronotrope
Useful in managing supraventricular tachycardia	Useful in managing supraventricular tachycardia
Treatment of hypertension	Treatment of hypertension (amlodipine)
Reduced myocardial oxygen demand	Reduced myocardial oxygen demand
Possible cardioprotective role	Cardioprotective role not reported
	Positive lusiotrope (enhances relaxation)
	May produce neuroendocrine activation
	Licensed for use in cats

ORGAN SYSTEMS

ORGAN SYSTEMS

β-Blockers
- Widely used in cats with apparently few side effects.
  ○ Most commonly prescribed in cats with severe dynamic LVOT obstruction not in CHF.
- Valuable effects on rate reduction.
- Atenolol preferred to propranolol as requires once daily dosing and is cardioselective (β_1).
- Clinical experience has suggested that atenolol is more effective in the management of cardiomyopathy in cats than calcium channel antagonists.
- May take up to 8 weeks to reach full efficacy in stable CHF cases.
- However, some evidence suggests a poorer outcome than the use of furosemide alone.

Diltiazem
- Licensed for treatment of HCM.
- Some evidence that reduces hypertrophy.
- Needs to be given three times daily, so long-term compliance issues:
  ○ Slow-release versions are available for use in man but may cause hepatopathy in cats.
- Clinical efficacy has been variable.
- Most valuable in concentric hypertrophy.

Improving systolic function
- Evidence of systolic failure in DCM, some cases of unclassified cardiomyopathy (UCM) and increasingly being demonstrated in moderate-to-severe RCM and HCM.
- Options:
  ○ Short-term fluid therapy, especially if over-diuresed.
  ○ Positive inotropes may worsen outflow obstruction but may be necessary in severe hypotension or low output failure:
    ▪ Dobutamine.
    ▪ Pimobendan.
    ▪ Digoxin.

Pimobendan
- Increasingly being used in cardiomyopathy cases where systolic dysfunction is evident.
- Inodilator with minimal increase in myocardial oxygen demand.
  ○ Calcium sensitization of myocard; vasodilation via phosphodiesterase III activity.
- Good clinical success reported in some case; no published evidence of efficacy.
- Appears safe (side effects seen in about 3% of cats).
- Dose rate 0.625–1.25 mg/cat q12h.

Dobutamine
- Acute output failure.
- Needs to be given by CRI.
- Potentially arrhythmogenic.
- Can cause seizures.
- Dose rate initially 1–5 μg/kg/minute but titrate to effect.
  ○ Some cats require >10 μg/kg/minute before positive effect on BP seen.

Digoxin
- Very rarely used in cats:
  ○ Unlikely to have significant positive inotropy.
  ○ Cats sensitive to toxicity.
  ○ Dose rate – 0.005 mg/kg PO q12–48h.

Management of arrhythmia (also see Section 2.3 and 4.2.4)
- Usually associated with underlying primary or secondary cardiomyopathy.
- Cats generally tolerate arrhythmias well – treat only if significantly affecting CO.
- Management aimed at underlying problem.

Summary of therapeutic options
Cardiomyopathy
- Asymptomatic – little current justification to treat.
  ○ Value of ACEi, β-blockers or diltiazem unknown.
  ○ Potential risk of harm has to be considered.

- CHF – furosemide ± spironolactone if oedema/pleural effusion.
- Thromboembolic risk – aspirin or clopidogrel.
- β-Blockers are most widely used in non-congested obstructive disease.
- Pimobendan if there is evidence of systolic failure.

Acute pulmonary oedema
- Cage rest.
- Oxygen.
- IV furosemide.
- Opiates
- Glyceryl trinitrate.
- Thoracocentesis.

Acute output failure (DCM, cardiogenic shock)
- Cage rest.
- Oxygen.
- Cautious i/v fluids.
- Dobutamine infusion.
- Diuresis/thoracocentesis.

Feline arterial (aortic) thromboembolism

Pathophysiology
- Most commonly associated with underlying cardiovascular disease and the presence of a ball thrombus in the left atrium.
- Can be associated with
  - Hypercoagulable states, e.g. nephrotic syndrome, pancreatitis, neoplasia.
  - Blood hypoviscosity (anaemia) and hyperviscosity (polycythaemia, hyperglobulinemia).
  - Idiopathic cases are reported but are uncommon.
- Altered blood flow and stasis releases serotonin and thromboxane resulting in vasoconstriction of adjacent collateral blood vessels and serotonin-induced platelet aggregation.
- Usually affects aortic trifurcation causing bilateral hindlimb involvement, but unilateral hindlimb and single forelimb involvement can occur (approximately 10% of cases).

Clinical signs
- Sudden, severe muscle pain (intermittent claudication).
- Paralysis.
- Dyspnoea and other signs of CHF.
- Vocalisation.
- Characteristics of affected limb(s):
  - Muscles firm, painful and in contracture.
  - Loss of arterial pulse.
  - Limb cold.
  - Pads pale.
  - Nail beds cyanotic.

Diagnosis
- Clinical signs.
- Failure of nail bed to bleed.

NB – *Other low output states or shock/ hypovolaemia associated with marked peripheral vasoconstriction can cause very slow bleeding of clipped nail bed.*

- Radiology and echocardiography ± ECG are valuable in assessing the extent of underlying cardiac disease, presence of a ball thrombus and the presence of CHF.
- CPK and AST increased.
  - Other common biochemical/haematologic change – azotaemia, increased ALT and LDH, hyperglycaemia, DIC, lymphopenia.

Further assessment
- Doppler echocardiography of affected artery.
- Non-selective angiography also details extent of obstruction and collateral supply.

Major differential diagnosis
- Spinal cord lesions, e.g. RTA.

ORGAN SYSTEMS

Treatment
- Every effort should be made to identify and manage the underlying disease.
- Opiate pain relief, e.g. methadone.
- Fluid and nutritional support.
- Vasodilators have not been shown to be of value and may be contraindicated in a shock patient with cardiac disease.
- Anticoagulants – reduce clot extension/further clot formation:
  ○ Benefit of anticoagulant therapy have not been demonstrated.
  ○ Aspirin – 2 mg/kg q24–48h.
  ○ Heparin given to prolong APTT by 1.5–2 times.
    ▪ Sodium heparin – 200–300 iU/kg s/c q6–8h.
    ▪ Dalteparin sodium – 100 iU/kg s/c q12–24h.
  ○ Clopidogrel – 18.75 mg/cat q24h.
  ○ Coumarin – may be effective but the patient then has to be kept as an indoor-only cat due to the risk of haemorrhage.
- Thrombolytics:
  ○ Streptokinase, urokinase, tissue plasminogen activator.
  ○ Safety of rapid thrombolysis unknown.
  ○ Efficacy of streptokinase in improving circulation vs. risks of inducing a generalised lytic state.
  ○ Tissue plasminogen activator is likely to be safer, but is significantly more expensive.
- Surgical removal of clot – significant risks of anaesthesia associated with underlying disease, benefit not demonstrated in improved medium to long-term survival.

Prognosis
- Recanalisation occurs in most cases in 2–4 days.
- Recurrence common.
- Residual peripheral neurological damage is common.
- Underlying heart disease persists.
- Median survival time in cats with underlying heart disease is 6 weeks.

Good prognostic indicators
- Resolution of CHF and control of arrhythmias.
- Lack of left atrial thrombus.
- Return of appetite.
- Renal function preserved.
- Return of limb function and arterial pulse.
- Lack of self-mutilation.
- Owner commitment.

Poor prognostic indicators
- Refractory CHF.
- Acute reperfusion hyperkalaemia.
- Poor limb viability – hardened gastrocnemius.
- Multi-organ embolisation.
- Neurologic signs.
- Left atrial thrombus.
- DIC.
- Arrhythmias.
- Owner financial constraints.

4.2.8 Pericardial disease
- Parietal (thicker) and visceral layers.
- Pericardium continuous with great vessels and sternopericardial ligament.
- 0.25 ± 0.15 ml/kg fluid concentrated at heart base.

Function
- Protects heart from adjacent infection.
- Protects from malignancy.
- Fixes heart within thorax.
- Reduce friction of beating heart.
- Restrains cardiac filling.
- Enhances diastolic ventricular coupling – balances left- and right-sided output.

Congenital disease
Absence
- Very rare.
- Defects more common and can be multiple – risk of herniation or entrapment.

Pericardioperitoneal diaphragmatic hernia

- Common in cats.
- Females and Persians possibly being over-represented.
- Often adult when diagnosed.
- Occurs alone as a failure of unification, or in conjunction with other deficits, e.g. perineal hernia.

Clinical finding

- Depends on what organs are in the sac:
  - Asymptomatic.
  - Torsion.
  - Strangulation.
  - Respiratory compromise.
  - Cardiac restriction of filling or tamponade.
  - Muffled heart sounds.
  - Lack of abdominal organs.
  - Poor appetite, emaciation, stunting.

Radiography

- Apparent cardiomegaly.
- Gas/fat in pericardium.
- Silhouetting of cardiac and diaphragmatic borders.

ECG

- Small complexes.
- Deviation of mean electrical axis.

Echocardiography

- Incomplete pericardium with abdominal organs in direct contact with the epicardium.

Therapy

- Surgical correction in most but not all cases.

Acquired pericardial disease

Pericardial effusion

- Reduces compliance.
- Small PE are not uncommonly seen in cats; the majority do not require direct intervention (drainage).

- Causes:
  - 75% associated with CHF.
  - 12% aetiology unknown (including idiopathic).
  - Remainder – neoplasia, hyperthyroidism, fluid overload, uraemia, FIP, Toxoplasma, FPV, coagulopathy, trauma, hypoalbuminaemia.

Cardiac and intrapericardial neoplasia

- Rare in cats (<5% cases of PE).
- Usually haemorrhagic.
- Atrial haemangiosarcoma, lymphoma, mesothelioma.
- Diagnosis on ultrasound or biopsy.

Pericarditis

- Exudate.
- Usually sterile.
- Secondary to FIP, Toxoplasma, FPV.

Clinical signs

- Depends on the speed of effusion accumulation.

Acute

- Severe hypotension.
- Cardiogenic shock.
- Weakness and collapse.
- Usually associated with trauma, sudden tumour bleed, coagulopathy.

Chronic

- If sufficient fluid then signs of right heart failure.

ECG

- Alternans uncommon in cats.
- Small complexes.

Radiography

- Enlarged, rounded heart silhouette.

Echocardiography

- Separation of wall from the pericardium by hypoechoic fluid.
- Mass.
- Diffuse thickening in lymphosarcoma.

ORGAN SYSTEMS

Treatment
- Only if affecting output.
- Pericardiocentesis.
- Diuresis and management of underlying disease.
- Fluid should be submitted for culture and cytology.
- Pericardiectomy if recurrent.

Constrictive pericarditis
- Not reported in cats.

4.2.9 Heartworm disease
- Caused by *Dirofilaria immitis*.
- Not seen in UK, other than in cats that have been abroad (southern Europe, USA).
- Incidence may increase with PETS travel scheme.
- Cats less susceptible than dogs.
- Clinical presentation very variable and may be transient/non-specific:
  - Thromboembolic disease signs.
  - Dyspnoea, coughing, collapse, vomiting, seizures, neurologic signs.
- Tachycardia, gallop sounds, harsh dry lung sounds.
- Diagnosis difficult as
  - Cats usually amicrofilaraemic.
  - Haematological and biochemical changes are non-specific.
  - Radiographic changes are variable and non-specific.
  - Echocardiography – right-sided enlargement, visualisation of worms.
  - Serological testing may confirm diagnosis:
    - Antibody tests are fairly sensitive but not very specific.
    - Antigen tests are highly specific but poorly sensitive.

- Treatment difficult as
  - Adulticide therapy associated with frequent, severe complications without clear evidence of increased survival.
- Prophylaxis is the most effective method of control, and clients taking their cats abroad should be advised accordingly – selamectin, ivermectin, milbemycin oxime.

4.2.10 Blood pressure monitoring and hypertension

Measurement and reference range
- Doppler technique – systolic BP 120–160 mmHg.
  - Systolic pressure seems to be clinically more relevant in cats.
- BP measured in awake cats is influenced by many external factors including
  - Measurement method – oscillometric methods are generally less reliable in cats.
  - Cuff size (approximately 40% of the diameter of limb/tail site).
  - Cuff position (should be at the level of the right atrium).
  - The 'white coat' effect (stress associated with BP measurement).
- To make valid assessments, BP should be measured 5–7 times discarding the first 1–2 readings:
  - If variation is >10 mmHg between measurements procedure should be repeated.
  - Diagnosis of hypertension requires persistent elevation of BP measured on more than one occasion.
- Diastolic BP is extremely difficult to reliably measure in awake cats.

Anaesthetic intervention criteria
See Table 39

Table 39 BP intervention guidelines during anaesthesia in cats

mmHg	Normal	Treat Outside range	Critical Outside range
Systolic BP (Doppler)	120	90–170	80–200
Mean BP (oscillometric)	100	70–130	60–150

Causes of hypertension

- Primary (essential) hypertension is thought to be rare in cats – <10% of cases.
- Usually secondary.
  - Hyperthyroidism.
  - CKD.
  - DM.
  - Hyperadrenocorticism.
  - Phaeochromocytoma.
  - Hyperaldosteronism.
  - Hyperparathyroidism (secondary to hypercalcaemia).
  - Acromegaly.

Importance

- Recognition of hypertension allows early intervention in underlying disease.
- Part of cardiac investigation.
- Introduction and monitoring of therapy in heart disease.
- Prognostication – very hypotensive cats have a poor prognosis regardless of the cause of their disease.

Clinical consequences

- Visual defects and blindness due to retinal detachment and haemorrhage.

- Neurological signs – ataxia, seizures, dementia, coma as a result of cerebrovascular accidents.
- LV hypertrophy – new murmur or gallop.
- Decreased renal function, proteinuria, glomerulosclerosis.

Management (Figure 21)

- Treat underlying disease where possible.

Hypotensive agents

- Calcium channel blockers:
  - Amlodipine is the drug of choice in cats – appears effective and safe.
  - At 0.625–1.25 mg/cat q12–24h.
  - Start on low dose and monitor changes.

Also consider

- Reduce sodium intake – diet 0.1–0.3%.
- Diuresis – furosemide.
- β-Blockers
  - Decrease CO.
  - Inhibit β-receptor-mediated release of renin from JGA.
  - Useful in hyperthyroidism where hypertension is due to excessive adrenergic stimulation.

ORGAN SYSTEMS

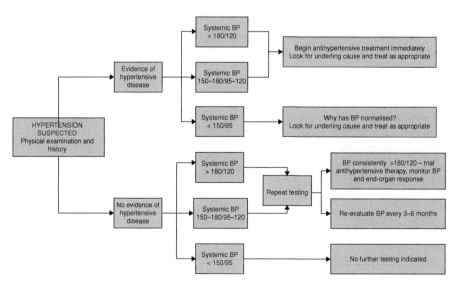

Figure 21 Algorithm for the approach to management of hypertension in cats. First published in Sturgess: *Pocket Handbook of Small Animal Medicine* (Manson Publishing, 2012). Reproduced by permission of the publisher.

- α-Adrenergic blockers, e.g. prazosin.
- ACE inhibitors:
  - Variable effects on BP.
  - Often insufficient as a sole agent.
  - Most useful if proteinuria.

4.3 GASTROINTESTINAL TRACT (GIT) DISEASE

4.3.1 Introduction

Gastrointestinal disease is a common reason for a cat being presented for veterinary intervention. Cats are often secretive about their signs, so disease may be relatively advanced at the time of presentation – 10% of cats with IBD have weight loss as their only reported presenting complaint.

Dental disease is seen in many cats over 3 years of age with the prevalence increasing with age and is a common reason for routine anaesthesia in an older cat as well as a cause of inappetence, anorexia, ptyalism and halitosis. Systemic ramifications of periodontal disease are well documented and thought to be associated with chronic low-grade bacteraemia causing a persistent inflammatory response. Periodontitis has been associated with increased rates of CKD, liver disease, insulin resistance, endocarditis and potentially airway disease.

Recent advances in diagnostics have highlighted the frequency of pancreatitis as a primary and secondary disease in cats and should be considered as a differential diagnosis for a number of presentations including non-specific anorexia, lethargy and depression as well as more expected GIT-associated signs of vomiting and jaundice.

4.3.2 Oral disease

Presenting signs
- Anorexia/inappetence.
- Halitosis.
- Dysphagia.
- Ptyalism.
- Bleeding from the mouth.
- Difficulty eating.
- Clawing at mouth.

Diagnosis
- Laboratory evaluation to rule out systemic disease.
- Virology – respiratory viruses, FeLV, FIV.
- Thorough oral examination (may require sedation/anaesthesia).
- Radiography.
- Biopsy of lesions.

Eosinophilic granuloma complex
- Ulcers, plaques and granulomas.
- Miliary dermatitis (papulocrusting dermatitis) is now considered a cutaneous reaction pattern that is not just associated with allergic and parasitic aetiologies but also bacterial and fungal pyoderma.

Eosinophilic ulcers
- Commonly on upper lip can be uni- or bilateral.
- Chronic, slowly progressive, erosive.
- Firm, non-painful, ulcerated mass.
- Most commonly adult female cats – possible genetic predisposition.
- Aetiology is unknown – hypersensitivity suspected but can occur secondary to focal insults such as foreign bodies or ticks.
- Biopsy essential to exclude neoplasia (SCC).
- Neutrophilic rather than eosinophilic infiltrates are common.
- Some cases will respond to antibacterial therapy alone.
- Short-term glucocorticoid therapy is required for the remainder.
- Recurrent or persistent lesions suggest ongoing triggers such as atopy or food allergy.

Cowpox
- See infectious diseases (section 5.14).

Gingivitis/stomatitis
- Plaque-induced gingivitis is a common reversible problem in many adult cats. Once periodontitis has developed then changes become irreversible.
- Many other potential causes:
  - Viral infection.
  - Periodontal disease.
  - Systemic disease.
  - Thermal trauma.
  - Immune-mediated disease.
  - Genetic predisposition.

Chronic lymphoplasmacytic gingivostomatitis
Clinical syndrome of focal or diffuse inflammation of the gingiva and/or oral mucosa.
- Cause is thought to be immune mediated.
- Suspected triggers include viral disease and Gram-negative anaerobic bacteria.

Presentation
- Halitosis, dysphagia, pain, ptyalism.
- Occurs despite good dental care.
- Hyperaemia and swelling of the gingival margin.
- Ulceration of the oral mucosa.
- Affects areas where there are no teeth, e.g. fauces.

Investigation and treatment
- Investigation should centre on defining underlying cause and treating where possible.
- In the absence of underlying cause then
  - Thorough tooth cleaning including subgingival area.
    - 3 weeks of post-operative antibacterial use with twice weekly chlorhexidine.
    - From 3 weeks daily brushing ± mouthwash and diet.
  - If this fails then medical management can be attempted but long-term success is often disappointing. Chronic, oral interferon may be of value.
    - Chronic antibacterial therapy, e.g. clindamycin – week on; week off basis.
    - Chronic glucocorticoids – often associated with an initial favourable response but poor long-term control.
  - Dental extraction – initially all molars and premolars – good response in about 80% of cats.
  - Total dental extraction ± intermittent antibacterial treatment ± interferon.

Gingivitis/stomatitis of young cats
- Common in some pedigree cats from 4 to 6 months of age.
- Usually mild-to-moderate severity.
- Most cases are self-limiting.

Periodontal disease
- Accumulation of plaque and calculus results in gingivitis and retraction of the gingival margin.
- Irreversible.
- Forms a gingival pocket.
- May eventually lead to loss of teeth.
- Management with
  - Descaling, curettage of periodontal pockets, removal.
  - Home care reduces recurrence rates.
  - Diets can help to reduce the rate of build-up.

Feline odontoclastic resorptive lesions (FORL, cat neck lesions)
- Erosion of the tooth at the cementoenamel junction.
- Occurs in the absence of significant periodontal disease.
- Higher incidence in FCV-positive cats.
- Extremely painful.
- Aetiology unknown.

ORGAN SYSTEMS

- Only effective treatment is removal.
- Radiography (especially small dental cassettes) is significantly more sensitive than visual examination in identifying the affected teeth.
- Premolars most commonly affected.

Palate defects
- Congenital midline defects in kittens.
- Affects hard ± soft palate.
- Rarely soft palate alone.
- Clinical signs:
  - Variable depending on the extent of the defect.
  - Nasal regurgitation of milk, most common sign.
- Can be both hereditary and non-hereditary.
- Management is by surgical closure.
- Acquired disease occurs secondary to head trauma.
  - RTA.
  - Fall from a height.

Oral neoplasia
Squamous cell carcinoma
- Most common oral tumour.
- Risk is increased in cats wearing flea collars, fed primarily canned, especially tuna food, or exposed to tobacco smoke.
- Sublingual, most common site.
- Locally invasive.
- Recurrence following local excision is common.
- Radical resection, often difficult margin of >20 mm recommended – hemimandibulectomy.
- Radiation is an alternative option.
- Piroxicam and other COX-2 inhibitors not shown benefit.
- Prognosis tends to be poor:
  - Median survival time 3 months with local resection; 14 month with mandibulectomy.

Fibrosarcoma
- Second most common tumour.
- Usually involves gingiva.
- Approach similar to SCC.
- Survival time appears better.

Other
- Odontogenic tumours – uncommon.
- Malignant melanoma – rare.
- Epulides – rare.
- Tonsillar neoplasia:
  - Associated with urban living.
  - SCC most common, lymphoma are rarely seen.

4.3.3 Oesophageal disease
Clinical features
- Regurgitation is the cardinal sign.
  - Tends to occur very suddenly, usually with no prior warning as a passive process although some cats will look 'uncomfortable' due to the accumulation of food prior to regurgitating.
- Needs to be differentiated from a number of other signs – vomiting in particular (see section 2.36).
  - Vomiting, which is active, involving vigorous abdominal effort often associated with some distress and following a prior phase of retching and nausea.
- Some diseases such as pyloric dysfunction and hiatal hernia present with both vomiting and regurgitation.
- Severe vomiting can lead to oesophagitis and secondary regurgitation.
- Paroxysmal coughing ending in retching producing white phlegm can be confused as vomiting or regurgitation by owners.
- Other indicators of oesophageal disease:
  - Hypersalivation.
  - Reluctance to eat, pain on eating, inappetence and anorexia associated with oesophagitis.
  - Gagging and retching with repeated attempts to swallow associated with oesophageal foreign body.

- Most cats with oesophageal disease (other than oesophagitis) initially have a good appetite.
- Respiratory signs – secondary to reflux rhinitis or aspiration pneumonia, although cats seem relatively less likely to develop clinically evident aspiration pneumonia than dogs with oesophageal disease.

Congenital disorders

- There are several congenital disorders that present as regurgitation in the young kitten. These generally first become apparent as the kitten begins to take solids at 3–6 weeks, but signs may pass unnoticed until the kitten goes to its new home and is kept on its own.

Primary megaoesophagus

- Congenital megaoesophagus is a rare disorder seen most often in mixed breed cats.
- It involves a failure in neurogenic control of oesophageal function resulting in dilation of the oesophagus throughout its length, although the exact level of failure of neurogenic control is not known.

NB – *This is distinct from oesophageal achalasia, a condition in humans in which there is failure of opening of the gastro-oesophageal sphincter. Achalasia is very rare in cats and is not involved in most cases of megaoesophagus.*

Diagnosis

- Generally readily recognisable on plain radiography taken under sedation.
- In a few cases, delineation using contrast techniques may be necessary.
- Fluoroscopy ideal to assess functional ability (if any).

NB – *Examine the radiograph for evidence of aspiration pneumonia – usually dependent cranial lung lobes, changes can be subtle despite significant clinical signs.*

Management

- Postural feeding may benefit some cats.
  - Raise the height of the cat's feeding bowl.
  - Holding the cat in an upright position whilst feeding.
  - After feeding the owner should walk around with the cat upright on their shoulder (like a baby).
- Feeding smaller meals more frequently.
- Experimentation to establish what type of diet suits the cat best.
- Therapy with motility modifiers such as ranitidine, metoclopramide or cisapride has had little success and could worsen signs by increasing the time of the gastro-oesophageal sphincter.

Prognosis

- Guarded.
- In many cases, the regurgitation cannot be managed successfully with consequent poor growth, etc.
- Secondary rhinitis and aspiration pneumonia.

Megaoesophagus associated with pyloric dysfunction

- The main sign is usually vomiting related to the pyloric dysfunction, but affected kittens may be presented with a history of regurgitation (see gastric disorders).
- More common in Siamese.

Hiatal hernia

- More common in Siamese and related Oriental cats.
  - Intermittent or persistent.

Clinical signs

- Can be suggested by either regurgitation or vomiting, or a combination of both ± hypersalivation.
- May not appear until adulthood. (Are these cases truly congenital or acquired?)

ORGAN SYSTEMS

- The nature of the defect is variable and may involve
  - Para-oesophageal herniation of the stomach through the phrenico-oesophageal ligament or intus-susception of the stomach into the oesophagus.
  - Herniation of the cardia through the oesophageal hiatus.

Diagnosis
- Radiography but the defect may occasionally be intermittent (sliding) particularly for the latter form of hiatus hernia; barium contrast may be helpful.
- Fluoroscopy may be required to demon-strate the defect in such cases of sliding hiatus hernia.

Management
- Medical management of oesophagitis (see page 196).
- Some cases may show improvement using a conservative approach, as for megaoesophagus, but this approach is unlikely to provide adequate long-term control of clinical signs.
- Best treated surgically.
  - Gastropexy will also help to prevent herniation through fixing the position of the stomach.

Vascular ring strictures
- Rare, congenital vascular anomalies that can lead to persistent regurgita-tion associated with poor growth in young kittens due to compression of the oesophagus.
- Persistent right aortic arch is the most common (though still rare); there may be a predisposition in Siamese.

Clinical signs
- Regurgitation as the kitten starts to take solid foods.
- Stunted growth.

- Secondary respiratory tract infection.
- Large pouch-like dilatation of the oesoph-agus may arise, just cranial to the stric-ture, resulting in a swelling appearing at the thoracic inlet when the kitten eats.
- Can be a long delay between eating and regurgitation.

Diagnosis
- Confirm radiographically, showing the megaoesophagus is present only cranial to the base of the heart often with a dilated pouch.
- Exact nature of defect requires echo-cardiography or angiography although endoscopy can be helpful demonstrat-ing a pulsating area of the wall beneath the vascular anomaly as it constricts the oesophagus.

Management
- Early surgical resection of the vascu-lar ring stricture as soon as the kitten's general condition permits:
  - Response to surgical treatment may be disappointing with regurgita-tion persisting, particularly if a large oesophageal pouch is present.
  - Supplementary gastrostomy tube feeding prior to surgery may be necessary.

Acquired oesophageal disorders
Secondary megaoesophagus
Anterior mediastinal lymphoma
- Particularly in younger cats, usually under 3 years of age and often under 1 year of age.
- More prevalent in Siamese and related Oriental cats.
- Suspected familial form of the disease has been seen in these same breeds.
- Previously most cats with mediastinal lymphoma have been positive on rou-tine FeLV testing, but the proportion of persistently viraemic cases has declined.

- Usually cause dyspnoea but in some cases a smaller, more localised tumour occurs that may cause regurgitation due to external pressure on the oesophagus with or without associated oesophageal dilation developing.
  - Mediastinal lymphoma is a common cause of pleural effusion especially in young cats.

Other mediastinal masses

- Thymomas and thymic cysts may also cause regurgitation through pressure on the oesophagus.

Diagnosis

- Radiographic demonstration of an anterior mediastinal mass.
- FNA/biopsy to confirm the diagnosis.
  - Often immunohistochemistry required to differentiate thymic lymphocytes from lymphoma.
- Some non-lymphomatous masses may require surgical biopsy.
- L-Asparaginase test – single injection of L-asparaginase will cause a marked reduction in clinical signs or measurable shrinkage of the mediastinal lymphoma within 48–72 hours.

Management

- Chemotherapy (see Section 4.12)

Dysautonomia ('Key-Gaskell' syndrome)

- Megaoesophagus is a prominent feature.
- Prevalence of this disorder has decreased considerably and it is restricted to certain countries.
- Occurs sporadically in the UK, incidence may be increasing.
- Clinical signs – regurgitation with a variety of other clinical signs associated with autonomic dysfunction such as constipation, dry mouth.

Other neuromuscular disease

- Megaoesophagus can occur in association with neuromuscular disorders such as myasthenia gravis.
- Much less common than in dogs, probably because of the difference in the type of musculature of the oesophagus.

Polyneuropathies

- Megaoesophagus has been seen as a feature of polyneuropathies.
- Generally rare in cats, but occasional clusters have occurred related to toxicity – previous cases been linked to compounding errors in commercial diets.
- Other signs of polyneuropathy will normally be more prominent in the presentation.

Oesophagitis and ulceration

Cause

- Often unclear.
- Reflux of gastric acid or persistent vomiting.
- Post-anaesthetic.
- Associated with hiatal hernia.
- Speculation over the role of the spiral organisms (*Helicobacter* spp.), but there is no convincing evidence.
- Ingestion of irritants (usually occurs during grooming, following contamination of the coat).
- Drug associated – doxycycline, clindamycin.
- Gastric heterotopia has been reported in Siamese cats in which ectopic gastric tissue capable of producing acid is found in the terminal oesophagus.

Clinical signs

- Inappetence.
- Repeated swallowing efforts when eating.
- May show evidence of discomfort or nausea, excessive salivation and spontaneous retching.

ORGAN SYSTEMS

ORGAN SYSTEMS

Diagnosis
- Clinical signs.
- Endoscopy.

Management
- Protection of lesions from further damage.
- Reduction of exposure to gastric acid.
- Appropriate dietary therapy:
  - Soft food will help to minimise mechanical irritation of the oesophagus.
  - Maintenance of feeding *per os* may reduce the likelihood of stricture development.

Sucralfate
- Mucosal protectant – a form of aluminium hydroxide and sucrose that binds to the surface of the damaged oesophagus protecting it against further damage. It may also stimulate mucosal healing. Sucralfate ideally needs to be given every 2 hours. It can be used prophylactically where reflux of gastric acid during anaesthesia is suspected.
- Dose rate – 50 mg/kg.

H_2 receptor antagonists and proton-pump inhibitors
- Increases gastric fluid pH by reducing acid secretion.

Prostaglandin analogues
- See gastric ulcers.

Prokinetics
- Metoclopramide (0.5 mg/kg PO q8h) or ranitidine (3.5 mg/kg PO q12h):
  - Cisapride (2.5 mg/cat PO q12h) appears to have better activity but is no longer easily obtained.

Oesophageal stricture
- Potential complication of any case of oesophagitis.
- Seen most often following anaesthesia or use of doxycycline or clindamycin.

Clinical signs
- Apparent within a few days to a few weeks of anaesthesia.
- The cat may be in considerable distress with almost immediate return of any food ingested.
- ± Ingesta streaked with blood.
- Painful retching.
- Initially the cat will usually be keen to eat, but may soon become inappetent resulting in weight loss.

Diagnosis
- Clinical signs and appropriate history.
- Contrast radiography preferably 24 hours before any endoscopic procedure to demonstrate the extent of the lesion if the stricture is severe.
- Endoscopy is most informative although bleeding from the lesion may hamper image quality.

Management
- Balloon catheter to dilate the stricture is preferred to bougienage.
  - With any dilation procedure, there is a risk of oesophageal perforation.
- Will need to be repeated several times at 2–3 day intervals.
- Administration of corticosteroids may help to minimise the risk of the stricture recurring.
  - Intralesional injections have been used.
- Nutritional support is especially important due to the repeat anaesthetics. Ideally food should be given orally but if the cat refuses or is unable to eat/retain food eaten, gastrostomy feeding is appropriate.
- Oesophageal stents have been used in some cases and may prove a better though costly solution.

Prognosis
- Guarded.
- Some cases show a complete resolution.

- May be possible to achieve sufficient improvement in some cats to allow long-term management with a liquid or semi-liquid diet.
  Poor prognostic indicators
- Duration of stricture.
- Extent.
- Severity.
- Degree of re-stricturing following dilation.
- Severe mucosal damage (either primary or as a result of attempts at dilation).

Oesophageal foreign bodies, fistula and diverticuli
- Cats are much less likely to acquire oesophageal foreign bodies than dogs due to their more discriminatory feeding behaviour.
- Bones, string/thread and needles are most commonly seen.
- Endoscopic retrieval or pushing the foreign body into the stomach is preferred.
- Surgical oesophagostomy is associated with significant post-operative complications mainly due to wound breakdown and subsequent mediastinitis.
- Stricturing following removal of a foreign body that has caused significant mucosal damage can occur but is rare.
- Fistula and diverticuli are very rare in cats, may occur secondarily to foreign body obstruction.

Oesophageal neoplasia
- SCC is the most common oesophageal tumour, but is still rare.
  ○ Benign polypoid masses can occur.
- Regurgitated material may be streaked with blood and there may be considerable distress to the cat as it regurgitates.
- Clinical signs are usually associated with a mass effect causing partial obstruction.

- SCC can interfere with the normal process of vomiting of fur balls, and the initial reason for presentation may be an impacted gastric fur ball.
- It is usually located at the terminal oesophagus and can be identified on radiography or endoscopy.
- Prognosis is very poor as it is unlikely to be resectable.
- Slow-growing masses may be managed by gastrostomy feeding in the short term.

4.3.4 Gastric disease

Clinical features

Vomiting (see Section 2.42)
- Differentiate from regurgitation.
- Important to establish that vomiting is a significant problem that warrants further investigation and management.
- If the cat has been vomiting infrequently for less than 24 hours and is not showing other significant signs, the vomiting is likely to have resulted from an isolated incident or insult to the GIT and will therefore be self-limiting. Extensive investigation is often not indicated in such cases and symptomatic treatment may be more appropriate.
- Vomiting centre of cats is sensitive and they vomit readily.
- Occasional vomiting in an otherwise healthy cat may not represent a significant problem.
- Symptomatic treatment of chronic vomiting is often ineffective.
- Vomiting can be a sign of extraintestinal disease (see Section 2.42 for differential diagnosis).
- Nature and the pattern of the vomiting does not often facilitate identification of the underlying cause.
- Frequent vomiting (in excess of 4–6 times daily) irrespective of its duration and the presence/absence of other clinical signs necessitates a more aggressive approach

ORGAN SYSTEMS

since it may rapidly lead to dehydration and electrolyte disturbances.

- Small amounts of fresh blood in the vomit are not necessarily a cause for concern. It may be a non-specific finding associated with any cause of vomiting and, whilst it may reflect more serious underlying gastric diseases, such as ulceration and neoplasia, these are uncommon in cats.
- Partially changed blood (coffee grounds) is a more serious and a cause for concern.
- In general, the relationship of vomiting with feeding is often inconsistent and can be misleading.
- Persistent, delayed vomiting over 24 hours after eating may indicate outflow obstruction, particularly if the vomitus has a foul smell ('faecal' vomiting) – the obstruction could be located in the antrum or proximal small intestine.
- Vomiting is often a more prominent sign in cats with intestinal disease than diarrhoea.

Abdominal palpation

- Most cats are good subjects for thorough evaluation of the abdomen; the stomach is not usually palpated unless there is gross distension or marked hepatomegaly.
  - Evidence of abdominal mass causing a secondary gastric outflow obstruction may be appreciated.

Diagnosis

Vomitus

- Can be examined for evidence of *Ollulanus tricuspis*, a nematode that can cause acute and chronic gastritis and vomiting.
  - The parasite has a worldwide distribution.
  - Treatment with 7 days of fenbendazole recommended but efficacy unknown and other parasiticides may be as or more effective.

- pH can be determined to establish that the material is gastric (acid pH) rather than oesophageal (alkaline pH).

Clinical pathology

- The main value of laboratory tests is to establish if the vomiting is secondary to another systemic disease and if metabolic complications have developed. In the majority of vomiting cats, significant haematologic or biochemical changes are not present.
  - In severely vomiting cats, evaluating electrolyte and acid–base status helps direct fluid choice for IVFT.

Imaging

Radiography

- Generally a low-yield procedure.
- Very helpful when radiographic changes are present:
  - Megaoesophagus.
  - Gastric dilation.
  - Gastric foreign body.
  - GI obstruction.
  - Gastric calcification.

Contrast radiography

- Liquid barium (10 ml/kg) preferably given via a naso-oesophageal tube can demonstrate gastric lesions.
- Liquid barium and barium mixed with food are of limited value as a way of examining gastric function as there is a wide range of normality (up to 13 hours for gastric emptying times). Repeat radiographs of cats can present technical problems.
- Barium can be useful to demonstrate the position of the stomach.
- Barium impregnated polyspheres (BIPS) can also be used to assess gastric emptying. The small BIPS are designed to simulate liquid phase emptying and the large BIPS solid phase. However, gastric emptying times measured using

this technique are extremely variable in normal cats, ranging from 2 to 8 hours.

- BIPS are perhaps more valuable for identifying intestinal obstructions (especially partial obstructions) in cats.

Ultrasound

- Also tends to be a low-yield procedure in gastric disease.
- Used to assess gastric size and contents, local or diffuse thickening of the gastric wall, ulceration or evidence of a loss of layering or lymphadenomegaly of the gastric lymph nodes.
- Gives a general impression of gastric motility.

NB – *Inter-rugal gastric wall thickness is reported to be ≤2 and ≤4.5 mm for rugal folds but is variable depending on the degree of gastric distension. Mass lesions of the wall are rare and false-positive ultrasound findings do occur.*

Fluoroscopy

- May be valuable in the investigation of gastric function.

Endoscopy

- Allows direct examination of the gastric mucosa and pylorus.
- Few lesions are pathognomonic for a disease, so biopsies are always required.
- May allow some foreign bodies to be removed.
- Limited value in identifying intramural lesions.
- Also allows evaluation of the upper small intestine.

Surgery

Laparotomy or laparoscopy may be necessary in some cases.

Acute vomiting

- Most cases of acute vomiting are related to relatively trivial isolated gastric insults and will generally resolve spontaneously within a short time – dietary factors are probably most often responsible.
- Acute gastritis is uncommon in cats and is most often associated with exposure to a chemical irritant ingested inadvertently through self-cleaning of contaminated fur.
- Acute vomiting is frequently associated with ingestion of grass or other plant material; the reason for this behaviour is uncertain although many cats are regular 'grazers' and appear to enjoy this.
- Hair balls are rarely a cause of non-specific vomiting. It is a normal physiological process for fur to accumulate in the upper GIT and occasionally be vomited.
  - Serious or persistent gastric impaction with hair may be an indication of a more fundamental underlying problem with gastric motility and emptying.
- Gastric foreign bodies are less common in cats than dogs. Bones are seen surprisingly infrequently as foreign bodies considering the ardent predatory behaviour many cats show. String, thread and occasionally toys may be involved.

Intoxication

Plants

- A number of houseplants which contain oxalates may cause vomiting, such as 'dumbcane' (*Dieffenbachia* spp.), philodendron and ivies (which also contain saponins). These have an irritant effect, which may be evident on oral examination in the form of glossitis and stomatitis. Other toxins which can cause GI upsets, with vomiting and diarrhoea, are mistletoe, some species of mushrooms and some bulbs.

Chemicals and drugs

- Heavy metal salts (most notably lead and zinc).
- Detergents.

ORGAN SYSTEMS

- Boric acid compounds.
- Strong acids and alkalis.
- Organophosphorus compounds still used in some non-prescription ectoparasiticide preparations and other household products, e.g. fly sprays, fly strips, can lead to cumulative toxicity.
- NSAIDs including home dosing by the owner.

Management

- Symptomatic management is appropriate for the majority of cases of acute vomiting.
- Dietary manipulation will suffice in many cases.
- Starve for 24 hours, provide water.
  - Although electrolyte solutions are potentially more appropriate, many cats will refuse to drink them.
- Feed a single-source protein, gluten-free, highly digestible, low-fat diet – given as frequent small meals, e.g. skinned chicken and rice

Anti-emetics

- Appropriate in many cases as they will improve the cat's well-being and reduce nausea; however, they should be viewed as symptomatic relief with the potential to mask worsening of the underlying disease.
- Metoclopramide has little central activity compared to dogs and neurologic side effects appear to be more common, nevertheless it is still a useful antiemetic.
- Maropitant is a very effective.
- Chlorpromazine (alpha-2 adrenergic antagonist) makes a useful additional choice of anti-emetic since it has a 'broad-spectrum activity' operating at the level of the chemoreceptor trigger zone and the emetic centre.

NB – *Chlorpromazine is hypotensive and should be used with care if the cat is dehydrated.*

- Mucosal protectants, antacids and H_2-blockers though not specifically indicated for the treatment of non-specific acute vomiting are appropriate in some cases.

Chronic vomiting

Congenital disorders

Pyloric dysfunction

- Pyloric dysfunction has been reported largely in Siamese cats and appears to have a familial basis.
- Clinical signs usually become evident at the time of weaning.
- Some affected kittens show dramatic, projectile vomiting which may be delayed occurring sometime after feeding.
- Megaoesophagus is also frequently present and the return of food may be more indicative of regurgitation.
- Secondary complications seen in kittens with persistent regurgitation, such as stunting and respiratory tract infections, are often evident.
- Appears to involve a functional abnormality as there is usually no evidence of physical stenosis.
- The major differentials are other congenital causes of regurgitation (see section 2.36).

Diagnosis

- Radiography.
- Gastric dilation may be seen on plain radiographs.
- May be an evidence to indicate very prolonged gastric emptying with food material still present in the stomach even though the kitten may have been starved for a prolonged period prior to radiography.

- Contrast radiography may help to confirm gastric distension and an abnormally slow passage of small boluses of stomach contents through the pylorus into the duodenum.

Management
- In most cases, pyloromyotomy or pyloroplasty is the treatment most likely to have a beneficial effect, despite the absence of any physical abnormality of the pylorus.
- Some cases show an initial improvement, but then recurrence of clinical signs as the pylorus heals.
- Medical management using manipulation of dietary consistency and administration of drugs to aid pyloric function, such as anticholinergics and prokinetics, are usually ineffective.

Chronic gastritis

Inflammatory bowel disease
- Chronic gastritis most often occurs as part of IBD.
- The small intestine is usually the site most severely affected and persistent or intermittent vomiting is often one, if not the most important, sign in these cases.
- Infiltration of the stomach may also be present contributing to the tendency to vomit.
- Rarely the stomach may be the only site showing lesions.
  - In cats with lesions restricted mainly to the stomach, the infiltrate is more likely to be predominantly eosinophilic (compared to lymphocytic/plasmacytic in primarily small intestinal cases), and this may be a feature of more widespread, pathological eosinophilic infiltration – associated with the hypereosinophilic syndrome.
- Diagnosis depends on histological demonstration of the inflammatory infiltrate in biopsies, collected most conveniently by endoscopy.
- Management – see small intestinal diseases.

Gastric ulceration
- Gastric ulcers are rare in cats.
- There are a variety of possible underlying aetiologies.
- Ingestion of an irritant or caustic substance.
- Therapeutic preparations can be implicated.
- Secondary to hypergastrinaemia.
  - Hypergastrinaemia can be associated with renal or liver failure; rarely caused by histamine release secondary to mastocytosis and very rarely gastrinoma.
- Late complication in seriously ill cats – stress, hypovolaemia and shock may be factors involved in the pathogenesis of these cases.
- Clinical features and the approach to investigation are very similar to that for all forms of gastric disease.
- Abdominal pain or discomfort particularly on palpation may be a prominent sign.
- Perforation is a potential complication of gastric ulcers that will rapidly lead to peritonitis.

Management
- Treatment of the underlying cause where this is appropriate.
- Sucralfate will help to protect the surface of the ulcer from further erosion.
- Oral H_2 receptor antagonists are an important element of treatment:
  - Cimetidine is commonly used at 5–10 mg/kg q8h.
  - Ranitidine is used at 3.5 mg/kg q12h.
  - Famotidine at 0.5 mg/kg q12–24h.

ORGAN SYSTEMS

- Omeprazole is a proton-pump inhibitor given at 0.5–1 mg/kg q24h but takes several days to reach full efficacy.
- IV preparations are also available and should always be given *slowly*.
- Misoprostol, a prostaglandin E_2 analogue, is particularly useful in cases of gastric ulceration caused by administration of NSAIDs.
  - Dose rate of 1–3 µg/kg PO q8h – tablet size is 200 µg, which makes dosing difficult.

Hypertrophic gastritis

- Rare.
- Extensive hypertrophy of the rugal folds visible on direct examination of the stomach lining or on radiography.
- May interfere with normal gastric outflow.
- Cause of this hypertrophic response is not known, but may relate to hypergastrinaemia.

Atrophic gastritis

- Reported in people and dogs associated with prolonged use of proton-pump inhibitors.

Helicobacteriosis

- A number of Helicobacters have been identified in the stomach of cats.
- *Helicobacter pylori* is uncommon and *H. felis* more commonly found in the stomach of cats.
- *Helicobacter bizzozeronii* can be isolated in most if not all cats, even if showing no vomiting or evidence of gastric disease, raising the questions of *Helicobacter*'s clinical significance.
- Diagnosis is usually on identification of spiral organisms on biopsy but can be inferred by putting a biopsy in urea broth and looking for colour-linked pH change associated with urease production.

- Management of *Helicobacter* may be considered in cases of gastritis where no other underlying cause has been identified – 14–28 day course of a combination of oral amoxicillin (15–20 mg/kg q12h), metronidazole (20 mg/kg q24h) and an antacid (famotidine or omeprazole) is recommended but the efficacy of treatment is unknown.
- There is no evidence to support *Helicobacter* in cats being a zoonosis.

Gastric neoplasia

- Gastric tumours are rare in cats, much less common than in dogs.
- Lymphosarcoma is the most common gastric tumour diagnosed.
  - Can be solitary or part of multisystemic disease.
- Adenocarcinomas and benign adenomas are very rarely seen.
- Chronic vomiting often with evidence of fresh or partially changed blood, anorexia and some accompanying weight loss are the most common clinical signs.
  - Clinical signs often occur when the tumour causes gastric mucosal ulceration.
- The progress of the disease can be quite slow and some cases show a surprisingly long history.
- Main differential diagnosis is gastric ulceration of other aetiology.
- Imaging may help to identify the presence of a gastric mass but lymphosarcoma can be diffused causing a more generalised wall thickening and loss of layering.
- Biopsy is necessary for definitive diagnosis.
  - Endoscopy provides a convenient method of collecting biopsies, but care is necessary to ensure that biopsies are deep enough and representative of the lesion. The periphery of the lesion should be biopsied, and repeated biopsy from the same site

will help to ensure a deep enough biopsy is obtained. Care is also required to avoid accidental perforation of the lesion. In some cases full-thickness biopsy following gastrostomy is required for diagnosis.

- Prognosis for gastric tumours is generally poor.
- Spread of the tumour, particularly to the local lymph nodes or adjacent organs, may limit the value of surgical excision.
- Benign tumours should be amenable to surgery.
- Chemotherapy is a possible option for lymphosarcoma, but there is a risk of gastric rupture if the wall has been substantially replaced by tumour cells.

4.3.5 Small intestinal disease

Clinical features

- Major presenting signs with small intestinal disease are generally diarrhoea, vomiting and weight loss.
- Diarrhoea is a sign that may frequently go unobserved in cats unless the cat uses a litter tray.
- The main reason for presentation is often, therefore, weight loss ± vomiting.
- Chronic vomiting can be a feature of partial intestinal obstruction.
- Most cats with chronic, primary intestinal disease are initially bright and alert.
- Appetite is often retained or even increased which can be a pointer to the presence of a primary intestinal problem rather than another systemic disorder.
  ○ Some cats show waxing and waning appetite going from being ravenously hungry to inappetent.
- Defaecatory pattern and the nature of the diarrhoea may occasionally give clues to the underlying cause, but frequently owners are unable to provide information on these aspects and

there tends to be less clear demarcation between features indicating small vs. large intestinal diarrhoea.

- Evidence of melaena, usually recognisable in the form of dark discoloration of the faeces, may suggest intestinal neoplasia or infection with protozoal parasites.
  ○ A lack of visible melaena does not rule out intestinal bleeding.
- Bulky, pale, malodorous faeces of fatty appearance suggest some form of malassimilation, such as malabsorption or maldigestion.
- Abdominal palpation is important in cats with possible intestinal disease, particularly to check for evidence of intestinal masses, thickening associated with infiltration, obstructive lesions and enlargement of abdominal lymph nodes. Small mobile lesions may be difficult to identify and repeated examination, using different approaches to palpation, may be necessary for detection and to enable differentiation from faecal material.
  ○ Intestinal loops in thin cats will often appear prominent which may be due to a lack of abdominal fat rather than pathological change within the intestines.

Pathophysiology of diarrhoea

There is some value in chronic diarrhoea of understanding the likely pathology underlying the diarrhoea as this may help with directing suitable dietary or therapeutic management.

Increased osmotic pressure

- May be caused simply by dietary factors in individuals with essentially normal intestinal function.
- Incomplete digestion allows an increase in food particles that have an osmotic effect increasing the water level of the luminal contents.

ORGAN SYSTEMS

- Carbohydrates are most often incriminated in other species, but may be less important in cats since they are usually an insignificant dietary constituent.
- Maldigestion and malabsorption can lead to osmotic diarrhoea.
- Pancreatic insufficiency is rare in cats, but maldigestion can occur through deficiency of specific brush border enzymes, most notably lactase leading to milk intolerance.
- Decreased bile production can also lead to fat maldigestion.
- Infiltrative disease (most commonly IBD, more rarely neoplasia) is the major cause of malabsorption.

Failure of permeability

- Failure of retention of electrolytes, which is necessary for maintenance of an osmotic gradient across the gut and regulation of water content.
- Usually results from the effects of endotoxins or enterotoxins produced by enteropathogenic bacteria.
- Can also arise if unconjugated bile acids and hydroxylated fatty acids accumulate, e.g. secondary to viral causes of diarrhoea such as coronavirus that inhibits absorption of conjugated bile acid.

Secretory effect

- Primarily caused by invasive bacteria.
- Effects on ion absorption, as well as secretion, caused by cAMP and other secretagogues.
- Secretory mechanisms are also involved in diarrhoea associated with protein-losing enteropathy, although this is not generally important in cats other than as a secondary effect of intestinal lymphosarcoma.
- The role of enteropathogenic *E. coli* as a cause of secretory diarrhoea in cats is unclear as isolation rates in diarrhoeic cats are similar to those from normal cats.

Motility disorders

- Hypo- or hypermotility can cause diarrhoea, e.g. hypermotility associated with hyperthyroidism in the absence of any primary structural disease of the bowel.

Investigation

Laboratory tests

- Frequently unproductive in cats especially with chronic intestinal disease.
  - Understanding the metabolic consequences of acute diarrhoea.
  - Eliminating systemic extra-intestinal disorders.
  - Excluding additional intercurrent disease.
- Intestinal infiltrates may be reflected in haematologic changes but these changes are inconsistent and generally not specific.
- Biochemical parameters are usually normal, as cats seem able to maintain blood albumin and cholesterol even in the face of severe weight loss.
- Retrovirus serology is important both as a potential cause and prognostically.
- Cobalamin is worth assessing as they are often low, and the failure to replete cobalamin has been associated with poor response to other therapies.
- Folate is usually measured in conjunction with cobalamin but the interpretation of increased folate in cats is unclear.
- Faecal testing is essential prior to other investigations, but is frequently unremarkable.
  - Pathogenic bacteria (*Salmonella*, *Campylobacter*, clostridia).
  - Parasites (helminths, *Giardia*, *Cystoisospora*, *Cryptosporidia*, *Tritrichomonas foetus*).
  - False-negative faecal results for Giardia are common – treatment with a benzimidazole before further investigation is advisable.

- Pancreatic testing (see section 4.3.7).
- Breath hydrogen and sugar absorption tests – not in routine clinical use.

Imaging
- Imaging of the intestine is a low-yield procedure in the majority cases, but is particularly important in cats suspected of obstructive lesions.
  - May give little further information than thorough abdominal palpation in a cooperative or sedated patient.
- Contrast techniques using liquid barium, usually mixed with food or BIPS may aid identification of obstructions but are otherwise of limited value.
  - Technical difficulties of administering barium and obtaining serial radiographs for barium studies.
  - BIPS have the advantage in that only one or two sets of radiographs are required.
- Ultrasonography may be useful in identifying.
  - Intestinal thickening (see Figure 22).
  - Loss of intestinal layering.
  - Intestinal masses.
    - Other abdominal masses related to the intestine particularly involving the mesenteric lymph nodes.
  - Pancreatic architecture.
  - Small-volume peritonitis.

  - Changes suggestive of IBD such as mucosal speckling, changes in blood flow.
  - Involvement of hepatobiliary system in 'triaditis'.
- Ultrasound can also be used for percutaneous sampling of indentified lesions.

Visual examination and biopsy
- Endoscopic, laparoscopic or at laparotomy.
  - Biopsy is essential.
  - Serious complication rates for full-thickness biopsies in cats occur in approximately 15% of cases.
- Endoscopy is less invasive and is associated with more rapid recovery although only obtains superficial mucosal biopsies.
  - Complication rates are low in the region of 0.3%.
  - Recently it has been suggested that obtaining ileal biopsies can be important via a colonic approach as pathology can be more severe in the distal small intestine.
- Exploratory laparotomy is routinely performed; indications and contraindications for the procedure should be borne in mind (Table 40).

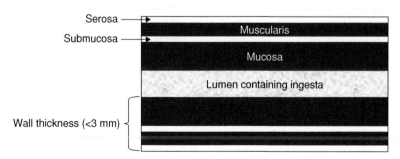

Figure 22 Intestinal layering identified on ultrasound of a longitudinal bowel segment

Table 40   Indications and contraindications for exploratory laparotomy

Indications	Contraindications
Rapid decline in patient condition	Diagnosis can be obtained non-invasively
Suspected intestinal perforation	Unacceptable anaesthetic risk
Lesion likely to be in jejunum/ileum	Delay in commencing immunosuppressive
Disease of associated lymph nodes, pancreas, liver	therapy
Lesions not involving the mucosal surface	Increased likelihood of wound dehiscence, e.g. recent glucocorticoid administration,
Disease likely to be resolved surgically, e.g. foreign body	protein losing enteropathy (PLE), cachexia
	Coagulopathy present

Infectious diseases
- Also see Section 5.13.

Viral infections
- Feline infectious enteritis.
- FeLV.
- FIV.
- Coronaviruses, astrovirus, reovirus and rotavirus.
- Generally cause mild diarrhoea, which is self-limiting.
- Specific diagnosis is unlikely largely due to the lack of availability of convenient diagnostic tests.
- Further investigations based on electron microscopy of faeces and attempts at isolation may be indicated in multi-cat households, particularly breeding catteries, where recurrent diarrhoea occurs especially in young kittens.

Nictitating membrane protrusion/ diarrhoea syndrome
- Chronic diarrhoea.
- Specific syndrome including persistent bilateral protrusion of the nictitating membranes.
- Affected cats are usually quite bright in themselves and do not lose significant body condition although they may show dullness and mild pyrexia for the first few days that signs become apparent.

- Cause of the syndrome is uncertain but a link has been found with torovirus infection.
- Seems to be a motility problem associated with autonomic dysfunction.
- Treatment is usually ineffective, but the condition is self-limiting, although in some cases signs may persist for some time, up to months in certain instances.
- Can be very persistent in breeding catteries and may appear repeatedly in successive new litters as they are weaned.

Bacterial infections
- Some specific bacterial enteropathogens may cause enteric infections and acute diarrhoea.
- Cats show a degree of natural resistance to some potential enteropathogens such as *Salmonella* spp., and others such as *Campylobacter* spp. may sometimes represent part of the indigenous intestinal flora, without significant pathogenic effects.
  - A variety of species of *Campylobacter* have been isolated from cats with *C.upsalensis* being the most common commensal (60% of cats).
  - *C.jejuni* is more frequently associated with clinical signs.
- Factors such as stress associated with overcrowding, poor hygiene that increases environmental exposure and

the presence of other infectious diseases may be important in contributing to the development of clinical disease associated with enteropathogens.

- Clinical signs are more likely in young animals.
- Clostridial species are also suggested as potential enteropathogens. These organisms can produce potent toxins that are implicated as a cause of diarrhoea in other species. However, *Clostridium perfringens* is a normal inhabitant of the intestinal bacterial flora in the cat as a carnivore. Isolation of *Clostridium perfringens* from the faeces is expected and therefore does not indicate that it is acting as a pathogen. The presence of clostridial spores may be more significant.
  - Although PCR techniques can show there is the genetic capability for toxigenic production they do not demonstrate toxin production is occurring.

Parasitic infections

Giardia lamblia

- Potential cause of chronic diarrhoea.
- Prevalence varies greatly between geographical areas.
- Has been found in clinically normal, usually adult cats.
- Young cats are at increased risk and most clinical disease occurs in cats under a year of age.
- Identification of oocysts in the faeces is complicated by intermittent excretion but this remains the most satisfactory diagnostic test.
  - At least three separate faecal samples should be collected although they can be pooled for analysis and should be examined whilst reasonably fresh will identify 95% of infected cases.
  - Faecal ELISA is sensitive (95%) but of low specificity.

Management

- Metronidazole at 25 mg/kg q12h for 5 days.
  - Side effects of GI irritation and neurological signs are possible at such high dosages – efficacy is slightly less than benzimidazoles.
- Fenbendazole 50 mg/kg q24h for 3–5 days is now frequently used as an alternative treatment.
  - Albendazole 25 mg/kg q12h for 2 days is also effective but is teratogenic, hepatotoxic and causes bone marrow suppression.
- All cats in the household should be treated.
- Second treatment after 3 weeks recommended.

Cystoisospora felis

- Recognised with increasing frequency as a cause of diarrhoea.
- Young kittens are most often affected and there may be copious amounts of blood in the faeces.
- Diagnosis can easily be achieved by faecal parasitology.
- Sulphonamides (e.g. trimethoprim sulphur at 15 mg/kg q12h PO for 7–14 days) are indicated for treatment but supportive care can be important, and the prognosis in very severe cases may be guarded.

Cryptosporidia pavum

- Rare infection in cats.
- Specific flotation methods or PCR required for diagnosis.
- Clinical signs similar to cystoisosporosis.
- Clinical effectiveness of treatment unknown – tylosin, clindamycin or azithromycin been used.

Tritrichomonas foetus

- Flagellate protozoan.
- Mainly causes very malodorous, colitis-like diarrhoea that can last for months.

ORGAN SYSTEMS

- More common in multi-cat households.
- Diagnosis – fresh wet preps, culture, PCR.
- Prognosis – good.
- Treatment – difficult.
  - Ronidazole current treatment of choice but efficacy unknown.
    - Not licensed for use in cats and there is limited toxicity data on potential hepatotoxicity.
    - 30–50 mg/kg once to twice daily for 2 weeks.

Inflammatory bowel disease

- Multifactorial syndrome with an inflammatory infiltrate within the intestine as an endpoint.
- Most common cause of chronic vomiting and diarrhoea in adult cats.
- Small intestine is usually the primary site for the inflammatory infiltrate, but lesions may also be present in the stomach or large intestine as well as, or instead of, in the small bowel.
- The infiltrate most commonly involves lymphocytes and plasma cells but, in a minority of cases, may be principally eosinophilic, granulomatous or suppurative in nature.
- The nature of the lesions suggests some immune dysregulation.
- Dietary hypersensitivity is believed to play a role in some cases and dietary management is often an important factor in successful treatment.
- Small intestinal bacterial overgrowth may occur in IBD in dogs, but its association with IBD in cats is more controversial.
- In some cases a link is found between the development of IBD and some specific disease problem, e.g. giardiasis or hyperthyroidism.

Presentation

- No obvious predispositions for this syndrome.
- Seen in cats of any age.

- Most consistent sign is weight loss which can be rapid and severe.
- Usually accompanied by vomiting and/or diarrhoea.
- Vomiting may be very intermittent in nature, typically with bouts of frequent vomiting for a few days interspersed by periods without vomiting for a week or more.
- Nature of the vomitus is also very variable and may consist of undigested food, froth or bile.
- Faeces may be bulky, semi-solid or of watery consistency.
- Frequently accompanied by noticeable polyphagia or cyclical polyphagia → anorexia.
- Intestinal thickening is occasionally detectable on palpation.
- May also be a mild enlargement of the mesenteric lymph nodes or a more generalised, mild peripheral lymphadenopathy.
- Up to 10% of cats with IBD show skin lesions, typically facial in distribution and suggestive of a hypersensitivity reaction.

Disease index

- A variety of scoring systems based on history, physical examination and results of diagnostic tests have been developed.
  - These indices have no value in differentiating IBD from other causes of the presenting signs.
  - They have some value in monitoring response to treatment.

Diagnosis

- No abnormalities are usually evident on routine blood tests and faecal screening.
  - Hyperglobulinemia and increased liver parameters present in some cats.
    - Feline pancreatic-specific lipase (fPLi) elevated in some cases associated with pancreatitis/triaditis.

- A small proportion of cases show haematological changes.
  - Circulating eosinophilia may accompany the eosinophilic form.
  - A neutrophilia with left shift that can be of striking magnitude of up to $50 \times 10^9/l$ or more is present occasionally in cats with lymphocytic/plasmacytic IBD.
  - B_{12} levels are low in some cats.
- Imaging often unremarkable.
  - Ultrasound may show subtle mucosal changes and lymphadenopathy.
  - Biliary and pancreatic changes may be present.
- Definitive diagnosis depends on histological assessment of intestinal biopsies collected either via endoscopy, laparoscopy or laparotomy.
  - Biopsy results should be reported according to the WSAVA GI standardisation group criteria.
- Rarely the inflammatory lesions are restricted to the submucosa or lower down the intestinal tract in which case endoscopic biopsies may miss the diagnosis and/or severity of the disease.
- Differentiation of severe IBD from low-grade alimentary lymphoma (LGAL) may require immunohistochemistry although treatment and prognosis for these two states are not very different.

Management

Diet

- Ideally, use alone before immunosuppressive therapy.
- Most cats that are going to respond will show improvement within 2 weeks.
- Owner education is important to ensure that diet is initially fed to exclusion.
- If signs resolve then re-challenge to prove sensitivity (often owner resistance).
- Some cats do not relapse following re-challenge – described as *diet responsive*.

- For cats that do respond, new ingredients should be introduced slowly one at a time for 2–3 weeks before the next ingredient is added.
- Some cats require a combination of dietary and immunosuppressive therapy.

Sacrifice diets

- An initial suitable diet (sacrifice) is fed for 4–6 weeks whilst the intestinal inflammation is being controlled by medication. It is assumed that because there is inflammation the cat may become sensitive to this diet over the period. A second new diet is then introduced when inflammation is no longer present that can be used long term. Clinical benefit of sacrifice diets is unproven.

Diet types

- Single-source protein, highly digestible, low residue, gluten free.
- Hydrolysed.

Immunosuppression

Initial management

- Prednisolone is usually the first choice for the lymphocytic/plasmacytic form, at an initial dosage of 1–2 mg/kg q12h. Where satisfactory clinical progress is maintained, with resolution of the GI signs and gain in body weight, the dosage is reduced by 25–50% every 10–20 days.
- Metronidazole can be used alone or in combination with prednisolone. Efficacy may be due to its immunomodulatory activity and/or an effect on the bacterial flora. Dose rate 10 mg/kg q12h for 1 month.

Refractory cases

- Other immunosuppressive agent such as cyclophosphamide, chlorambucil, ciclosporin or (azathioprine).
  - NB – Cats lack the enzyme pathways to metabolise azathioprine efficiently, hence other agents should be used first.

ORGAN SYSTEMS

ORGAN SYSTEMS

- Budesonide can be considered for cats that respond to but do not tolerate oral prednisolone.
- Eosinophilic forms of IBD generally prove much more refractory to treatment and may not respond to corticosteroids. Hydroxyurea may be effective but, for safety reasons, there are problems in dispensing this cytotoxic drug.
- Granulomatous and suppurative forms suggest further investigation to rule out infectious agents should be undertaken.

Adjunctive therapy
- A variety of other treatments have been used indicated by laboratory results or in poorly responsive cases including tylosin, motility modifiers e.g. loperamide, metoclopramide, maropitant, cisapride, cobalamin, vitamin K_1, glutamine, probiotics, vitamin A, C and E, zinc and n-acetyl glucosamine.

Prognosis
- Variable but generally good in the medium term depending on presence of concurrent and intercurrent disease.
- Treatment may be required lifelong.

Small intestinal bacterial overgrowth
- Cats have a particularly large number of both aerobic and anaerobic bacteria in the small intestine.
- Clear cases of SIBO are rare and likely reflect other underlying disease that prevents normal immune system regulation of bacterial numbers.
- Changes in the subpopulations may be more significant but are difficult to quantify.

Intestinal neoplasia
A variety of intestinal tumours are described in cats including mast cell, plasma cell and histiocytic types as well as leiomyosarcoma. Benign polyps are also reported.

Alimentary lymphoma
- Most common intestinal neoplasm in cats.
- Two forms exist in cats (Table 41):
  ○ Low-grade alimentary lymphoma (LGAL) mostly small cell lymphoma.
  ○ High-grade alimentary lymphoma (HGAL) that are more often large cell lymphoma.
  ○ Lymphoma are uncommon in younger cats.
  ○ Siamese over-represented.

Table 41 Comparative features of high- and low-grade alimentary lymphoma

	HGAL	LGAL
Median age	12 years	13 years
FeLV status	>70% negative	>99% negative
Form	More commonly focal/segmental	More commonly diffuse
Phenotype	B cell	T cell
Therapy	IV multi-agent	Oral prednisolone/chlorambucil
Median survival time for remission cases	8 months	19–29 months

○ An important differential diagnosis to consider in the older cat presented with progressive weight loss.

○ May be accompanying diarrhoea and vomiting.

○ Appetite is variable but cats may become finicky.

○ In some cases enlargement of the mesenteric lymph nodes is evident on abdominal palpation.

○ Infiltrate can be localised in a mass (HGAL) or appear as a more subtle diffuse thickening of the intestine (LGAL).

○ Mass lesions, intestinal thickening, loss of layering and focal necrosis/ulceration, lymph node enlargement and peritonitis may be appreciated on ultrasound examination.

○ If mesenteric lymphadenopathy is present, the collection of needle aspirates is possible using ultrasound guidance and may yield diagnostic information.

○ Intestinal biopsy for histopathological examination may prove necessary for definitive diagnosis in these cases but there is a significant risk of dehiscence if the lymphoma occupies the full thickness of the intestinal wall.

○ Routine blood tests frequently reveal a mild non-regenerative anaemia and there may be a lymphopenia.

Management (see Table 41)

• Surgical resection of mass lesions with adjunctive chemotherapy.

○ Response to treatment is variable.

○ HGAL: COAP or COP protocols have limited success and complications such as intestinal rupture or peritonitis can occur.

• Adjunctive therapy including nutrition, antacids, vitamin B_{12} is appropriate in many cases.

Carcinomas

• Second most common intestinal tumour.

• Predisposition in Siamese and related Oriental breeds.

• Tend to be localised lesions with a segmental or annular nature.

• Clinical features are frequently related to partial or total intestinal obstruction and delayed vomiting is the most prominent presenting sign.

• Ultrasound is usually the most efficient diagnostic technique as well as allowing FNA of the mass to distinguish carcinoma from lymphoma.

○ Thoracic radiographs should be taken to exclude lung metastasis.

○ Plain abdominal radiographs are of low sensitivity; contrast techniques to demonstrate wall thickening/obstruction are often required.

• Some carcinomas may be surgically resectable but metastasis, particularly to the local mesenteric lymph nodes, may have occurred before a diagnosis has been made.

• High mortality rate within first 2 weeks post surgery.

○ Survival beyond 2 weeks carries reasonable 1 year survival times.

○ Clear benefits of adjunctive chemotherapy have not been shown.

Foreign bodies

• More often of a linear nature in cats.

• Causes partial obstruction and sometimes creates a particular diagnostic challenge if not radiopaque.

• Thread/string is the most common foreign body.

• Physical examination should always include careful examination under the base of the tongue.

• Linear foreign bodies can become embedded in the intestinal wall, plicating the intestine around the thread.

ORGAN SYSTEMS

- Vomiting is usually the most prominent sign, but may be intermittent if only partial obstruction is present.
  - Cases will often appear to respond to conservative medical management.
- A barium meal may help to identify wool or thread linear foreign bodies, as the barium becomes trapped in the fibres of the material. A 24 hour film post barium film should always be obtained.

Intussusception

- Most often in young kittens, less common than dogs.
- Possible predilection in Siamese and Burmese cats.
- Occasionally more than one kitten is affected in the same litter – which may reflect some common enteric infection, or other cause of diarrhoea.
- There may be an absence of faeces, but if present, there may be diarrhoea with evidence of blood.
- Vomiting is usually a prominent feature.
- Affected kittens are very dull and depressed.
  - Severity of signs depends on duration, site (more proximal intussusceptions generally more severe signs) and whether the bowel is completely obstructed.
  - Endotoxic shock may be present
- Usually readily palpable as a sausage-like swelling on abdominal palpation.
- Additional diagnostics:
  - Haematology and biochemistry if systemically unwell.
  - Radiography – dilated loops of small intestine.
  - Ultrasound – dilated proximal bowel terminating in a section with too many layers in an onion-ring arrangement on cross section.
- Most common site for intussusceptions is at the ileocolic junction, but they can occur higher up the small intestine.

- Recent cases are readily reducible at laparotomy but, if the intussusception has been present for some time, there may be significant adhesions and necrosis of gut tissue requiring resection.
- Recurrence is quite common after surgical reduction of intussusception and cases should be monitored carefully following surgery.
  - Plication of the mesentery may reduce the recurrence rate.
- Care must also be taken to prevent post-operative stricture, particularly in small kittens.

4.3.6 Large intestinal disease

- Constipation is the most common reason for cats to present with large bowel disease.
- Colitis is relatively uncommon in cats compared to dogs.
- Often in combination with small intestinal disease.

Clinical signs of large bowel disease

- Changes in the nature and pattern of defecation.
- Dyschezia, haematochezia, tenesmus, vocalisation.
- Digital rectal examination may be difficult, due to size, but can be used to identify possible neoplastic lesions or strictures in the terminal colon.

Diagnosis

- Clinical pathology usually unremarkable.
- Faecal examination is unlikely to be helpful since *Trichuris* spp. are not considered to be important in cats.
- Imaging, including barium enema, may help to identify more cranial lesions – particularly neoplasia and strictures that may not be accessible via endoscopy.
  - Allows extent and severity of constipation and integrity of the pelvis to be assessed.

Colonoscopy

- Rigid colonoscopes of appropriate size can be used but limit access to transverse and descending colon.
- Flexible endoscope is generally preferable.
- Careful patient preparation is important.
- Iso-osmotic bowel cleansing solution based on polyethylene glycol (e.g. 'Klean Prep' at 30 ml/kg) is given by naso-oesophageal tube twice within 24 hours of the procedure.
  - Patients should be starved for 24–48 hours prior to colonoscopy.
- Residual faecal material is often present and can be removed with a warm water enema.

Inflammatory bowel disease/colitis

- Large intestine may be affected as part of more widespread IBD also affecting the small intestine, but occasionally lesions are restricted to the colon.
- Inflammatory infiltrate may be predominantly lymphocytic/plasmacytic, as usually occurs in the small intestine, but may be of a granulomatous nature.

Clinical signs and diagnosis

- Usually increased frequency of defaecation.
- Straining ± appearance of fresh blood and mucus in the faeces.
- Appearance of the faeces can be very variable and at times they may be normal.
- Cats may be otherwise clinically well.
- No or minimal weight loss.

Colonoscopy

- No gross lesions are evident in many cases.
- Specific ulcerative or raised lesions that can be hyperaemic may be present.
- A general increase in the granularity of the mucosal surface that may appear proliferative.

- Increased tendency to bleed.
- Biopsies should be collected from regions that look abnormal and every 3–5 cm along the length of the large intestine regardless of gross appearance.

Management

- Prednisolone is the most useful drug for therapy given at an initial dosage of 1–2 mg/kg BID, gradually reducing as for IBD of the small intestine.
- Other forms of prednisolone may be appropriate for cats that require long-term high dose therapy, such as prednisolone enemas.
- Sulphasalazine can be used for the anti-inflammatory effect of the salicylate fraction, which is not released until the large bowel is reached which avoids significant absorption and potential problems with toxicity. It is given at a dosage of 10–20 mg/kg q8–12h.
- Metronidazole is an alternative given at 10 mg/kg q12h and may prove beneficial.

Dietary management

- Novel protein diet if enterocolitis is present.
- Modification of dietary fibre content.
- Some cats respond to a low fibre, low residue diets; others respond better to increased fibre; excessive fibre levels will, in themselves, lead to softening of the faeces.

Neoplasia

- Uncommon site for neoplasia in cats.
- Lymphosarcoma, carcinomas and other tumours may occur.
  - Prognosis for colonic adenocarcinoma with adjunctive doxorubicin seems better than small intestinal adenocarcinoma.
- Considerable amounts of blood may be present in the faeces.
- Dyschezia may be severe.

ORGAN SYSTEMS

- Caudal tumours may be palpable on digital examination.
- Colonoscopy and biopsy is usually necessary.

Strictures

- Neoplasia, particularly carcinoma, may cause stricturing of the colon; other causes may rarely be involved.
- May only be able to pass small quantities of misshapen, thin, thread-like faeces.
- May even appear like diarrhoea with small amounts of watery faeces being all that can pass the obstruction.
- Cause considerable pain and discomfort to the cat.
- Diagnosis by colonoscopy or barium enema.
- In some cases surgical resection may be feasible.
- Conservative medical management using faecal softeners may help the cat to defecate more easily. Lactulose can be given to effect (usual dosage of 0.5–1 ml/kg q8–12h), together with a highly digestible, low residue diet.

Irritable bowel syndrome

- Some cats show signs typical of large bowel disease with frequent passage of mucoid, bloody faeces, often associated with straining, suggesting colitis.
- Gross appearance, seen at colonoscopy and biopsies are normal.
- Underlying cause is speculative, but may be similar to irritable bowel syndrome in man.
- May be related to stress and psychogenic factors.
- Some cases improve using the treatment regime recommended for IBD of the colon.

Constipation and megacolon (see Section 2.11)

- Chronic or recurrent constipation is a common problem in cats.

- May be associated with megacolon.
- Occurs most frequently in older cats.
- Megacolon can occur in very young kittens and may involve a congenital problem in the failure of neurogenic control. This can be associated with spina bifida, particularly in cats carrying the Manx gene.
- Check for pelvic deformities associated with previous traumatic injuries or severe nutritional osteodystrophy, which may be predisposing factors.
- In older cats, large quantities of fur may accumulate in the impacted faeces; this may predispose long-haired cats to megacolon.
- Constipation and faecal retention can be prominent signs of dysautonomia.

Management

Mild cases

- May be managed successfully once the obstructing faeces have been removed with conservative treatment.
- Faecal softeners – lactulose.
- Other proprietary faecal softeners based on lubricants are unlikely to achieve effective control.
- Cisapride can be used as a prokinetic to promote colonic motility, at a dosage of 0.5 mg/kg q8–12h but is no longer easy to obtain.
  - Metoclopramide and ranitidine are of limited efficacy as colonic prokinetics.
- Stimulate colonic activity by using a parasympathomimetic such as bethanechol at an initial oral dosage of 2.5 mg/cat q8h. The dosage may require adjustment to achieve a therapeutic effect, and avoid the adverse effects of parasympathetic over stimulation. This treatment can be particularly effective for dysautonomia.
- Dathron (2.5–5 ml q12h) is sometimes used as a stimulant laxative and comes in a combined preparation with a faecal softener (Docusate – 'Normax').

Severe cases

- Enemas will be necessary to relieve recurrent impaction.
  - NB – Take care with the choice of enema; high phosphate and glycerine enemas can be toxic to cats.
- Colectomy may be considered for non-responsive cases, prognosis is better if performed in the first 6 months.
  - Diarrhoea can persist for up to 6 weeks post colectomy
- Pelvic surgery may be beneficial where there is an anatomical deformity narrowing the pelvic canal.

Diet

- Very rarely effective in treating established constipation, but can be useful to prevent or reduce recurrence.
- Increasing the fibre content of the diet, and regular grooming to minimise ingestion of fur.
  - 1–2 tsp of psyllium/meal or 1 tsp wheat bran/meal.
- Some cats seem to respond better to a low residue, single-source protein/hydrolysed diets.

Rectoanal disease

- Rectal prolapse is common in kittens secondary to chronic tenesmus.
  - Small prolapses can be replaced manually, if a recurrent loose purse-string suture can be used.
  - Topical local anaesthetic or corticosteroid ointments may be helpful.
  - Surgery may be necessary if the bowel is devitalised or replacement not possible.
  - Medical causes of tenesmus should be addressed.
- Perineal hernias are uncommon in cats.
- Atresia ani is a rare congenital defect in kittens.
  - Management depends on type – imperforate anus → significant segment of bowel missing.
  - Rectovaginal or rectourethral fistula may be present.

- Rectal neoplasia is uncommon; lymphoma will occur.

Anal sac disease

- Abscessation, impaction and sacculitis are infrequent.
  - Differential diagnosis is a perianal bite wound.
- Anal sac adenocarcinoma very rare in cats.

4.3.7 Pancreatic disease

Exocrine pancreatic insufficiency

- Rare disease in cats.
- Can occur as a result of long-standing, chronic pancreatitis.

Clinical signs

- Polyphagia.
- Weight loss.
- Steatorrhoea.
- DM.

Diagnosis

- Feline trypsin-like immunoreactivity assay (fTLI).
  - Appears to be specific.
    - False elevation in fTLI occurs in renal disease.
  - Sensitivity is unknown but probably good.
- Imaging of limited value.

Management

- Fat restricted diet.
- Pancreatic enzyme supplementation – raw pancreas (10–20 g/feed) is generally more effective than powdered products.
- Parenteral vitamin $B_{12.}$
- Chronic antibacterial treatment may be necessary – metronidazole or tylosin.

Pancreatitis

- Anatomically different from dogs, pancreatic duct fuses with bile duct before opening into the duodenum.
  - Anatomic differences may be associated with an increase in incidence of chronic disease allowing easier access to ascending bacterial infection.

ORGAN SYSTEMS

ORGAN SYSTEMS

Causes
- Majority of cases – underlying cause is unknown.
- Suggested risk factors:
  - Hyperlipoproteinemia.
  - Drugs/toxins.
  - Furosemide, azathioprine, sulphona-mides, tetracycline, L-asparaginase, corticosteroids.
  - Hypercalcaemia.
  - Pancreatic duct obstruction.
  - Duodenal/biliary reflux.
  - Pancreatic trauma/surgery.
  - Pancreatic ischaemia/reperfusion (including anaesthetic associated).
  - Severe systemic disease.

Acute pancreatitis
- Mild–to-severe clinical signs.
- Initiating causes:
  - Hypothermia, hypovolaemia, sepsis.
  - Virulent strain FCV.
  - Neoplasia.
  - Ascending bacterial infection.
  - Toxoplasmosis.
  - Abdominal trauma.
  - Organophosphate intoxication.

Clinical signs (moderate-to-severe disease)
- Poorly defined – reflect a shocked animal.
- Despite the 'acute' signs many cats will have a prior history of days–weeks of depression and anorexia.
- Collapse, lethargy and dehydration.
- Hypothermia.
- Tachycardia and hypotension.
- Abdominal pain/abdominal mass.
- Vomiting in about one in three of cats.
- Ascites due to peritonitis.
- Dyspnoea.

Diagnosis
- Clinical signs.
- Numerous non-specific biochemical changes.
- Amylase and lipase of no diagnostic value.
- fPLi (fTLI has been used in the past but is less specific).
- Pancreatic ultrasound is a sensitive imaging modality.
  - NB – Identification of a mass lesion is not synonymous with neoplasia.
- Biopsy is definitive but consideration must be given to the surgical risk.

Management
- Non-specific.
- Shock treatment – maintenance of BP and pancreatic perfusion.
- Pain relief – opiates usually required.
- Management of DIC.
- Antibacterials may be indicated – fluo-roquinolone.
- Plasma transfusion to replete pancreatic protease inhibitors.
  - Large amounts of plasma may be required.
- Optimal nutritional approach unknown – moderate fat diet is reasonable.
- Surgery should be considered if there is gross necrosis, marked exudative peritonitis or the patient is failing to improve with aggressive conservative management.

Prognosis
- Guarded in moderate–to-severe disease.
- Significant mortality approaching 100% in some studies of acute necrotis-ing pancreatitis.

Chronic pancreatitis
- Common postmortem finding.
- Diagnosis rates have increased since wide access to fPLi.
- Pancreatitis is often associated with other diseases, particularly as part of a syn-drome involving IBD and cholangitis/cholangiohepatitis often termed 'triaditis'.
- In the UK, Burmese cats may be predis-posed.

Clinical signs
- Typically middle-aged to older cats.
- Often vague as can be a chronic, recurrent disease.
- Intermittent anorexia.
- Weight loss.
- Variable GIT signs – vomiting, diarrhoea.
- Abdominal pain is NOT a consistent finding.
- Associated IBD and cholangitis.
- DM (PU/PD).

Diagnosis
- Routine laboratory tests are non-specific.
  - Neutrophilia, hyperglobulinemia, increased bilirubin and liver enzymes.
- Amylase and lipase (section 3.6) are of no value – the value of including these tests in a feline profile is questionable.
- Increase in feline TLI is insensitive and has poor specificity.
- fPLi is now available both as a quantitative external laboratory test and an in-house ELISA that gives a positive, equivocal or negative result.
  - NB – fPLi test is relatively sensitive and specific for pancreatitis BUT this may be secondary to another underlying condition, e.g. hypovolemia.
  - Correlation between the in-house and laboratory-based test is good.
- Ultrasound changes are present, but do not distinguish ongoing disease from past episodes.
- Definitive diagnosis at laparotomy/laparoscopy and biopsy.
- Biopsies of small intestine and liver should be considered at the same time.

Management
- Dependent on severity.
- No specific treatments have been shown to directly influence pancreatitis:
  - Chronic antibacterials such as metronidazole may reduce episodes of ascending infection.
  - Vitamin B_{12} if deficiency is documented.
  - Antioxidants, e.g. vitamin E, may be helpful.
  - Vitamin K_1 may be deficient due to reduced fat absorption – 0.5 mg/kg s/c q24h weekly.
  - Low-fat diets have not been shown to be beneficial.
  - Value of pancreatic supplements unknown.
  - Starvation to allow pancreatic rest is likely to be ineffective.
- Maintenance of hydration to ensure adequate perfusion and oxygenation, particularly of the pancreas is important.
- Pain relief – opiates are the drugs of choice if necessary.
- Increased risk of gastroduodenal ulceration if NSAIDs are used.
- Anti-emetic/prokinetic drugs and gastric protectants may help inappetent cats that are nauseated.
- Corticosteroids if evidence of concurrent cholangitis/IBD.

Prognosis
- Many cats with smouldering pancreatitis have minimal signs and treatment is unlikely to be helpful; survival time for these cats can be many years..
- Chronic pancreatitis can eventually lead to secondary DM ± EPI.

Pancreatic neoplasia
- Pancreatic acinar cell adenocarcinoma is very rare in cats.
- Highly malignant and rapidly metastasise.
- Insulinoma is rare in cats.

NB – *Not all pancreatic masses are neoplastic; benign fibrotic masses, as a consequence of chronic pancreatitis, look very similar at laparotomy.*

ORGAN SYSTEMS

4.3.8 Peritoneal disease

For causes of peritoneal effusion see sections 2.1 (also section 2.4) – ascites and 5.6 – FIP

Peritonitis

- Primary peritonitis is uncommon (except in FIP).
- Secondary peritonitis occur due to
  - Trauma.
  - Surgery.
  - Necrosis and rupture of intra-abdominal vesicle (intestine, gall bladder, urinary bladder, etc.).
  - Pancreatitis.

Clinical signs

Acute peritonitis

- Vomiting.
- Anorexia.
- Pyrexia.
- Abdominal pain and distension.
- Shock – dull, depressed, poorly responsive, hypothermic.

Chronic peritonitis

- Signs can be more subtle associated with low grade GI signs, inappetence and depression.
- Abdominal pain may not be present.

Diagnosis

- Neutrophilia with left shift.
- Neutropenia in acute disease.
- Hypoglycaemia can be significant.
- Radiography is usually non-specific.
  - Global or regional loss of abdominal detail.
  - Ileus.
  - Abdominal fluid.
  - Free gas.
- Ultrasound is more useful especially with focal peritonitis, can be used for guiding aspiration.
- Abdominal paracentesis essential; submit for cytology and culture.

Treatment

- Aggressive treatment is necessary in acute disease.
- Fluid – colloid, crystalloid, plasma.
- Broad spectrum IV antibacterial.
- Opiate pain relief.
- Exploratory laparotomy is usually necessary when the patient has been stabilised.

4.4 HEPATOBILIARY DISEASE

4.4.1 Introduction

Clinical signs of liver and biliary system disease in cats are similar regardless of cause. Many cats will present with non-specific signs of anorexia/inappetence, weight loss and lethargy. The most consistent hepatobiliary-related signs are jaundice and hepatomegaly. Less commonly vomiting, diarrhoea, pyrexia effusion and CNS signs lead to presentation. Congenital hepatobiliary disease, apart from PSS, is rare in cats.

Like any organ hepatobiliary signs secondary to primary disease elsewhere primarily neoplasia, thyrotoxicosis, DM, right CHF, hypoxaemia, FIP and toxoplasmosis will occur.

WSAVA International Liver Standardisation Group has published guidelines for the diagnosis of liver disease in dogs and cats dividing liver disease into four groups:

- Vascular liver disorders.
- Biliary tract disorders.
- Parenchymal disorders.
- Neoplasia.

4.4.2 Functions of the liver

The liver has a wide variety of functions; clinical signs will be modified by the function that is most affected by the disease process. As cats have evolved, they have developed a number of unique adaptations in liver function tailored to their lifestyle that renders them more or less susceptible to disease.

Primary liver functions are –

- Carbohydrate – gluconeogenesis, glycogen storage.
- Lipids – fatty acid cycling, energy metabolism.
- Protein – synthesis, albumin homeostasis.
- Production of clotting factors.
- Bile acid production.
- Vitamin metabolism and storage.
- Detoxification and excretion.
  - ○ Bilirubin conjugation.
  - ○ Hormone excretion.
  - ○ Drug metabolism.
- Immune function – removal of bacteria in portal blood.
- Extra-marrow haematopoiesis.

Idiosyncrasies of feline hepatic metabolism

- High protein requirement for gluconeogenesis.
- Decreased ability to down-regulate nitrogen catabolic enzymes if intake is reduced.
- Limited conjugation ability – important pathway for solubilisation and excretion of drugs.
  - ○ Glucuronidation pathways particularly affected.
  - ○ Reduced ability to excrete salicylates, morphine derivatives, diazepam, phenols, benzoic acid and chloramphenicol.
  - ○ BUT this does not affect all drugs and toxins; some are excreted more rapidly.
- Only able to conjugate cholic acid with taurine.
- Limited ability to synthesise taurine.

4.4.3 Laboratory tests for liver disease

Liver enzymes (also see 3.12)

- ALT is a useful marker of hepatocellular damage.
- Alkaline phosphatase (ALKP; ALP; SAP) has a short half-life in cats and there is no steroid-induced isoenzyme

in the cat; hence elevations of ALP are generally much more indicative of cholestasis than in the dog.

- Gamma-glutamyl transferase (γ-GT) is also increased in cholestasis, though rarely in hepatic lipidosis – it has a greater sensitivity but lower specificity than ALKP for liver disease.

Bilirubin

- Differential bilirubin estimations are of limited value in assessing the origin of the jaundice for several reasons, but particularly because the traditional tests do not reliably discriminate between the different forms of bilirubin.
- Pre-hepatic jaundice is relatively rare in cats.

Ammonia

- Particular care is required in the collection and handling of blood samples for ammonia estimation.
- Samples can be chilled on ice for rapid transport to a local laboratory for assessment.
- Generally on-site measurement required that limits the practical value of the test in practice.
- Useful; if signs are suggestive of hepatic encephalopathy.
- Ammonia tolerance tests are potentially risky in cats.

Bile acids

- Most valuable marker of liver function.
- Maximum value may be obtained from a dynamic bile acid test.
- Mild-to-moderate increases in bile acids can be associated with a variety of non-hepatic diseases.
- Reliability affected by jaundice.
- Magnitude of increase does not accurately reflect the degree of hepatic dysfunction.
- A change in level in the same cat likely indicates a change in function.

ORGAN SYSTEMS

Cholesterol and triglycerides
- Liver is central in metabolism of lipids.
- Liver disease can result in both increases (cholestasis) and decreases (portosystemic shunting) in cholesterol levels.

Urea/albumin
- Manufactured in the liver.
- Tend to fall in dogs with severe chronic liver disease.
- Decreases in cats are less consistent, and therefore of limited value in assessing liver function.

Clotting factors
- The liver produces a number of clotting factors.
- Severe liver disease results in reduced synthesis and may lead to impaired clotting function.

Haematology
- Check for regenerative anaemia, which may indicate a haemolytic cause of jaundice.
- Screening for FIA should also be considered.
- Mild-moderate non-regenerative anaemia does occur as a feature of some hepatic conditions causing other types of jaundice, and is relatively common in cats with chronic, systemic disease.
- WBC changes may be useful in some cases of liver disease for differentiation of the underlying cause.
- Lymphocytic cholangitis is frequently associated with a lymphopenia and sometimes neutrophilia, although FIP produces similar haematological changes.
- Marked leucocytosis with a left shift reflecting an infective process is common in ascending bacterial infection.

Urinalysis
- Identification of ammonium urate crystals may indicate liver disease (including the possibility of a PSS).

4.4.4 Diagnostic imaging

Abdominal radiography
- Size – based on silhouette and gastric angle.
  - Gastric barium may aid in the appreciation of liver size which is usually bounded within the costal margins.
- Position.
- Shape.
- Most useful in demonstrating hepatomegaly.
- Reduced liver size even with severe disease is uncommon in cats.
- Portovenography to identify presence and position of abnormal blood vessels in vascular anomalies.

Ultrasound scanning
- Assessment of changes in liver texture which may occur in several hepatic diseases.
  - Diffuse or focal disease.
- Ultrasound has a high degree of sensitivity for focal changes.
- Less sensitive if there is a diffuse, even, change in echogenicity.
- Poor specificity for identifying aetiology of the changes seen.
- Enables the biliary tree including the gall bladder to be assessed, and any retention of bile or dilation of biliary ducts to be seen.
  - Differentiation of hepatic and post-hepatic obstructive disease.
- Allows imaging of the pancreas – a frequent cause of post-hepatic obstruction.
- Ultrasound guided procedures – liver aspirate/biopsy and bile aspiration.
- Identification of the presence and position of abnormal hepatic vessels (PSS).

Advanced imaging
Scintigraphy
- Technetium scintigraphy can be used to
  - Identify the existence of an abnormal vessel.
  - Calculate the fraction of the blood that is bypassing the liver (shunt fraction).

CT and MRI

- Limited diagnostic advantage vs. costs in hepatobiliary disease.

4.4.5 Tissue sampling

Liver aspirates

- Can be performed in conscious/sedated cat.
- Delivers a relatively small number of cells without architecture.
- Most useful in diagnosis of diffuse disease.
  - Inflammation.
  - Lipidosis.
  - Lymphoma.
- Value in focal disease dependent on level to which tissue can be exfoliated.

Bile aspiration

- Should be performed in conjunction with most aspirates or biopsies.
- Can be performed in a conscious/sedated amenable cat.
- Sample submitted for cytology and culture.
  - Bile culture more sensitive than liver biopsy culture for ascending bacterial infection.
- Risk of bile peritonitis low.

Liver biopsy

- Histological examination necessary to make a definitive diagnosis in many cases of liver disease.
- Careful patient selection and preparation important.
- Assess clotting function prior to biopsy should be performed BUT poor predictor of risk of bleeding post biopsy.
- Anaesthesia is required in almost all cases.
  - Choice of anaesthetic agents and premedicants in a cat known to have impaired hepatic function.

- Samples should be submitted for histology.
  - Frozen samples retained for further analysis, e.g. immunohistochemistry, copper level, mycobacterial culture.
- Limited value in the diagnosis of PSS.

Techniques (see Table 42)

- Blind biopsy is possible but not recommended.
- Complication rates are strongly associated with the experience of the clinician performing the procedure.
- With all techniques, multiple biopsies are recommended.
- DO NOT USE biopsy gun-type devices as these have been associated with post-procedural fatalities.
- Percutaneous sampling use 14–18g biopsy needle.

4.4.6 Portosystemic shunts

- Congenital PSS is uncommon; incidence 0.25% in referral population.
  - Acquired shunting occurs secondary to portal hypertension.
- Approximately 75% of shunts are extrahepatic.
- Variety of anomalies described.
- Most commonly reported in domestic short hair (DSH), Persian; Himalayan, Siamese and Burmese – partly reflects breed prevalence.

History and presentation

- Signs usually first exhibited at 10–14 weeks of age.
  - Will wax and wane.
  - Can be precipitated by another disease or stress, e.g. neutering.
- Poor growth and body condition but can be relatively normal.
- Variable appetite.
- Hypersalivation (antimicrobial responsive) in the absence of oral lesions.
- Exaggerated chewing movements.

ORGAN SYSTEMS

- Intermittent neurological signs – stupor, apparent blindness, seizures, head pressing.
  - Encephalopathic crisis – seizuring, coma.
- GIT signs – vomiting, diarrhoea, inappetence.
- Dysuria and haematuria associated with ammonium urate urolithiasis.
- PU/PD and renal enlargement uncommon compared to dogs.

Clinical examination
- Often relatively unremarkable apart from stature.
- Copper coloration to irises.
- Soft I–II/VI systolic murmur.

Diagnosis
- Urea/albumin is often normal rather than low.
- Liver enzymes – slightly low → normal → mild elevation.
- Microcytosis relatively common.
- Mild non-regenerative anaemia uncommon (<15%).
- Hyperammonaemia very common but not all cases.
- Elevated bile acids (pre-prandial can be normal):
  - High post-prandial bile acids is nearly 100% sensitive but not diagnostic (specific), i.e. a good negative rule out.
- Urate urolithiasis/crystalluria.

Radiography
- Liver and kidneys usually within normal limits on radiography.
- Portovenography to confirm presence, position and number of shunt vessels.

Per rectal portal scintigraphy
Ultrasound
- Reduced hepatic vascularisation.
- Identification of shunting vessel very operator dependent.

Treatment
Medical management
- Prior to surgery.
- Long term.
- Medium protein diet – added cottage cheese may be beneficial in young kittens to meet protein requirement.
- Small frequent meals.
- Antimicrobial – neomycin or ampicillin.
- Lactulose – 0.5–1 ml/kg q8h.

Encephalopathic crisis
- Diazepam.
- Fluid support.
- Lactulose or povidone iodine enema.
- i/v antimicrobials.

Surgical management
- Treatment of choice where feasible (surgically or financially).
- Partial or full occlusion – many cases require a second procedure for full ligation.
  - Follow-up bile acid stimulation testing at 1 and 3 months.
- Intrahepatic shunts are technically more demanding.
- Prolene suture, ameroid constrictor, cellophane banding.
- Anaesthesia demanding:
  - Severe hypothermia.
  - Hypoglycaemia.
  - Fluid balance.
  - Pain management.
- Medical management continued post surgery.

NB – *Cats with PSSs can be very sensitive to sedative, anaesthetic or analgesic agents that undergo hepatic metabolism.*

Post-surgical complications
- Ascites.
- Intestinal necrosis.
- Thromboembolism.

- Neurologic complications – variety reported (15–30%).
- Mortality – primarily due to neurologic complications up to 20% reported.

Prognosis
- Median survival time 1–2 years for medical management.
- Full ligation at surgery may lead to a better long-term prognosis.
- Post surgery – gradual withdrawal of therapy and a return to a standard diet.
- Re-canalization of ligated vessel can occur.
- Development of acquired shunts due to portal hypertension can occur following surgery.

4.4.7 Hepatic lipidosis
- Relatively common in the USA, becoming increasingly common in the UK, probably associated with changes in lifestyle (more indoor cats) and body weight.
- More common in middle-aged to older, obese, female cats.
- Begins with a period of anorexia often following a stressful event, e.g. house moving, infection, pancreatitis.
  - Period of anorexia variable – usually a number of days or weeks, but can occur only after 24 hours.
- Progresses to severe weight loss and marked anorexia and depression.

Table 42 Comparison of liver biopsy techniques in cats

Percutaneous Tru-cut	Laparotomy	Laparoscopy
Small sample – can limit diagnostic accuracy	Larger samples – maximises diagnostic accuracy	Intermediate sample size
Highest risk of iatrogenic damage to associated structures	Low risk of iatrogenic damage to associated structures	Moderate risk of iatrogenic damage to associated structures
No further information on liver architecture delivered	Allows visual inspection of the liver	Allows visual inspection of the liver
Limited ability to control post-procedure haemorrhage	Haemorrhage can be easily controlled	Haemorrhage can be easily identified but less easily controlled
Other abdominal organs cannot be examined and biopsy of the organs can be problematic, e.g. pancreas	Other abdominal organs especially pancreas can be sampled	Other abdominal organs especially pancreas can be sampled
Can be directed towards focal change	Focal lesions may not be easily accessible	Focal lesions may not be easily accessible – less access than laparotomy
Short procedure time	Moderate procedure time	Moderate procedure time
Small set-up costs	Small set-up costs	Set-up costs relatively higher
Rapid post-procedural recovery	Slower recovery	More rapid recovery/lower morbidity than laparotomy
Moderate clinician experience required	Standard clinician experience required	Greater clinician experience required
Low-moderate procedural costs	High procedural cost	Moderate-high procedural costs
No treatment delay	Treatment may have to be delayed until surgical wound has healed	No treatment delay

ORGAN SYSTEMS

Clinical presentation

Commonly

- Period of anorexia.
- Dehydration.
- Jaundice.

Less commonly

- Hypersalivation.
- Neurological signs.
- Vomiting.
- Constipation.
- Ascites.
- Fever.

Diagnosis

- Marked increases in the liver enzymes ALT and ALKP.
- γ-GT levels usually normal.
- Hyperbilirubinaemia.
- Raised bile acids and hyperammonaemia.
- Hypokalaemia.
- Hyperglycaemia.
- Neutrophilia, lymphopenia, mild non-regenerative anaemia.
- Coagulopathy in >50% cases.
- Diffusely hyperechoic liver on ultrasound.
- Grossly the liver appears rounded at the margins, yellow and friable.
- Liver aspirate or biopsy (more definitive) reveals hepatic vacuolation due to lipid.
  - Consider risks of procedure especially bleeding.
  - Relatively poor correlation between cytology and histology.

Treatment

- Aggressive supportive therapy is necessary.
- Initially rehydration ± potassium.
- Water-soluble vitamins.
- Parenteral vitamin K_1 at 5 mg/cat and B_1 (thiamine) at 50–100 mg/cat.
- Control vomiting and nausea.

- Ursodeoxycholic acid.
- Nutritional support – 65–90 kcal/kg/day.
  - May need to be prolonged (4 months).
  - Gastrostomy or oesophagostomy tube is ideal.
    - In cats that are too sick at presentation to risk anaesthesia initially place a naso-oesophageal tube.
    - Supplementation with L-carnitine (150–250 mg/cat) and arginine (1000 mg/cat) is suggested.

Prognosis

- Early diagnosis is crucial.
  - Evaluate for concomitant disease especially pancreatitis.
- Greater than 60% survival rate can now be expected with aggressive nutritional support.

4.4.8 Inflammatory hepatopathies

Inflammatory hepatopathies are the most common group of diseases affecting the feline liver. It remains unclear whether the conditions are distinct entities or a spectrum with a common pathogenesis. Pathogenesis remains poorly clarified.

Based on the WSAVA standard classification they are divided into five classes:

- Acute neutrophilic form of cholangitis/cholangiohepatitis.
- Chronic neutrophilic form of cholangitis/cholangiohepatitis.
- Lymphocytic cholangitis/cholangiohepatitis.
- Lymphocytic portal hepatitis.
- Liver fluke.

Neutrophilic disease

- Ascending infection of the biliary duct is considered to be the most likely aetiology.
- Bacteria isolated from the bile are usually of an enteric nature.
- Associated with IBD and pancreatitis (50% of cases) (triaditis).

ORGAN SYSTEMS

- Common opening of the bile and pancreatic duct into the duodenum may make it easier for infection to ascend.
- Level of concurrent lymphoplasmacytic cholangitis is variable.

Clinical signs
- Acute disease in young to middle-aged cats.
- Chronic disease more frequently in middle to older-aged cats.
- Frequently severely ill when first presented.
- Marked malaise, pyrexia, inappetence, vomiting, diarrhoea, weight loss and dehydration.
- Most cases are jaundiced (may be absent in the very early stages).

Diagnosis
- Moderate to marked increase in liver enzymes.
- Hyperbilirubinaemia.
- Raised post-prandial bile acids.
- Inflammatory leucogram ± mild non-regenerative anaemia.

Imaging
- Radiography often unremarkable.
- Ultrasound:
  - Diffuse multifocal, hyperechoic areas on liver ultrasound.
  - Bile duct distension.
  - Gall bladder wall thickening.
  - Pancreatic changes.
  - Regional lymphadenopathy.

Biopsy
- FNA is suggestive.
- Histology provides more definitive diagnosis.
- Bile culture.
- Severity of signs shown by affected cats may deter the use of invasive diagnostic procedures at initial presentation.

Management
- A significant proportion of cases are treated after making a presumptive diagnosis based on clinical signs, laboratory results, radiography and USG.
- Intravenous fluid therapy (IVFT) and opioid pain relief.
- Long-term antibacterial treatment minimum of 2 weeks but may be required for months.
  - Choice of antibacterial based on culture and sensitivity, but potentiated amoxicillin with metronidazole makes a good empirical choice.
  - Decision on the length of treatment difficult – based on follow-up blood work and imaging.
- Prednisolone may be required in some cases balanced against its immunosuppressive effects.
- Adjunctive treatment:
  - Ursodeoxycholic acid – improves bile flow at 10–15 mg/kg q24h.
  - S-Adenosyl methionine (SAMe) elevates liver glutathione, which may have a protective effect on hepatocytes at 90 mg/cat/day.
  - Silymarin, vitamin E may be beneficial.

Prognosis
- Guarded in acute severe disease with pancreatitis.
- Chronic disease usually responsive to treatment but recurrence is common.

Lymphoplasmacytic disease
- Lymphoplasmacytic infiltrate around the bile ducts.
- Portal fibrosis and biliary hyperplasia markers of chronicity.
- Primarily in the younger to middle-aged cats.
- Long-haired cats may be over-represented in our series of cases.
- Condition has been seen in more than one, sometimes closely related cats

ORGAN SYSTEMS

from the same household suggesting a potential genetic predisposition or that environmental/managemental factors may be of importance.
- Immune-mediated possibly autoimmune pathogenesis.

History and presentation
- Very variable.
- Can be insidious with gradual weight loss.
- Intermittent lethargy, fever, anorexia.
- Vomiting.
- Polyphagia in some cats.
- Signs can appear acutely – jaundice and collapse.
- Ascites associated with portal hypertension.
- Hepatomegaly.
- Mesenteric or generalised lymphadenopathy.
- Major differential is FIP as many cases will have positive coronavirus titres.

Diagnosis
- Inflammatory leucogram.
- Raised globulin.
- Increased ALT, ALKP and γ-GT.
- Hyperbilirubinaemia.
- If ascites is present, examination of abdominal fluid will enable differentiation from most other causes of ascites, but may be indistinguishable from FIP.

Imaging
- Radiography of limited value.
- Ultrasound:
  ○ Hepatomegaly ± mesenteric lymphadenopathy.
  ○ Diffuse/patchy increase in echogenicity.
  ○ Portal tracts prominent and echogenic.
  ○ Variable changes in extrahepatic bile ducts.

Liver biopsy
- Confirm diagnosis and differentiate from FIP.
- Can be difficult to distinguish severe lymphocytic disease from a mature cell lymphoma.

Management
- Immunosuppressive agents provide the basis for treatment.
  ○ Prednisolone is given initially at a daily dosage of up to 2 mg/kg q12h.
  ○ Maintain initial dose for several weeks and then gradually reduced over a period of several months.
  ○ Other immunosuppressive agents may be necessary – chlorambucil.
- Ursodeoxycholic acid – has anti-inflammatory and immunomodulatory activity as well as choleresis.
- Metronidazole may also be helpful.
- If extensive ascites is present and this is causing discomfort or distress, the distension should be relieved by abdominocentesis and diuretic (spironolactone) treatment to help minimise further accumulation of fluid.
  ○ Depending on the amount of fluid removed, IVFT may be necessary especially if there is rapid re-accumulation of the peritoneal fluid.

Prognosis
- Some cases respond well to treatment which can be completely withdrawn eventually.
- Recurrence does occur.
- Mild cases may resolve spontaneously without treatment.
- If severe cirrhosis has developed, the condition is likely to become refractory to treatment.

Lymphocytic portal hepatitis
- Lymphocytic infiltration around portal triads with less biliary involvement.

- Older cats.
- Often incidental finding in biopsies taken for GI disease.

Liver fluke
- Several species reported to infect cats (not UK).
- Usually young adult hunting cats.
- Anorexia and lethargy.
- Diagnosis of histology; faecal flotation usually unhelpful.
- Praziquantel variably successful treatment – surgical intervention often necessary.

4.4.9 Gall bladder and extrahepatic biliary duct disease

Gall bladder
- Anatomic abnormalities of the gall bladder are common in cats but rarely clinically significant.
- Common bile duct joins the major pancreatic duct before entering the duodenum.

Cholelithiasis
- Contain cholesterol, bilirubin derivatives and calcium.
- Incidental finding in many cats unless infected or obstructive.

Cholecystitis
- Inflammation of the gall bladder wall.
- Usually associated with ascending bacterial infection.
- Asymptomatic if mild → anorexia, fever, vomiting and abdominal pain.
- Low risk of rupture and bile peritonitis.
- Diagnosis by ultrasound – thickened wall.
- Treatment:
  - Antibacterials (based on culture results), IVFT, pain relief.
  - Surgical cystectomy.

Extrahepatic biliary obstruction

Cause
- Bile duct carcinoma.
- Pancreatic neoplasia, fibrosis, cyst.
- Choledocholith (stone in common bile duct).
- Inspissated bile.
- Bile duct stricture.

Clinical findings
- Anorexia, fever and weight loss.
- Vomiting.
- Jaundice.
- Acholic faeces.

Diagnosis
- Hyperbilirubinaemia.
- Elevated ALKP, γ-GT, ALT.
- Hypercholesterolaemia.
- Ultrasound:
  - Dilation and tortuous ducts of the biliary tree.
  - Gall bladder enlargement is an inconsistent finding.
  - Choledocholith cause shadowing (+ radiodense on radiography).

Treatment
- Medical management of pancreatic disease, inspissated bile.
- Surgical relief of obstruction.
  - May require biliary diversion procedures.
  - Mortality rates in sick cats undergoing biliary surgery are high (25– 50%).

4.4.10 Hepatic neoplasia
- Not a common site for primary tumours in cats (1–3%).
  - Account for 7% of non-haematopoietic tumours.
- Lymphoma occasionally affects the liver and must be differentiated from lymphocytic cholangitis.

ORGAN SYSTEMS

ORGAN SYSTEMS

• Primary hepatic lymphoma is rare in cats and other sites of lymphomatous involvement are frequently present, which may be identified on clinical investigation.
• Primary tumours more common than metastatic tumours to the liver in cats.
• Relatively benign tumours are more common than malignant tumours in cats.

Primary neoplasia

• Usually older cats (except bile duct carcinoma).
• Biliary duct adenoma (>50% of all hepatobiliary tumours in cats) and carcinoma.
  ○ Adenoma usually large before causing clinical signs.
• Hepatocellular adenoma or adenocarcinoma.
• Rare – carcinoid neuroendocrine tumours, myelolipoma and sarcomas.

Clinical findings

• Chronic debilitation – inappetence, weight loss and lethargy.
• Vomiting, PU/PD, ascites.
• Non-regenerative anaemia.
• Palpable abdominal mass.
• Jaundice.
• Elevated liver enzymes– may not be present if the mass is slow growing.
  ○ Biliary carcinoma induces ALKP production.
• Elevated bilirubin and bile acids.

Diagnosis

• Imaging particularly ultrasound.
  ○ Staging – local extension and regional metastasis.
• Biopsy and histopathology.

NB – *Not all focal spherical changes in the liver of cats are necessarily neoplastic, e.g. nodular change.*

Management

• Symptomatic and supportive.
• Surgical resection may be possible for lobar masses, e.g. hepatocellular adenoma.
• Biological activity of adenomas may be more aggressive than histologic classification.
• Response to chemotherapy and radiation therapy is poor.

4.4.11 Toxic hepatopathy

• Many causes – bacterial, fungal, plant, chemicals, drugs, heavy metals.
  ○ Drug toxicities – amiodarone, aspirin (>33 mg/kg/day), clonazepam, diazepam, diltiazem slow release, glipizide, griseofulvin, ketoconazole, methimazole, nitrofurantoin, paracetamol (120 mg/kg) (acetaminophen), stanozolol (not UK), tetracycline.
  ○ Environmental – pine oil, amanita mushrooms, aflatoxin, dry cleaning fluid, wood preservative, toluene, phenols, heavy metals, chlorinated compounds.
• Both acute and chronic hepatic injury.

Acute disease

• Severe depression and jaundice.
• Affected cat may still be in good bodily condition due to the acute nature of the problem.
• Extreme abdominal pain may be shown.
• Marked increases in liver enzymes, particularly ALT, and hyperbilirubinaemia.
• Imaging non-specific – normal-to-mild generalised hepatomegaly.
• Often hepatotoxin not determined.
• Management:
  ○ Prevention of further absorption – activated charcoal, demulcents, gastric lavage, induction of emesis.
  ○ Symptomatic and supportive, including IVFT, SAMe, alpha-tocopherol (vitamin E), antibacterial cover due to reduced reticuloendothelial activity, silymarin, nutritional support.

- If ingestion is very recent then activated charcoal or cholestyramine and warm saline enema may be helpful.
- A significant number of cases will, however, die from acute liver failure.

4.4.12 Other hepatopathies

Telangiectasis and peliosis hepatica
- Telangiectasis – dilation of hepatic sinusoids.
- Peliosis – blood-filled spaces within hepatic parenchyma.
- Can cause major intra-abdominal haemorrhage.
- Rare – Siamese may be over-represented.
- Few cases have a more chronic disease – anaemia and abdominal distension.
- Suggested link to Bartonella infection.

Amyloidosis
- Rare, usually as part of systemic amyloidosis.
- Familial in Abyssinians, Siamese, oriental shorthair, Devon rex, Burmese and DSH cats.
- May very closely mimic signs of FIP affecting the liver.
- Increased organ fragility and coagulopathy can cause catastrophic abdominal haemorrhage.
- Ultrasound – diffuse hypoechoic liver ± focal lesions associated with haematoma.
- Diagnosis on histopathology.
- Treatment is palliative immunosuppression – prednisolone ± cyclophosphamide.

Other
- Familial lipoprotein lipase deficiency.
- Hepatic toxoplasmosis.
- Biliary cysts.
- Congenital biliary atresia.

4.5 RENAL DISEASE

4.5.1 Introduction

Renal disease is particularly common in cats; it is estimated that around 16% of cats over the age of 15 years have a significant degree of CKD, making it the most common cause of death in old cats.

Functions of the kidney
- Water balance.
- Acid–base balance.
- Electrolyte balance.
- Hormonal – erythropoietin, calcitriol and renin production.
- Metabolic – activation vitamin D_3.
- Excretion of peptide hormones, e.g. gastrin.

Definitions
- *Renal insufficiency* – renal damage has occurred, but routine clinical and laboratory changes are absent; glomerular filtration rate is however normal.
- CKD – progressive loss of functional renal mass to the point that there is clinical or routine laboratory evidence of renal dysfunction.
- International renal interest society (IRIS) classifies CKD into four phases (see section 4.5.6).
- *Azotaemia* – increase in blood urea ± creatinine.
- Pre-renal (reduced perfusion).
- Renal (intrinsic renal disease).
- Post-renal (obstructive disease, rupture of bladder/urethra).
- *Uraemia* – this is the spectrum of clinical signs associated with a loss of renal function caused by a build-up of uraemic toxins together with the loss of metabolic and endocrine functions.

4.5.2 Physical examination
- Abdominal palpation to assess size, shape and position of the kidneys.
- Evidence of renal pain.
- Bladder size.
- BP.
- Other evidence of renal disease.
- Pallor – associated with anaemia and/or dehydration.

ORGAN SYSTEMS

- Dehydration.
- Halitosis associated with uraemia.
- Uraemic ulceration of the lingual or buccal mucosa.
- Loss of bone rigidity (rubber jaw).
- Ocular examination indicating hypertension.
  - Tortuous retinal vessels.
  - Retinal haemorrhage.
  - Retinal detachment.
  - Haemorrhage into the aqueous or vitreous humour.
- Coat quality and grooming.
- Body condition score.
- Muscle stiffness/pain – associated with hypokalaemia.

Differential diagnosis of renomegaly

- Physiologic.
- Hydronephrosis.
- PKD.
- FIP.
- Pyelonephritis.
- Acute nephrosis.
- Peri-renal pseudocysts.
- Amyloidosis.
- Renal neoplasia.
- Acromegaly.
- Unilateral renal agenesis.
- PSS (uncommon).

4.5.3 Laboratory investigation of renal disease

Urinalysis (also see section 3.16)

- Frequently overlooked but central to the investigation of disease.
- Preferably cystocentesis to allow culture otherwise voided (into clean litter box with aquarium gravel, polystyrene, plastic beads [e.g. Katkor]).

Physical properties

- Assess whether urine concentration is appropriate or inappropriate.

- Most normal cats have hypersthenuric urine (>1.030).
  - USG persistently below 1.025 indicates problems with urine concentrating ability.

Biochemistry

- Significant changes can occur within 30 minutes of sampling. If immediate analysis is not possible, the sample should be stored in the dark and preferably refrigerated. Any form of storage renders the presence of crystalluria unreliable.

Protein

- Ideally use UPC ratio as dipstick protein levels are not particularly accurate and are unreliable in dilute urine seen with CKD.
- Always in conjunction with sediment analysis to aid characterisation of any proteinuria as pre-renal, or renal (or post-renal if voided).
  - <0.2 – normal.
  - 0.2–0.4 – equivocal.
  - >0.4 – proteinuria.

Blood

- Need to distinguish whole red cells from haemoglobin or myoglobin.

Fractional excretion of electrolytes

- Spot measurement of the relative concentration of serum and urinary electrolytes.
- Used to assess renal tubular function.
- Accuracy is questionable, but it can be of value in investigation of specific cation abnormalities, e.g. unexplained serum hypokalaemia or hypercalcaemia.
- FE of phosphate has been used as an indicator of success in the dietary management of CKD.

Sediment analysis

Casts

- Significant numbers indicate tubular involvement.
- Absence is not a rule out for active renal tubular disease.

Urine changes in renal disease

- Cats with established CKD usually have USG in the isosthenuric range.
  - Around 40% of cats with CKD have hypersthenuric urine, rarely above 1.035.
- Marked hypersthenuria ⇒ pre-renal azotaemia.
- USG cannot be interpreted in the face of fluid loading, or following the use of diuretics.
- Proteinuria is a common feature of renal disease, but can have other causes, e.g. cystitis.
- Glycosuria occurs in around 20% of non-diabetic, sick cats, sometimes due to hyperglycaemia, but often secondary to tubular dysfunction.

Haematology

- Limited value in AKI or glomerular disease.
- Changes in CKD are non-specific but typically include.
  - Non-regenerative anaemia as a result of multiple mechanisms that can be moderate – severe in some cases and a significant cause of the presenting clinical signs.
    - Lymphopenia.
    - Leucocytosis; a mature neutrophilia sometimes found with pyelonephritis.

Biochemistry
See Section 3.7 and Table 43.

Urea

- Can be elevated due to pre- and postrenal factors, e.g. hypovolaemia, catabolic disease, GIT haemorrhage, high protein diet/recent meal, hypoadrenocorticism.
- Level can be falsely low in anorexic animals, or in the face of significant hepatic dysfunction/PSS.

Creatinine

- Can be affected by age, sex, muscle mass and diet.
- Less affected by pre-renal disease or a recent meal.
- Excreted by glomerular filtration, so rough estimate of GFR.

Protein

- Serum protein levels reflect glomerular function.
- Other proteins, besides albumin, which have important functions, e.g. ATIII or lecithin cholesterol acetyl transferase (LCAT), may also be lost.

Table 43 Typical biochemical and haematologic changes in cats with CKD with reported frequency of occurrence

Raised urea	99%	Other changes	<20%
Raised creatinine	97%	Hyper/hypocalcaemia	
Hypercholesterolaemia	73%	Hyper/hyponatraemia	
Hyperphosphataemia	64%	Hyper/hypochloraemia	
Lymphopenia	57%	Hyper/hypoalbuminaemia	
Hyperproteinaemia	49%	Hyperkalaemia	
Anaemia	37%	Hypomagnesaemia	
Hyperamylasaemia	31%	Acidosis	
Hyperglycaemia	28%		
Leucocytosis	28%		
Hypokalaemia	23%		

ORGAN SYSTEMS

Sodium and potassium
- Regulation is primarily a renal function although level also reflects dietary intake.
- A fall in the number of nephrons leads to an increase in the FE of individual nephrons, and a reduced ability to cope with changes in dietary intake.
- Hyponatraemia and hypokalaemia occur most commonly.

Calcium and phosphorus
- Reduced renal phosphate excretion leading to hyperphosphataemia.
- Causes:
  - Increased PTH production.
  - Decreased vitamin D_3 conversion.
- Calcium levels are variable in CKD reflecting the balance between intestinal absorption, bone resorption and renal excretion.
  - Correlation between total and ionised calcium is poor; measure ionised calcium where possible.

Acid–base balance
- Acidity increases with CKD.
- Proximal tubular deficits result in a failure of bicarbonate resorption causing a metabolic acidosis.

Measurement of glomerular filtration rate
A variety of techniques (exogenous creatinine, inulin, iohexol, technetium) have been developed to measure GFR in cats usually using a plasma clearance methodology. For accuracy, repeat blood samples are required limiting their use in many cats. A rough estimate of GFR can be obtained using a single time point measurement, e.g. inulin level at 180 minutes post i/v injection.

4.5.4 Imaging of the kidneys
Imaging of the kidneys primarily provides information on structure but will also give a general indication of function.

Table 44 Differential diagnosis of uni- and bilateral renomegaly

Unilateral	Bilateral
Primary renal tumour[a]	Renal lymphoma (rarely unilateral)
Compensatory hypertrophy	Acromegaly
	FIP
Peri-renal pseudocyst[a]	Acute nephritis, e.g. ethylene glycol
Hydronephrosis	PKD
Pyelonephritis	Pyelonephritis
	Hydronephrosis

[a]rarely bilateral

Radiology
- Renal size can be estimated relative to L_2.
  - $2.4–3.0 \times L_2$ in cats.
  - Differential diagnosis of renomegaly – Table 44.
- Normal renal outline is smooth and regular.
- Shrunken irregular kidneys evident in about one-third of cats with CKD on radiography.
- Normal or even enlarged kidneys do not rule out CKD.
- Changes of size and shape on plain radiographs rarely give any indication of the pathology.
- Plain radiographic changes are unusual in AKI or glomerular disease.

Intravenous urography
- Low volume rapid injection technique is the most common.
- Water soluble iodine-based contrast agents.
- Starved overnight, and faeces removed using an enema/laxative.
- 600–800 mg iodine/kg.
- Films taken at 0, 1, 5, 10, 15 and 20 minutes – VD and lateral images.

Potential side effects
- Bradycardia and hypotension.
- Tachycardia and hypertension.

- Allergy/anaphylaxis.
- Acute renal failure.
- IV haemolysis.

Renal changes seen on intravenous urography
See Table 45.

Ultrasonography
- Right and left sublumbar views with the cat in dorsal, sternal or lateral recumbency.
- Scan in longitudinal (sagittal) and cross-sectional (transverse) planes.
- Variation in the amount of fat within the kidney can cause significant changes in echogenicity.

Normal appearance
- Smooth oval or bean-shaped.
  - Reference range for renal length 30–45 mm.
- Thin echogenic capsule.
- Hypoechoic, finely granular cortex.
  - Similar echogenicity to the liver and obviously less than the spleen.
- Anechoic medulla with echogenic arcuate vessels.
- Irregular echogenic pelvis.
- A medullary rim sign can be seen in normal, especially male cats.

Pathological changes
Focal
- Renal cysts (anechoic).
- Abscesses (variable).
- Neoplasia (only if large, appearance variable – hypoechoic, homogeneous if lymphosarcoma).
- Haemorrhage (anechoic).
- Ischaemia (hypoechoic).
- Infarcts create a wedge-shaped hypoechoic (acute) to hyperechoic (chronic) region pointing towards the corticomedullary junction. Retraction of the renal surface occurs with chronicity.

Diffuse parenchymal
- Ultrasound is of limited value.
- Many cases have no obvious changes.
- Interpretation of reduction in corticomedullary definition is very subjective unless marked.
- Exceptions include:
  - Generalised enlargement in diffuse neoplasia.
  - Increased echogenicity, particularly at the corticomedullary junction with calcification.

Collecting system
- Progressive change to an anechoic area continuous with the ureter.
- Calculi are strongly echogenic.

Table 45 Interpretation of changes seen on intravenous urography

Large smooth	⇒	Inflammatory, neoplastic or amyloid infiltrate, hydronephrosis, renal cyst/abscess, hypertrophy, subcapsular urine/blood
Large irregular	⇒	Focal – tumour, abscess, cyst or haematoma Multifocal – cysts, lymphosarcoma, FIP
Normal size and shape	⇒	Normal, amyloid, glomerulonephritis or acute pyelonephritis
Normal size, irregular	⇒	Focal – infarct, inflammation, abscess or cyst Multifocal – polycystic or chronic pyelonephritis
Small smooth	⇒	Hypoplasia, amyloidosis or chronic glomerulonephritis
Small irregular	⇒	End stage, amyloidosis or infarct

ORGAN SYSTEMS

- Blood clots are hypoechoic and vary with the positioning of the cat.
- Pyelonephritis may cause minimal ultrasound changes when acute.
  - Chronic pyelonephritis leads to mild pyelectasia and hyperechogenicity of the renal crest and wall of the pelvis. Often associated changes consistent with CKD.
- Hydronephrosis – initially seen as dilation of the pelvis.
  - Mild pelvic dilation can occur with PU/PD or IVFT.

Ultrasound changes associated with CKD
- Small size.
- Irregular outline.
- Increased cortical echogenicity (present in some normal cats associated with renal fat) progressing to loss of corticomedullary definition and generalised increase in echogenicity.
- Distortion of the collecting system.
- If urea/creatinine are elevated changes would be bilateral.
- Unilateral changes suggest previous ureteric obstruction; often associated with hypertrophy of contralateral kidney.

Renal biopsy
- Consider renal aspirate if diffuse disease, e.g. lymphoma suspected.
  - May be sufficient to establish a diagnosis of ethylene glycol toxicity.
- Allows investigation of early renal disease.
- Limited value in established renal failure.
- 95% accuracy of diagnosis compared with histology results from post-mortem for diffuse lesions.
- *Diagnostic yield is poor if lesions are focal.

Indications for biopsy
- No specific diagnosis has been made.
- Morphological abnormalities have been demonstrated.
- Chronic renal proteinuria or haemorrhage.

Contraindications for biopsy
- Pyelonephritis.
- Pyonephrosis.
- Renal abscessation.
- Hydronephrosis.

Method
- Ultrasound, mini-laparotomy or laparoscopy guided wherever possible.
- General anaesthesia, avoiding renally excreted or nephrotoxic agents.
- Caudal pole of left kidney is usually the easiest target.
  - Feline kidneys are very mobile and if there is fibrosis it can be difficult to penetrate the capsule into the cortex.
- Biopsy along cortical profile (although some clinicians advocate a transmedullary approach, there is a risk of damage to arcuate artery and infarction of a renal segment as it is an end arteriole system).
- 16g Tru-cut needle.
- Withdraw and apply gentle pressure to the kidney.
- Samples should be sent for light and electron microscopy to an experienced nephropathologist using appropriate technique and transport media.

Complications
- Complication rate strongly associated with clinician experience with technique.
- Urinary tract obstruction, secondary to clot formation.
- Haemorrhage especially if hypertensive.
- Ischaemia/infarction.
- Thromboembolism.
- Precipitation of renal failure.

4.5.5 Acute kidney injury
- AKI rapid onset (hours to days) – intrinsic dysfunction.
- Usually associated with tubular necrosis, secondary to an ischaemic or toxic event as
  - Kidneys account for 0.5% of body mass but receive 20% of CO.

Table 46 Estimated survival rates depending on the cause of AKI

Category	Obstructive FLUTD	Infectious	Metabolic and haemodynamic	Other	Toxic
Survival (%)	90	80	66	50	45–70

- ○ They have high metabolic demands.
- ○ They will concentrate certain drugs and metabolites, e.g. potentiated sulphonamides, ethylene glycol.
- Prognosis for primary, intrinsic AKI is poor unless rapid aggressive treatment is instituted (see Table 46).
- It is a common, but potentially reversible, terminal event in significant numbers of sick, hospitalised cats.
- Important in oligoanuric cases to differentiate from post-renal obstruction.

Definition
- No precise definition in veterinary medicine.
  - ○ Sudden rise in urea/creatinine by >50%.
  - ○ IRIS type scheme being developed.

Risk factors
Certain patients are likely to be at increased risk of developing AKI and necessary measures should be taken prospectively to reduce this risk; risk factors are additive.
- Concurrent use of nephrotoxic drugs – NSAIDs are given to the majority of patients.
- Pre-existing renal, heart, pancreatic disease.

- Geriatric.
- Sepsis, fever, systemic disease, e.g. vasculitis, neoplasia.
- Muscular damage, e.g. trauma.
- DM.
- Hypoalbuminaemia, electrolyte and/or acid–base imbalance.
- Recent anaesthesia.
- Hypovolaemia.
- Hyperviscous states.
- Low protein diets?

Causes
Ischaemia
- Shock.
- Decreased CO.
- DIC.
- Excessive renal vasoconstriction or renal vascular disease (thrombosis).
- Hyperviscosity.
- NSAIDs.
- Deep anaesthesia.
- Transfusion reaction.
- Severe hypo-/hyperthermia.

Toxic (see Table 47)

Table 47 Potential toxins causing AKI

Therapeutic agents	Non-therapeutic
Antibacterials – aminoglycosides, sulphonamides, tetracycline, cephalosporins	Heavy metals – lead, mercury
Antifungals – amphotericin B	Organic compounds – pesticides, herbicides, ethylene glycol
Chemotherapeutic agents – doxorubicin, azathioprine,	Haemo- or myoglobin
NSAIDs (prostaglandin mediated)	Venom – bee
Intravenous contrast agents	Mushroom toxicity
Other – ACEi, cimetidine, ciclosporin, tricyclic antidepressants, penicillamine	Lilies
	Melamine adulteration of protein supplements
	Vitamin D_3 containing rodenticides
	Melamine/cyanuric acid (page 238–239)

ORGAN SYSTEMS

ORGAN SYSTEMS

Primary renal diseases
- Infectious – pyelonephritis, Leptospirosis, borreliosis.
- Immune mediated – glomerulonephritis, amyloid, SLE, vasculitis.
- Neoplasia.

Secondary to other systemic disease
- Infection – FIP, babesiosis, Leishmaniasis, bacterial endocarditis.
- Hypercalcaemia – parathyroid disease, neoplasia, vitamin D_3 analogues.
- Systemic inflammatory syndromes.
- Pancreatitis.
- Hepatorenal and cardiorenal syndromes.
- Hypertension.
- DM.

Phases of AKI
- Induction – initial insult to kidney.
- Extension – hypoxia and inflammatory response propagate damage.
- Maintenance – established damage to tubules lasting 1–3 weeks.
- Recovery – improvement of tubular function lasting weeks to months and can be associated with marked sodium loss.

  Central to the management of AKI is prompt intervention to interrupt the induction/extension phase limiting the number of nephrons that become damaged. Clinical detection is, however, difficult.

Diagnosis
- History of exposure to toxins, trauma, hypovolaemic episode, etc.
- Acute of chronic syndromes are common in cats where existing CKD decompensates.
- Distinction between acute and CKD as a cause of the azotaemia can usually be made on the basis of history, physical examination, blood, urinalysis and imaging.

- In general, AKI will lead to significant clinical signs with moderate azotaemia, potassium is typically increased, phosphate normal to mildly elevated and renal changes on ultrasound often minimal.
  - Pre-renal disease will typically result in urine of high SG unless pre-existing renal disease, sepsis, hepatic disease, recent fluid or diuretic use, (adrenal disease).

Clinical presentation
- Vomiting, anorexia, lethargy and dehydration.
- Polydipsia.
- Change in urine output – polyuria $\rightarrow$ oliguria $\rightarrow$ anuria.
- Uraemic signs – halitosis, oral ulceration, haematemesis, melaena, hypothermia, CNS depression.
- ± renal pain; ± renomegaly.

Laboratory findings
Typically:
- Azotaemia (often moderate for degree of clinical signs).
- Hyperkalaemia commonly.
- Hypokalaemia rarely (vomiting and diarrhoea, pre-existing CKD).
- Hyperphosphataemia and hypocalcaemia.
- Acidosis.
- Urine changes:
  - Sediment – presence of casts.
  - Urine biochemistry – ± alkaline urine, proteinuria, glycosuria.
  - High urinary sodium >25 mmol/l.
  - UPC ratio elevated but usually <1.0.

Imaging
- Often unhelpful – kidneys appear normal.
- Ultrasound look for
  - Evidence of nephroliths.
  - Renal pelvic dilation or pyelonephritis.
  - Evidence of pre-existing renal damage.
  - Ureteric dilation.

○ Bladder size.

○ Evidence of other underlying disease as a trigger.

Aspiration/biopsy

Value in establishing a diagnosis vs. risks of performing the procedure and the time before results are available.

Treatment

Goals

- Prevention of further renal damage – induce emesis, GI adsorbents, diuresis.
- Discontinue nephrotoxic drugs.
- Maintain renal perfusion with fluid therapy.
- Diuresis to maintain urine flow and limit rise in uraemic toxins but
  ○ Increased urine flow alone does not mean improved GFR.
  ○ Use with care if pre-renal issues.
- Correction of acid/base and electrolyte abnormalities.

NB – *electrolyte abnormalities can be associated with cellular shifts rather than absolute change and can therefore alter very rapidly.*

○ Primary correction of acidosis is rarely required if urine flow can be induced.
- Control uraemic damage to GIT – omeprazole, H_2 blockers and sucralfate.
- Control vomiting – metoclopramide (not in conjunction with dopamine), maropitant, α_2-adrenergic antagonists (with care as hypotensive), ondansetron/dolasetron.
- Antibacterial cover as uraemic patients are immunocompromised.

Failure to re-establish urine output over the first 24-hour period represents a very guarded prognosis.

Maintaining urine output

- Fluids and diuretics are the cornerstone of treatment.
- In oliguric or anuric states care must be taken to avoid over-hydration as pulmonary oedema can develop rapidly.
- Ideally fluid rates should be titrated to CVP, but this is not generally available; so an 'in and out' approach can be used.

In and out method (Box 4)

- Requires urinary catheter placed.
- Calculate the volume deficit (% dehydration – if no clinically detectable dehydration, assume 5%).
  ○ Aim to replace this over 2–4 hours with Hartman's or 0.9% NaCl.
    ▪ After rehydration, fluids lower in sodium are more appropriate, e.g. 0.45%NaCl + 2.5% dextrose.
  ○ Add 1 ml/kg/hour for insensible loss.
  ○ Add the urine output from the previous hour.
  ○ Add 2–4 ml/kg per episode of vomiting or diarrhoea.
- Regular monitoring of electrolytes, glucose and acid–base status should be undertaken.
- If urine output is not improving, safe volume expansion by 5% can be delivered.
- Aim for urine output above 1–2 ml/ hour.

Box 4

5 kg DSH with 8% dehydration (replaced over 4 hours); vomited once 5 hours after admission with a urine output of 3 ml/hour initially rising to 5 ml/hour

First 4 hours – 400 ml (deficit) + 20 ml (insensible loss) + 12 ml (urine) = 432 ml (108 ml/hour or 21 ml/kg/hour)

Hour 5 and 6 – no deficit + 10 ml (insensible loss) + 10 ml (vomit) + 10 ml (urine) = 30 ml (15 ml/hour or 3 ml/kg/hour)

ORGAN SYSTEMS

Diuretics
- Diuresis can accompany fluid loading if urine output is low.
- *Furosemide* is effective at low urine outputs within 20–60 minutes.
  - IV bolus 1–2 mg/kg q2h or
  - 2–6 mg/kg bolus followed by 0.25–1 mg/kg/hour as a CRI. This should result in increased urine output within 20–60 minutes.
  - Signs of toxicity can occur at doses of >10 mg/kg (apathy, anorexia, hypotension).
- *Mannitol* (10–20% solution)
  - 0.5 g/kg IV slow bolus over 15–20 minutes.
  - If mannitol is unavailable then 50% glucose can be used but is less effective.

NB – *Do not repeat if oliguria persists due to the osmotic effects of the mannitol which remains in the circulation.*

Renal replacement therapy
- TOC for patients that fail to respond to medical management.
  - Haemodialysis is currently not available in the UK.

Peritoneal dialysis
- Possible but is a complex.
- Expensive and time-demanding procedure that may need to be continued for days–weeks.
- Published recovery rate in cats – 5/6.

Renal transplant – unavailable in the UK.

Ethylene glycol poisoning
Relatively uncommon poisoning in the UK cats.

Prompt aggressive treatment is essential if ingestion has been documented.

If suspected ingestion has occurred, then fluid therapy and close monitoring (preferably via indwelling urinary catheter) may be sufficient.

Clinical signs
- Immediate (due to alcohol-like effects) – ataxia, incoordination, depression, tachycardia and hyperpnoea.
- Delayed signs (due to AKI) – uraemia, acidosis, anuria.
- Toxic dose requiring treatment is considered to be 0.1 ml/kg and minimum lethal dose 1.4 ml/kg of pure ethylene glycol (typical concentration in car radiators is 40–50%).

Treatment
Ethanol
- Needs to be administered within 6–12 hours of intoxication.
- 5 ml/kg q6h for five treatments then q8h for four treatments or as CRI.
- If medical alcohol unavailable use vodka.
  4-Methylpyrazole is a better alternative but not available in the UK.

Prevention
- Identify cases that are at risk and try to prevent the development of disease.
  - Low risk – no known risk factors evident.
  - Moderate risk – some risk factors present but no evidence of renal dysfunction.
  - High risk – multiple risk factors or known renal dysfunction.
- There should be a clear structured plan for monitoring urine output and an action plan should urine output start to fall.
- Better to assume that AKI is occurring and institute immediate treatment than adopting a waiting approach to see whether 'things will get better on their own'.

Melamine toxicity
- Melamine and cyanuric acid are of low toxicity separately.
- Melamine was used to adulterate protein supplements to increase the nitrogen levels.

- Manufacturing process led to cyanuric acid being produced.
- Compounds absorbed through the stomach and precipitated (re-crystallise) in the distal tubules of the kidney.
- Results in acute obstruction of the nephron and AKI.
- Renal interstitial oedema and corticomedullary haemorrhage also seen.

4.5.6 Chronic kidney disease
Recognised causes of CKD
- Chronic idiopathic interstitial nephritis (50%).
- Chronic pyelonephritis.
- Polycystic kidneys.
- Infectious – FIP/FeLV/FIV.
- Nephrotoxins.
- Renal lymphosarcoma.
- Hypercalcaemia.
- Hypokalaemia.
- Amyloidosis.
- Hydronephrosis.
- Chronic glomerulonephritis, usually membranous, resulting in nephrotic syndrome.

Presentation
Signalment
- Mid-to-old aged (though 10–15% of cases are less than 3 years old).
- Clinical signs.

Common signs
- Depression.
- Lethargy.
- Weight loss.
- Inappetence.
- PU/PD (only reported in 40% of cats).
- Dull hair coat.

Less frequent signs
- Vomiting.
- Diarrhoea.
- Blindness.

Clinical examination
Common findings
- Dehydration.
- Weight loss.
- Changes in renal size.

Less common findings
- Oral ulceration.
- Pallor.
- Pyrexia.
- Retinal changes.

Rare findings
- Renal secondary hyperparathyroidism.
- Oedema.

Laboratory changes (see Table 43)
- Management of CKD can be improved by full assessment of the haematologic, biochemical and urine changes beyond urea/creatinine increases.
  - Full urinalysis including UPC and culture.
  - Electrolytes, calcium and phosphorus.
  - Albumin.
  - Cholesterol.
  - Acid–base status.
  - PCV and erythropoietin level if PCV low.
  - CK and AST if potassium is low.
  - BP.
- Azotaemia.
- Hyperphosphataemia.
- Non-regenerative anaemia.
- Metabolic acidosis.
- Hypokalaemia.
- ± Hypocalcaemia.
- Isosthenuria with an inactive sediment.

NB – *Many cats with CKD retain some concentrating ability despite advancing azotaemia.*

Differential diagnosis
- Hyperthyroidism.
- Sepsis.

ORGAN SYSTEMS

Table 48 Distinguishing AKI from CKD

	AKI	CKD
Azotaemia	Rapidly progressive signs with moderate azotaemia	Stable/slowly progressive signs with marked azotaemia
Onset	Rapid	Insidious
Serum potassium	Tend to be hyperkalaemic	Tend to be hypokalaemic
PCV	Normal to mildly increased	Often low – non-regenerative
Previous PU/PD	No	Noted in 40% of cases
Weight loss	No	Yes
Osteodystrophy	No	Yes
Kidney palpation	Normal to large, may be painful	Tend to be small, irregular and non painful
Urine sediment	Casts commonly found	Usually inactive unless UTI
Biopsy	May be helpful	Rarely helpful

- DM.
- AKI (Table 48).
  - Most difficult to differentiate acute on chronic disease.
- Alimentary lymphosarcoma.
- Other neoplasia.
- IBD.
- Hypoadrenocorticism (rare in cats).

IRIS classification (Table 49)

- IRIS disease stage classification facilitates appropriate monitoring and therapy.
- Staging is based initially on fasting plasma creatinine in normovolaemic cats with stable disease.
- Note that creatinine value is irrespective of laboratory reference range, as cats in the upper reference range often have excretory failure and this extends into the mid-range in very thin patients.
- IRIS staging is subdivided according to the presence of
  - Proteinuria (non- (NP), borderline- (BP) and proteinuric (P)).
  - Persistent hypertension (see Table 49).
  - Evidence of end organ damage, coded as: nc – no complications; c – complications (end organ damage); RND – risk not determined.

Management

- Degree of compromise of the various renal functions will be different.
- Prioritise important problems that need treating.
- Consider how long-term management will work.
- Some problems will only require short-term treatment, e.g. nausea may need initial drug therapy, but will be controlled in the long term by reducing uraemia.
- Essential that the client understands that the treatment is aimed at managing their cat's disease, and will need to be lifelong.
- Appetite will tend to improve with a fall in uraemic toxins, which should enhance the acceptance of dietary changes.
- Dietary change as a part of intensive treatment may be inadvisable, as renal diets tend to be less palatable, and there is a risk of learned food aversion developing.
- Long-term dietary management is of paramount importance.

Options
- Correction of hydration and acid–base status.
- Reduction of hyperphosphataemia.

Table 49 IRIS classification for CKD based on creatinine and blood pressure measurements

Stage	Plasma creatinine (μmol/l)	Comments
1	<140	Non-azotaemic. Kidney abnormal based on urine concentration, palpation, proteinuria or biopsy
2	140–249	Mild renal azotaemia – clinical signs usually mild or absent
3	250–439	Moderate renal azotaemia – many systemic clinical signs may be present
4	>440	Severe renal azotaemia – many extra-renal signs present

Systolic BP (mm Hg)	Diastolic BP (mm Hg)	Substage risk
<150	<95	Minimal (N)
150–159	95–99	Low (L)
160–179	100–119	Moderate (M)
≥180	≥120	High (H)

ORGAN SYSTEMS

- Dietary protein restriction.
- Correction of potassium balance.
- Management of nausea and vomiting.
- Reduction in hypertension.
- Management of non-regenerative anaemia.
- Management of hypocalcaemia.
- Antibacterial therapy.
- Correction of hypernatraemia.
- Vitamins B and C supplementation.

Principles of dietary management
- Diet can have a significant effect in reducing medication requirements and significantly increase survival.
- In general, canned diets are preferred to dry diets and tend to be
  - Significantly higher in water content;
  - More palatable;
  - Provide calories through fats rather than carbohydrates.
- A significant number of cats will not tolerate such dietary modification.

- Dietary modification is best initiated in the owner's home once urgent medical needs have been addressed, e.g. dehydration, ulceration.
- Muscle metabolism has an important role in nitrogen homeostasis, hence the maintenance of body weight is important as it maximises non-renal management of nitrogenous waste.
- If the ideal cannot be achieved, the recommendations below provide the basic aims for dietary modification.

  It is vital that something is eaten, as body protein catabolism will have more serious adverse effects than almost any diet.

When to start dietary management?
- Opinions differ as to the best time to start dietary management.
- The value of dietary management in early stage 2 disease is not proven.
- Most cats require dietary intervention from late stage 2 onwards.

Rationale for dietary phosphorus restriction

- Hyperphosphataemia has been correlated with the progression of renal disease.
- Phosphate restriction has been shown to blunt renal secondary hyperparathyroidism and reduce the level of PTH (implicated as an important uraemic toxin).
- Phosphate restriction reduces mortality and improves well-being, but hyperphosphataemia can persist in the face of dietary restriction, so oral phosphate binders should be administered with food.

Oral phosphate binders

- Lanthanum carbonate (Renalzin) – 0.5 ml/day divided between meals.
- Aluminium hydroxide – 20–40 mg/kg PO q12h (available as liquid or tablets).
- Chitin-based products, e.g. ipakitine – have limited ability to reduce plasma phosphate.

Protein restriction

NB – *A fall in serum urea level associated with dietary protein restriction does not represent improved renal function, but is a reflection of the change in nitrogen balance.*

- Excessive protein restriction can have serious negative consequences leading to weight loss, hypoalbuminaemia, anaemia and metabolic acidosis.
- Balanced high protein diets do not lead to renal failure in cats.
- There is no clear evidence that feeding high protein diets in cats with renal failure leads to progression.
- There is some evidence to suggest that protein restriction may slow the rate of clinical deterioration in cats by controlling uraemia, thereby increasing their life expectancy by delaying the decision for euthanasia.

- Optimal protein requirements of uraemic cats are currently unknown.
- It is generally recommended that protein should be restricted to approximately 20% of the total calorie intake.
- Lowering protein is a practical way of reducing dietary intake.
- Low protein diets are less palatable to cats, but a higher fat content or increased flavouring (e.g. tuna juice, chicken broth) may help.
- Short-term use of appetite stimulants may be beneficial when a low-protein diet is being introduced.

Management strategy based on IRIS classification (see Table 50)

Management of acidosis

- Most renal diets are alkalinising in their action, and supplementation without measuring acid–base status is potentially dangerous.
- Metabolic acidosis may contribute to nausea, vomiting, lethargy, weakness, muscular wasting and weight.
- Chronically, acidosis may also promote the progression of renal failure.

Potassium citrate – 75 mg/kg q12h initially then adjust dose to maintain TCO_2 at 18–24 mmol/l.

Sodium bicarbonate – 8–12 mg/k q8h PO and adjust dose to TCO_2 as above.

Fatty acid supplementation

- Increased PUFA may lower the elevated cholesterol levels frequently seen in cats with CKD.
  - Reduced cholesterol levels have been associated with the preservation of renal function in dogs with experimental renal disease.
- Over-supplementation of diets with PUFA may increase renal damage associated with lipid peroxidation.

Table 50 IRIS recommendations for the management of according to CKD stage

Stage	Treatment
1	Discontinue any nephrotoxic drugs and rule-out treatable underlying disease, e.g. pyelonephritis Correct dehydration and other pre- and postrenal causes Treat hypertension if end organ damage otherwise monitor UPC >2.0: full investigation including renal biopsy, consider ACEi and aspirin/clopidogrel UPC 1.0–2.0: requires thorough investigation and close monitoring UPC 0.4–1.0: requires close monitoring
2	Treat as for stage I disease with additional treatment for proteinuria if UPC >0.4(C) Manage phosphate levels to between 0.9 and 1.45 mmol/l Consider dietary management even if phosphate within the range as hyperparathyroidism common Treat acidosis (blood bicarbonate or total CO_2 <16 mmol/l) with sodium bicarbonate/potassium citrate Potassium gluconate, if hypokalaemic
3	Treat as stage 2, target phosphate below 1.6 mmol/l Treat anaemia, if affecting quality of life (darbepoetin or erythropoietin, transfusion) Manage nausea/vomiting (antacids, mucosal protectants, anti-emetics) Maintain hydration with parenteral fluids if necessary
4	As stage 3, target phosphate below 1.9 mmol/l Intensify efforts to maintain body weight, nitrogen balance and hydration Consider chronic s/c fluid or PEG feeding Benefit of low dose calcitriol unproven in cats

ORGAN SYSTEMS

- Benefits over risks of increasing PUFA levels in the diets of cats with CKD have not been established.
- Omega-3 is thought to be more beneficial.
  - Prostaglandin and thromboxane-mediated effects on decreasing systemic hypertension and increasing renal blood flow.

Dietary fibre
- Reduced ability of the kidneys to excrete nitrogenous waste can be ameliorated by increasing the levels of fermentable fibre in the diet.
- Increase nitrogen in the faeces by around 10%.

- Increase in fibre is at the expense of digestibility, and may also reduce palatability.

Management of hypokalaemia
- Cats with CKD often waste potassium in the urine in order to conserve sodium and maintain hydration.
- Potassium wastage is further exacerbated by acidosis.
- Hypokalaemia may increase renal ammoniagenesis causing further damage to the kidneys.
- Hypokalaemia causes an inflammatory myopathy which is seen initially as a stiff, stilted gait (often put down to arthritis in old cats) and a poor hair coat.

- More extreme hypokalaemia presents as muscle weakness and ventroflexion of the neck.

When to start supplementation?

- Routine supplementation of all cats with CKD is not widely advocated.
- Generally supplementation is started when low serum potassium is demonstrated.

NB – *Serum potassium is a poor reflection of whole body potassium status, hence some cats that would benefit from supplementation, as they are whole body deficient, but are managing to maintain normal serum potassium, may be overlooked.*

What to use?

- Potassium gluconate is most commonly used as it is more readily accepted by cats.
- Potassium citrate can be used in cats that are acidotic as it is alkalinising.
- Potassium chloride should be avoided as it is very acidic and unpalatable.
- Supplementation rates will vary according to the individual, but are generally around 2–4 mmol (mEq) K^+/cat/day.

Management of hypocalcaemia

- In order to maintain a suitable calcium:phosphorus balance, most diets designed for the treatment of CKD have lower calcium.
- Hypocalcaemia is usually associated with hyperphosphataemia; hence, reduction in serum phosphate levels will naturally tend towards correcting the hypocalcaemia through reduced PTH levels.
- The value of ultra-low dose calcitriol unproven but increasingly being used where diet and phosphate binders is failing to control phosphate levels.

Management of hypernatraemia and hypertension

- Lowering dietary salt to reduce BP is unproven; if attempted it should be undertaken slowly as reduced renal adaption in CKD.
  - The risks of salt restriction have not been critically evaluated in cats with CKD as there is the potential for promoting pre-renal azotaemia as well as reducing palatability.
  - Enhanced omega-3:omega-6 fatty acid ratio may help to reduce hypertension.
- Cats with moderate–to-severe hypertension should be treated with
  - Amlodipine (0.625–1.25 mg/cat q12–24h).
  - If hypertension persists consider ACE inhibitors.

Vitamin supplementation

- Higher requirement for water-soluble vitamins (B and C) due to the increased turnover of water.
- Levels of supplementation tend to be increased in commercial diets. If such diets are not used then oral supplementation is appropriate.
- Care should be taken if a vitamin/mineral preparation is used, as many contain significant levels of calcium and phosphorus that may be undesirable.

Appetite stimulation

- May be appropriate in the initial management of disease.
- Mirtazapine is currently the drug of choice (3.75 mg/cat q48–72h).
  - Alternatives are cyproheptadine or benzodiazepines.
- There is little evidence that anabolic steroids or vitamin B_{12} are effective.
- Corticosteroids and progestogens are contraindicated.

Use of ACEi in the management of CKD

- Studies in man and dogs have suggested that ACEi use may ameliorate some of the effects of CKD.
- Some supporting evidence in cats.
- Most effective in the management of proteinuria.
  - Proteinuria can lead to renal inflammation and fibrosis, sodium retention, oedema, ascites, hypercholesterolaemia (nephrotic syndrome), hypertension, hypercoagulability, muscle wasting and weight loss.
- ACEi are indicated in cats with known proteinuria and/or hypertension.
- ACEi should be used with care in other forms of CKD.
  - Benazepril is licensed for the management of renal disease in cats.

Unresolved issues

- Is there a benefit only in cases with significant proteinuria?
- What is the optimal dose?
- When should therapy start?
- What are the potential risks associated with the use of hypotensive agents in normotensive animal – could this worsen pre-renal disease?

Pyelonephritis

- Similar organisms to those causing lower urinary tract infections.
- Requires long-term antimicrobial treatment preferably based on culture and sensitivity.
  - If culture negative, then empirical choices include fluoroquinolones and cephalosporins.

Acute

- Uncommon.
- Pain on palpation of kidneys, mainly present as apparent back pain when the cat is being stroked.

- Mild renomegaly.
- Pyrexia, lethargy, depression, inappetence.
- Urine culture is usually positive.
- Treat with fluids, opiate pain relief and, initially IV antibacterials.

Chronic

- Often no overt clinical signs.
- May be a significant cause of CKD in cats.
- Hyperechoic renal pelvis or pylectasia on ultrasound.
- Urine culture may be negative.

4.5.7 Glomerular disease

- Membranous glomerulonephropathy most common form described in cats.
  - Thickened glomerular basement membrane with little or no cellular infiltrate.
- Other forms are rare:
  - Amyloidosis.
  - Glomerulosclerosis.
  - Glomerulonephritis.
  - IgA nephropathy.
  - Hereditary nephritis.
  - Lupus nephritis.
  - Minimal change glomerulonephropathy.

Diseases associated with glomerular disease

- Chronic bacterial infection.
- Mycoplasma polyarthritis.
- FIV, FIP and FeLV.
- Pancreatitis.
- Inflammatory liver disease.
- Immune-mediated disease – polyarthritis, SLE.
- Neoplasia – lymphoma, leukaemia, mastocytosis.
- Acromegaly.
- Familial.
- Idiopathic.

ORGAN SYSTEMS

ORGAN SYSTEMS

Clinical presentation
- Asymptomatic proteinuria (See Section 3.16 for causes of proteinuria).
- Nephrotic syndrome.
- CKD (rarely AKI) secondary to glomerular disease.

Protein-losing nephropathy
- Continued protein loss leads eventually to nephrotic syndrome.

Nephrotic syndrome
- Proteinuria leading to hypoalbuminaemia
- Reduced oncotic pressure eventually causing ascites/oedema (albumin <10–15 g/l).
- Worsened by RAAS activation, expanding plasma volume and further dilution of proteins.
  - Diuretics can potentially make the ascites worse by causing increased urine output (and therefore increasing protein loss) together with further RAAS activation.

Clinical presentation
- Usually young to middle-aged adults.
- Common clinical signs.
  - Ventral oedema/ascites.
  - ± Anorexia and weight loss.
  - ± Poor coat, lethargy.
  - ± Polydipsia.
  - ± Azotaemia and uraemia.
  - Often insidious onset.
- May be hypercoagulable (due to renal loss of ATIII), so signs related to thromboembolism such as dyspnoea.

Diagnosis
- Oedema and ascites – fluid is a pure transudate.
- Hypoalbuminaemia.
- UPC usually >3; USG may be normal.
- ± Hypercholesterolaemia.
- ± Azotaemia.

- ± Hyaline urine casts.
- ± Evidence of hypertensive disease.

NB – *Cats with nephrotic syndrome may NOT be azotaemic.*

Management
- Look for and treat underlying cause wherever possible, renal biopsy may be appropriate.
- Use of natriuretic diuretics, e.g. furosemide in conjunction with a low salt diet, only if ascites is a clinical problem.
- ACE inhibitors.
- Corticosteroids – controversial, may promote urine protein loss and hypertension.
- Anticoagulants – warfarin, heparin or aspirin, clopidogrel.

NB – *Heparin may be ineffective due to the loss of ATIII.*

Prognosis
Asymptomatic
- Good (i.e. proteinuria without ascites/oedema, significant hypoproteinaemia or azotaemia).

Symptomatic
- Variable and difficult to predict.
- Remission between episodes may be prolonged and spontaneous.
- Some progress to CKD.
- If CKD is advanced at presentation, prognosis is poor.

Further tests
- Urine protein electrophoresis.
- Assay of specific proteins, e.g. lysozyme, ribonuclease in tubular loss.
- Urinary γ-GT as indicator of acute tubular damage released by the brush border.

Amyloidosis
- Usually cats over 5 years of age.
- Extracellular deposition of beta-pleated sheet protein.

- Cases in cats due to secondary (reactive) deposition of amino-terminal of acute-phase reactant serum amyloid A protein (SAA).
  - SAA is released by macrophages following injury.
  - Normally removed by proteases.
  - Chronic inflammation may inhibit these proteases, e.g. antitrypsin.
  - Reported in FIV positive cats.

Treatment options
- Focus on limiting the effects of hypoproteinaemia and the management of CKD.
- ACE inhibitors.
- Dimethyl sulphoxide (DMSO) – efficacy is unknown in cats.
- Colchicine – 0.02–0.04 mg/kg q24h PO – efficacy is unknown in cats.
  - Once the disease has progressed to the plateau phase, DMSO and colchicine are ineffective.

4.5.8 Renal neoplasia
- Primary renal neoplasia is relatively uncommon.
- Represent around 1% of neoplasms.
- Over 90% are malignant.
- Metastatic spread to the kidneys is more frequently encountered.
- Polycythaemia is the most commonly reported paraneoplastic syndrome.

Clinical signs
- Weight loss and haematuria.
- Palpable abdominal mass.
- Signs of CKD – suggests bilateral renal involvement or pre-existing renal disease.

Renal lymphoma
- Most common tumour in cats with bilateral renomegaly and CKD.
- FIV positive cats predisposed.
- High prevalence of spread to CNS.
- Treatment with standard chemotherapy protocols.

Renal cell carcinoma
- Rare.
- Management – survival following nephrectomy is 8 months, but there is high perioperative mortality.

Other renal tumours
- Renal transitional cell carcinoma.
- Renal SCC.
- Sarcoma – leiomyosarcoma, haemangiosarcoma.
- Renal adenoma/papilloma.
- Nephroblastoma.
  - Embryologic tumour with 60% of cases reported at <1 year.

4.5.9 Familial renal disease
- Juvenile nephropathy covers conditions affecting young cats that may or may not be heritable.
- Glomerular and non-glomerular pathology is equally common in cats <3 years.

Unilateral agenesis
- Relatively common in cats.

Renal hypoplasia and dysplasia
- Rare.
- Hypoplasia – all small kidneys regardless of aetiology. Usually occurs due to loss of nephrons and fibrosis or severe pyelonephritis.
- Dysplasia – disorganised development due to abnormal differentiation.

Polycystic kidney disease
- Multiple cysts replacing normal renal tissue.
- Very prevalent in Persian and exotics (around 45% of cats affected).
- Autosomal dominant.
- Genetic screening programme available.
- Varying severity with progressive cystic enlargement.
- Eventually leading to renal failure ± abdominal swelling.
  - Cause of renal failure in kittens or young adult cats.

ORGAN SYSTEMS

ORGAN SYSTEMS

- Diagnosis on ultrasound or IVU.
- Prognosis poor once clinical signs are seen.

Renal tubular defects
- Uncommon, congenital or acquired disease.
- Fanconi's syndrome.
- Nephrogenic DI (see endocrine disease).

Renal tubular acidosis
- Associated with
  - An inability to excrete H^+ ions into the urine.
  - An inability to reabsorb HCO_3^- from the filtrate into the tubule.

Cysts
Renal
- Dilated nephron segments, some of which are small and non-progressive.
- Others progressively enlarge eventually causing symptoms associated with CKD.
- Diagnosis based on repeat ultrasound examination.

Peri-renal pseudocysts
- Associated with abdominal distension, PU/PD and weight loss.
- 75% of cases concurrent CKD.
- Non-epithelial lined causing a separation between the kidney parenchyma and capsule.
- Contains serum, urine or blood.
- Diagnosis on ultrasound.
- Management with drainage if required – sterile technique vital.

4.5.10 Ureteric disease
- Most commonly reported is damage to the ureter during spaying.

Ectopic ureters
- Very uncommon.
- May be clinically silent.

- Urinary incontinence.
- Perineal scalding.
- Excessive washing of perineal area.
- May appear to urinate normally if unilateral.

Diagnosis
- IV urography.

Treatment
- Surgical relocation.

Ureteroliths
- Acute ureteral obstruction is an emerging syndrome in cats.
- Most common cause is nephroliths moving into and obstructing the ureter.
  - Other causes include stricture, trauma, mural or retroperitoneal neoplasia or non-mineralised material.
- Median age is 6 months.
- Most commonly clinical signs become evident when a previous episode has rendered one kidney dysfunctional (that becomes shrunken and fibrotic) and then a second ureterolith blocks the ureter of the functional kidney resulting in hydronephrosis and acute uraemia – 'big kidney–little kidney' syndrome.
- Clinical presentation is is of AKI.
- Abdominal discomfort is variable and 'renal colic' seen in man is rare.
- Definitive diagnosis is with imaging.

Management
- Medical – cautious IVFT and diuresis may dislodge the ureteroliths in 20% of cases.
  - Amitriptyline (1 mg/kg PO q24h) acting as a smooth muscle relaxant may improve success rates.
- Surgery – variety of techniques possible but small size of the feline ureter makes surgery technically demanding.
- Catheter-based techniques and lithotripsy are also available in a few centres.

Prognosis
- Depends on
  - Speed and success of intervention.
  - Degree of obstruction – partial vs. complete.
  - Availability of haemodialysis.
- As the cause of calcium oxalate nephrolith formation is usually difficult to treat recurrences will occur.

4.6 LOWER URINARY TRACT DISEASE

4.6.1 Introduction
- LUTD is a common presenting problem.
- Distressing and frustrating condition both for the cat and the owner.
- Clinical presentation is usually typical for LUTD.
- Treatment of FLUTD can be a challenge.
- In recurrent idiopathic cases it is important to emphasise that a multimodal approach is likely to be necessary and that the aim is towards control (reducing frequency and severity of episodes) rather than cure.

Definitions
- See dysuria and haematuria in Section 2.16 and 2.21.

  Additional definitions
- *Periuria* – inappropriate urination.

4.6.2 Clinical signs and diagnosis
Non-obstructed disease
- Typical clinical signs of cats with non-obstructed LUTD are well recognised:
  - Acute onset.
  - Restlessness.
  - Vocalisation.
  - Inappetence.
  - Lethargy.
  - Frequently asking to be let out, visiting the litter tray, urinating in the house (periuria).
  - Squatting and straining tending to produce small amounts of blood-stained urine often with mucus (dysuria, stranguria).
  - Rarely significant systemic signs.

  BUT the clinical dilemma is whether these signs could be associated with urethral obstruction.

Obstructed disease
- Initial clinical signs are similar.
- Squatting and straining.
- In some cases small volumes of urine are produced, in others the straining is unproductive.
- Unless the obstruction is relieved, cats quickly become systemically unwell.
- Some cats will stop attempting to urinate.
- Become very quiet, lethargic and inappetent.
- Temporary improvement may be associated with bladder rupture.
- Increasing numbers of cases do not have a physical obstruction but urethrospasm.

Predisposing factors
- Young to middle-aged.
- Persian and long-haired cats; Siamese at reduced risk.
- Male and female cats are equally affected with non-obstructive disease.
- Obstructive disease is more common in male cats.
- Obesity.
- Sedentary lifestyle and reduced urinary frequency.
- Low urinary output (usually associated with a dry diet).
- 'Stressors' – recent house moves, multi-cat household, rainy winter days, less freedom.
- Nervous, aggressive, fearful personality.
- Nutrition – feeding dry cat food (some studies), low fluid intake, portion feeding.
- Owner observed GI signs.

ORGAN SYSTEMS

Diagnosis

Non-urinary diseases causing similar clinical signs

- Few non-urinary conditions present with similar clinical signs, but the following should be considered:
  - Behavioural – urination in inappropriate sites (distinguish from urge incontinence by history and observation).
  - Colitis.
  - Reproductive tract disease.
  - Lumbar neuromusculoskeletal problems.
  - Anal gland infection/abscessation.

Causes of FLUTD

- Relative frequency of the various underlying causes of LUTD in cats is markedly different from dogs (and man).
- In a significant percentage of cases the underlying cause is not apparent; these cases have been variously called FUS (feline urologic syndrome), idiopathic FLUTD, and FIC – feline idiopathic cystitis or feline interstitial cystitis.
- A number of case series have looked at prevalence of various diagnoses; there is a relatively large range in some conditions but this often reflects the population studied and/or geographic region (Table 51).

Differential diagnosis

- Idiopathic.
- Obstructive:
  - Physical obstruction – urolithiasis, urethral plug, neoplasia (very rare).
  - Urethrospasm.

  - Urethral stricture:
    - Post catheterisation.
    - Post urethrostomy.
  - Urethritis (rare).
- Trauma:
  - LMN damage.
  - UMN damage.
  - Urethral rupture.
  - Bladder rupture.
  - Bladder displacement through body wall tear.
  - Foreign body.
- Reflex dyssynergia (<0.1%).
- Compression from prostate or uterus.
- Inflammatory:
  - Infectious – bacteria, *Candida*, *Capillaria feliscati*, (viral) (1%).
  - Chemical – cyclophosphamide, Walpole's solution.
  - Immune-mediated – granulomatous urethritis, role in FLUTD.
- Anatomic (10%):
  - Urachal anomalies.
  - Ureterocoele.
  - Phimosis, paraphimosis.
- Neoplastic:
  - Transitional cell carcinoma.
  - SCC.
  - Adenocarcinoma.
  - Leiomyoma, leiomyosarcoma.
  - Haemangiosarcoma.

Key history

- Age, breed, sex of cat.
- Is the cat neutered – recent oestrous or parturition?
- Current and recent diets.
- Have there been recent changes in household or other stressors?

Table 51 Published prevalence figures for various causes of FLUTD

iFLUTD	Urethral obstruction	Urethral plug	Uroliths	Behavioural	Incontinence	UTI	Anatomic	Neoplasia
55–64%	19–58%	10–21%	12–22%	0–9%	0–4%	1–15%	0–11%	0–2%

- People, pets, visitors, trips to the vet, building work, etc.
- How much is the cat drinking?
- How many times is the cat passing urine and what volume is being produced?
- Where is the cat urinating – all over the house or in a few specific places?
- Is the cat showing other signs of change in behaviour?
- Is the cat defecating inappropriately?
- Previous history of similar clinical signs.
- What clinical signs are being shown?
- Is the cat systemically unwell?
- Duration of clinical signs?
- History or evidence of trauma?
- History or evidence of exposure to toxins?
- If haematuria is present.
  - When does the blood appear during urination?
  - Is blood present every time the cat urinates – is it only associated with urination?
  - Has there been haemorrhage from any other sites – what colour are the faeces?

Physical examination
- Usually unrewarding, but is essential to establish whether there is urethral obstruction.
- Always examine the preputial and vulval area.
  - Look for evidence of excessive grooming.
- Where the bladder is small, thickening of the wall can sometimes be appreciated.
  - When the bladder is palpated are there reflex attempts to micturate indicating significant irritation to the bladder wall.
- In cases with significant haematuria; consider the possibility of a coagulopathy.

NB1 – *If the bladder cannot be palpated it is essential to rule out the possibility of rupture.*

NB2 – *An overfull bladder can also be associated with neurogenic disease.*

4.6.3 Laboratory investigation

Urinalysis (see Section 3.16)
- Essential diagnostic information.
- Full urinalysis including sediment analysis, UPC and culture for recurrent cases.

Urine collection
- Free-catch samples are notoriously difficult – consider a litter tray filled with fish-tank gravel, polystyrene packing or co-polymeric beads (e.g. Katkor), which is non-absorbent and sterile.
- Cystocentesis may be necessary as it
  - Saves cats having to be caged for long periods waiting for micturation to occur.
  - Allows culture results to be easily interpreted.
  - Is not influenced by disease of the urethra, vagina, vulva or prepuce.
- In acute/severe disease the collection of urine may be virtually impossible due to the frequency with which the cat is urinating resulting in the bladder being permanently empty.
- In some cats, palpating the bladder (prior to cystocentesis) will induce urination, so a collection dish should be available!

Technique for cystocentesis
- Quick, simple and minimally invasive procedure.
- Preferably with ultrasound guidance.
- 23 gauge/1 inch needle; 5–10 ml syringe.
- Standard position is dorsal recumbency with the bladder identified and stabilised, the needle introduced in the midline and directed caudodorsally.
  - There is a small risk of trauma to the aorta especially if ultrasound is not used; the bladder is small and the patient uncooperative and wriggly.

ORGAN SYSTEMS

- In many cases, cats tolerate a lateral approach better, with the cat standing or in lateral recumbency. The bladder is again identified and stabilised, and the needle directed caudomedially.

Routine haematology and biochemistry
- Generally unhelpful.
- May be necessary in order to
  ○ Exclude other causes (coagulation profile, renal/hepatic function).
  ○ Evaluate the degree of blood loss.
  ○ Explore the possibility of intercurrent disease (FIV/FeLV).
  ○ Assess metabolic consequences of obstructive disease.

4.6.4 Imaging of the lower urinary tract
Radiography
Plain
- Sedation usually sufficient.
- Mid-caudal abdomen.
- Legs pulled caudally.
- Minimise exposure time, avoid grid.
- Centre midway between the last rib and pelvic brim.
- Collimate to caudal two-thirds of abdomen.
  ○ Include the urethra in the radiographic field.
- Lateral view is usually the most informative.
- A VD view can give further information, particularly about the pelvis.

Check for
- Size, shape, position.
- Definition of outline of bladder and associated structures.
- Radio-opaque or lucent areas within the bladder.
- Sublumbar lymph node enlargement.
  ○ Urethra (not usually visible).

Contrast
- Allows more detailed evaluation of bladder wall, lumen and urethra.
- Both positive and negative (pneumocystogram) can be performed.
- Most information will generally be provided by a double contrast urethrocystogram.
- General anaesthesia is required in order to produce high-quality images.
- Lateral and VD views are mandatory.

Technique
- Plain radiographs first.
- Enema to remove faeces from descending colon.
- Introduce a urinary catheter (for female cats a 4FG Jackson catheter can be introduced blindly, taking care to remain in the midline and directing the tip of the catheter ventrally).
- Remove all urine from the bladder – save for urinalysis if not already performed.

Urethrography
Male cats
- Withdraw the catheter slowly and smoothly whilst injecting a few millilitres of contrast.
- The radiograph is taken just as the last few centimetres of the catheter are being withdrawn from the urethra.
- Water-soluble, iodinated contrast media are ideal – take care not to introduce air bubbles.
- If a filling defect or narrowing is seen the procedure should be repeated to make sure the change is consistent.

Female cats
- Vaginourethrography is the easiest technique.
- The catheter is withdrawn from the urethra to lie 1–2 cm within the vagina.

- The vulval lips will need to be clamped (tongue clamp, Allis tissue forceps).
- 1 ml/kg of contrast media is injected with the radiograph being taken just as the injection is being completed.

Cystography

- Following urethrography, more positive contrast can be introduced into the bladder, if required, until it is moderately distended (10–30 ml) and further radiographs taken.
- In many cases, this yields little further information, and a double contrast study can follow the urethrography.
- The majority of the contrast is removed and the bladder filled with air until it is moderately turgid.
- Injection should be made smoothly to prevent introducing air bubbles into the contrast media.
- Following insufflation, lateral and VD radiographs can be obtained and the bladder then deflated.

Ultrasound

- For the majority of cases this is the imaging of first choice as it does not generally require chemical restraint and provided more information than plain radiographs as it allows the bladder wall to be evaluated.
- Only the very proximal urethra can be evaluated unless it is abnormal.
- The entire bladder should be imaged in longitudinal and transverse planes.

Check

- Size, shape, position.
- Thickness and regularity of wall (can be difficult if the bladder has little urine inside).
- Material within the lumen.
  - Clots – similar to less echogenic than soft tissue may be adherent to the bladder wall.
  - Debris – usually echogenic and swirl on ballottement of the bladder.
  - Calculi – usually very echogenic with acoustic shadowing.
  - Masses – similar echogenicity to soft tissue, adherent to wall.
- Ureteric openings.
  - Ureteric jets can be seen in a cooperative patient using a high frequency probe especially if urine output is increased with a single injection of furosemide.
- Prostate, cannot be imaged transabdominally.

Cystoscopy

- Most applicable in female cats.
- Valuable technique to evaluate the mucosal surface of the bladder.
- Allows directed biopsies to be obtained.
- Direct view of ureters.
- 2.4 mm rigid arthroscope with sheath is appropriate for female cats.
- Limited availability of equipment for male cats – vision only.

Biopsy

Ultrasound guided aspirate

- Bladder masses can be easily aspirated.
  - There is a small risk in neoplastic disease of the tumour tracking along the needle path.
- Aspiration of a thickened bladder wall often does not deliver diagnostic quality samples.

Catheter

- Superficial samples of the mucosal surface can be obtained by placing a catheter into the bladder and applying negative pressure sucking the mucosal surface into the fenestrations of the catheter.
- Diagnostically valuable in focal, superficial lesions, but may require ultrasound to direct the catheter tip to the lesion.
- More successful in female cats, as a larger bore catheter can be used.

ORGAN SYSTEMS

Cystoscopic
- Small (1 mm) superficial biopsies can be obtained.

Laparotomy/laparoscopy
- Allows full thickness biopsies to be obtained.
- Value can be limited if diffuse, interstitial cystitis is likely to be the cause.
- Most likely to yield useful information in cases in which a focal lesion has been identified.

4.6.5 Managing the obstructed cat
- Medical emergency.
- Will die from acid–base and electrolyte disturbance.
- In UK cats, urethrospasm is more likely than urolithiasis or urethral plugs to be causing the obstruction.
- Stepwise approach.
- Place IV catheter.
- Obtain baseline blood – minimum PCV, total solids, electrolytes, urea and glucose ± calcium.
- ECG if arrhythmia.
- Start fluid therapy according to bloods.
- Relieve bladder distension – cystocentesis or catheter.
- Sedation or anaesthesia may be required.
- Post-obstructional diuresis will occur and potassium can fall dramatically.
- Maintain urinary catheter for 3–10 days.
- Start therapy directed at underlying disease process.

Cystocentesis
- Provides immediate decompression.
- Use a 22 gauge needle connected via a flexible extension tube to a 60 ml syringe (minimises the risk of bladder laceration if the cat moves).
- If the bladder is severely distended the needle should be introduced as smoothly as possible to reduce the risk of bladder rupture.

- Complete drainage is unnecessary and increases the risk of iatrogenic damage.

Biochemistry
- Metabolic changes secondary to lower urinary tract obstruction can be life-threatening, particularly hyperkalaemia and acid–base disturbances.

NB – *The effects of hyperkalaemia are worsened by low calcium/sodium or acidaemia.*

- ECG:
  - If facilities for measuring potassium are unavailable, ECG changes can provide useful diagnostic information.
  - ECG changes rarely occur until the potassium is significantly raised (>6.5 mmol/l), but depends on both the absolute value and rate of increase (see Box 5) and are not present in all cases.

Box 5 ECG changes accompanying hyperkalaemia	
5.5 mmol/l	Slowing of heart rate, peak T wave, shortened QRS
6.5–7.5 mmol/l	Widened QRS complexes, small R waves
7.0–8.5 mmol/l	Small but wide P waves, increased PQ interval
8.5–10.0 mmol/l	Loss of P, ST segment abnormalities
>10.0 mmol/l	Death

Therapy
- Sodium chloride is the initial fluid of choice.
- Hartman's solution following relief of the obstruction.

- Post-obstructional diuresis – increase fluid according to urine output – may be necessary for several days following.

Hyperkalaemia
- Severe hyperkalaemia (>7.5 mmol/l) should be managed before attempting catheterisation.
- If patient appears bright and stable then cystocentesis and fluid diuresis may be sufficient.
- Severe hyperkalaemia with evidence of cardiac changes.
  - 10% calcium gluconate – 50–100 mg/kg (0.5–1.0 ml) slow IV.
  - Short-acting (neutral) insulin (0.1–0.2 U/kg) AND glucose (2 g/unit of insulin).
- Sodium bicarbonate (1 mmol/kg) slow IV.
- Rarely necessary to actively treat acid–base disturbances, as these will resolve on fluid administration and relief of the obstruction.

NB1 – *There is a significant risk of hypoglycaemia so it is essential that the patient is closely monitored for 1–2 hours following insulin use – particularly during anaesthesia – in which case serial blood glucose measurements are recommended.*
NB2 – *Post-obstructional hypokalaemia can be a problem; potassium supplemented fluid (20–40 mmol/l) should be used once the obstruction has been relieved.*

Chemical restraint
- Passage of a urinary catheter using physical restraint and local anaesthetic is insufficient in the vast majority of patients and is potentially dangerous.
  - Increased stress in a metabolically unstable patient.
  - Increased risk of iatrogenic complications.

Sedation
- Oxygen by mask or flow by.
- Buprenorphine (0.01 mg/kg) or butorphanol (0.1 mg/kg) with ACP 0.01–0.02 mg/kg given IM.
- If insufficient then 1 iU medetomidine/kg IM.
- If still insufficient then diazemuls IV to effect.
- Ketamine is also used with midazolam 50:50 mix given slowly to effect IV. If IM start with 1–2.5 mg/kg ketamine with 0.125 mg/kg midazolam.
  - Ketamine is renally excreted and its use in obstructed cats controversial.

Anaesthesia
- Buprenorphine 0.01 mg/kg IM.
- Propofol or alfaxalone *slowly and incrementally* to effect.
- Maintain with CRI or sevoflurane.

Epidural

Relief of obstruction
- Urethral massage.
- Urohydropulsion.
- Catheterisation.

Tips on catheterisation
- Lubricate the catheter with sterile K-Y jelly or similar.
- Maintain sterility as far as possible.
- Make sure the penis is properly extruded from the prepuce.
- Choose the right catheter.
  - Polyamide catheters can be used but are relatively inflexible and traumatic especially for repeated use.
  - Female cats – 4–5Fr gauge, 11–30 cm silicone Foley catheters are best for indwelling catheters.
  - Male cats – 3–4Fr gauge, 11–14 cm (11 cm catheters can be too short for some large male cats).
- Sometimes gently rotating the catheter or flushing saline through the catheter as you insert can help.

ORGAN SYSTEMS

- If the catheter gets stuck be patient and do not push too hard as this will traumatise and potentially rupture the urethra.
- Some patients are masters at removing catheters even when stitched in so they may need an Elizabethan collar.
- Closed urine collection systems are preferred.
- Antibacterial cover is NOT recommended.

Successful
- Drain all the urine from the bladder.
- Submit for any necessary analysis.
- Flush the bladder repeatedly with warmed Hartman's solution.
- DO NOT use Walpole's solution.
- Leave an open, indwelling catheter in place for 3–5 days to maintain patency and allow the tight junctions to recover.
- Urine output should be measured if possible.

Unsuccessful
- Surgery.
- Perineal urethrostomy if lesion is distal to the bulbourethral glands.

4.6.6 Approach to idiopathic FLUTD (FIC)
- Approximately 60–70% of cats presenting with signs of LUTD will not have an identifiable underlying cause.
- Frustrating for the veterinarian and client as investigation costs can be significant, effective treatments are lacking and recurrence is likely.
- Crucial in such cases to spend the necessary time with the client to explore suitable management options for the individual cat/client temperament and lifestyle.
  ○ Management is likely to be multimodal.
- Also important to emphasise that this is a management strategy designed to

reduce the frequency and duration of recurrences, and is highly unlikely to lead to a long-term cure.
- iFLUTD is likely to have multiple aetiologies.

Natural history
- Most cases of iFLUTD will resolve in 3–7 days if left untreated
- Frequency of recurrence is variable
- The client should keep an accurate diary noting the date, length and severity of episodes in order for you and the client to effectively evaluate treatments.
  ○ Also helpful in recording the natural variations in the condition and the response to previous attempts at treatment.

Pathophysiology (see Figure 24)
- Complex interrelationship between a variety of patient and environmental factors.
- Psychoneuroendocrine dysfunction seems to be a crucial factor.
- Pain and discomfort of FLUTD is associated with an increased number of C pain fibres and substance P pain receptors.
  ○ When the C fibres are stimulated they release a variety of neuropeptides including substance P that causes pain, vasodilation of intramural blood vessels, increased vascular and bladder wall permeability, submucosal oedema, smooth muscle contraction and mast cell degranulation.
- Under normal conditions the urothelium is protected from direct contact with urine by a layer of hydrophobic glycosaminoglycans (GAG).
  ○ In FLUTD the GAG layer appears diminished allowing the urine (potassium, magnesium, calcium and hydrogen ions) to come into contact with and stimulate the nerve endings in the bladder wall.

- In some cats, where the disease has been long-standing and the episodes frequent, the bladder wall will be very thickened and the bladder difficult to distend, due to thickening and fibrosis. Such cases carry a very poor prognosis.

General approach (Figure 23)

Therapeutic options

- Despite episodes tending to be relatively short-lived with spontaneous resolution, it is a distressing condition for both the cat and the owner.
- In male cats, there is a risk of urethral obstruction, made worse by a tendency to over-groom the perineal area causing inflammation and effective narrowing of the urethra.
- Not providing treatment will tend to encourage clients to look elsewhere for possible solutions, with the associated risks of wasting money on ineffective and potentially harmful 'remedies'.
- Owners will quickly recognise the signs of an impending episode.
- There is some anecdotal evidence to suggest that early intervention can significantly reduce the severity and duration of an episode, in some cases.

- Early recognition of signs will also help to identify any common environmental themes that may precipitate an attack.
- ALL CURRENT TREATMENTS ARE PALLIATIVE.

Dietary recommendations

- Diets that encourage large volumes of dilute urine (wet diets) have been shown to decrease the recurrence of episodes (11% in cats on wet diets vs. 39% in cats on dry diets).
- There is no convincing evidence that diet type, e.g. acidifying diets, has any significant effect, and in some situations may predispose cats to other problems.
- Cats that will only eat dry diets should have water mixed in with the food (if they will accept this) or be provided with a ready supply of fresh water.
  - Discovering from where a client's cat will drink can be important, e.g. fountains vs. still water.
  - Increasing water intake not only increases urinary volume but also urinary frequency.
- Increasing salt levels within the diet will promote thirst and water turnover.
- Hypertension secondary to salt-supplement does not seem to be a significant issue in cats.

ORGAN SYSTEMS

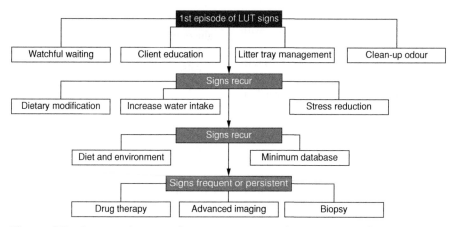

Figure 23 Sequential approach to investigation and management of iFLUTD

ORGAN SYSTEMS

Litter trays/access outside
- Litter trays should be made as comfortable and appealing as possible to encourage frequent use.
  - Separate litter tray from feeding area.
  - In multi-cat households provide one more litter tray than cats.
- For cats that urinate outside, whilst their ability to 'hold on' is legendary, efforts should be made to allow frequent outside access.
- Urination/defecation outside is a vulnerable time for many cats, and nervous cats may be going out but rarely passing urine; in these circumstances introducing a safe outside area or indoor litter trays may be worthwhile.

Medical treatment

Amitriptyline
- Tablets or syrup.
- 2.5–10 mg/cat PO once daily, best given in the evenings (if the cat is kept indoors at night) as it may cause mild sedation.
- Amitriptyline has been widely used in the management of FLUTD.
  - A number of short-term studies have not shown a positive benefit, and some have suggested that episodes are worsened.
  - One longer term study indicated possible improvement.
  - Contraindicated in cases with obstructive histories.
  - Reasonable time needs to be given before assessing efficacy of amitriptyline therapy, and should be based on good client record keeping.
- Amitriptyline is a tricyclic antidepressant that has anti-inflammatory, analgesic, anticholinergic and anti-alpha adrenergic properties.
  - For the drug to act as a tricyclic antidepressant, weeks/months of therapy are required to achieve full efficacy.

- It is thought to work by decreasing 'stress', stabilising mast cells and reducing degranulation and histamine release.
- Most commonly encountered side effects include dose-dependent sedation, urinary retention (due to anticholinergic activity) and elevated liver enzymes.
  - Liver function should be evaluated on initiation of treatment, 1 month into therapy and periodically thereafter.

Analgesia
- The use of NSAIDs is variably successful; it is often most effective given very early in an episode, and requires clients to have medication available at home.
- In severely affected cats short-term opioids may be required.

GAG supplementation
- Parenteral and oral GAG supplements have been used.
- Results of clinical trials have been variable and disappointing.
- Initial parenteral treatment can be followed with oral maintenance.
- Pentosan polysulphate (Cartrophen) – 3 mg/kg s/c on days 1, 2, 5, 10 and then every 5–10 days thereafter.
- N-acetyl glucosamine – variety of products available, all contain 125 mg glucosamine/capsule
  - Some contain additional nutraceuticals, e.g. hyaluronic acid and L-tryptophan a precursor or serotonin that may have a beneficial effect on behavioural/neurogenic aspects.
  - Orthopaedic supplements have not been optimised for FLUTD and are not recommended.

Antispasmodics (see Table 52)
- Following an episode of urinary obstruction or iFLUTD some cats

Table 52 Suggested drugs and dose rates of antispasmodics for use in cats with iFLUTD

Drug	Classification	Dose	Action	Side effects
Phenoxyben-zamine	α-adrenergic antagonist	2.5–7.5 mg/cat PO q12–24h	Decreases smooth muscle tone	Hypotension and GIT irritation
Prazosin	α-adrenergic antagonist	0.25–1 mg/cat PO q12h	Decreases smooth muscle tone	Hypotension – use with care if there is a risk of occult cardiomyopathy
Diazepam or midazolam	Skeletal muscle relaxant	1–2.5 mg/cat PO q8h	Decreases smooth muscle tone	Sedation, increased appetite, paradoxical excitement, rare hepatotoxicity
Dantrolene	Inhibits calcium release from the sarcoplasmic reticulum	0.5–2.0 mg/kg PO q12h	Skeletal muscle relaxant	Sedation, weakness, contraindicated in cardiac, pulmonary and hepatic disease

appear to have difficulty urinating, due to urethrospasm or reflex dyssynergia.

- Similarly pollakiuria is presumed to be the result of inflammation-induced stimulation of the bladder sacral sensory afferent nerves.
- Various drugs have been suggested aimed at improving urethral smooth muscle relaxation.
- These drugs can take up to 3–4 days to reach full efficacy.

Antibacterials

- Despite anecdotal support, there is no evidence that antibacterials are beneficial.

Corticosteroids

- The role of corticosteroids in the management of iFLUTD has not been investigated.
- In acute cases, corticosteroids may control inflammation and stabilise mast cells.

- Long-term use has not been shown to be effective, and is associated with many potential side effects.

Behavioural modification

- Increasing evidence suggests that cats with iFLUTD are hyperreactive and this may be a factor in their disease.
  - ○ Suitable questionnaires exploring a patient's home environment, diet, urination pattern are worthwhile.
  - ○ Behaviouralist input can be valuable.
  - ○ Stress reduction is an issue that is worth investigating to develop ways of minimising the problem.
  - ○ When stressful events are likely to occur prophylactic treatment should be considered.
  - ○ Environmental enrichment should be considered.

Behaviour modifying drugs

A variety of drugs have been used in more severe cases whilst behavioural and

ORGAN SYSTEMS

environmental modification has a chance to become effective. There efficacy is unproven.

- Clomipramine – 0.25–0.5 mg/kg PO q24h.
- Buspirone – 2.5–5 mg/cat PO q24h.
- Fluoxetine (Prozac) – 1 mg/kg PO q24h.

Feline facial pheromones
- Although no trials have been conducted, the use of appeasing pheromones in multi-cats households is a logical treatment option.

α-Casozepine (zylkene)
- Derived from milk with a benzodiazepine-like anxiolytic effect. There have been no clinical trials of this product but there have been no reported side effects; hence a-casozepine (<5 kg – 75 mg/cat PO q24h, >5 kg – 150 mg/cat PO q24h) may represent a useful initial adjunctive therapy.

4.6.7 Management of urolithiasis
- Successful management of urolithiasis depends on accurate identification of the liths involved.
- Significant numbers of uroliths are made up of several components, and are not necessarily of the same type as crystals that may be present in the urine.
- Calcium oxalate and struvite account for the vast majority of uroliths in cats (Table 53).

Diet
- Primary therapy is diet in many cases apart from calcium oxalate.
  ○ Diet is an important factor in trying to reduce recurrence rates.
- The aim of dietary management is to reduce the amount of precursors in the urine, preferably to below the solubility product allowing the uroliths to dissolve.
- A number of manufacturers now produce standard diets for general use designed to reduce the risk of both struvite and oxalate urolith formation through control of pH, solute concentration and water balance.

Diagnosis of urolithiasis
- Imaging, urine sediment microscopy, urolith analysis.
- Oxford Stone Analysis – chemical but fails to detect calcium, semi-quantitative.
- X-ray diffraction is better – section and analyse whole urolith, e.g. core calcium oxalate with shell struvite.

Causes of urolithiasis
- In many cats the cause of urolith formation is unknown; however, if an underlying cause can be identified then management of this cause is important to reduce recurrence rates.
- PSS.
- Hypercalcaemia.
- Urinary tract infection (UTI), e.g. urea-splitting bacteria altering pH.

Urinary acidification
- Urinary acidifiers – consider ammonium chloride, chlorethamine.
- Vitamin C and methionine are inadequate urinary acidifiers; high doses of methionine can induce Heinz body anaemia in cats, and bone demineralisation.
- Acidifying diets with high protein and marginal potassium have been shown to cause renal failure in cats.

(See Figure 24 and Table 53.)

Table 53 Composition, radiographic appearance, predisposing factors and nutritional management of feline uroliths

Urolith	Appearance	pH	Predisposing factors	Nutritional aims
Ammonium urate Amorphous urate	Radiolucent – smooth, round or oval	Any acidic	Increased urate excretion PSS UTI with urease producers	Reduce protein and nucleic acid (purine) intake Alkaline urine >pH 7 Diet alone may be inadequate, consider antibiotics if UTI and sodium bicarbonate
Calcium carbonate	Radiodense	Alkaline	Very rare	Not described
Calcium oxalate monohydrate	Very radiodense, rough, round to oval	Acidifying agents may increase bone release	Hypercalciuria (absorptive, renal leak, hypercalcaemia), M>F Low magnesium, acidifying diets	Generally necessary to remove surgically, and then avoid high salt, low or high phosphorus, high protein, high calcium diets that are adequate in magnesium. Alkalinising the urine may decrease formation (e.g. potassium citrate). Acidifying diets increase bone resorption and tubular reabsorption of calcium and should be avoided.
Calcium phosphate (Cal. hydr phos)	Very radiodense, smooth, round or faceted	Alkaline	Minor component of other liths, metabolic disorders – primary hyperparathyroidism, renal tubular acidosis	Not described
Cystine	Relatively radiolucent	Inhibited by very alkaline	Rare in cats	Low protein and salt-restricted diets. The value of urine alkalising diets (maintain urine pH >7.5) is not proven.
Struvite	Radiodense (variable), smooth, round or faceted	Favoured by alkaline	Urease-producing bacteria Usually sterile in cats	Reduce magnesium (<20 mg/100 kcal diet) and phosphate (ash <3%), energy-dense diet, protein reduced (to decrease urea level) and increased salt to stimulate thirst. Diets should produce an acidic urine pH <6.5 (high cation:anion ratio, increased sulphur amino acids). Should be obvious radiographic change within 60 days. Continue diet 4 weeks after disappeared radiographically. Surgical removal when been on struvite diet more difficult as liths become soft. Once dissolved maintenance diet may be required
Silica	Relatively radiodense – Jack stone shape	Less soluble in acid	Corn gluten free or soybean hull diet. Pica and ingestion of soil	Surgical removal, avoid plant protein-based diets, increase urine volume.

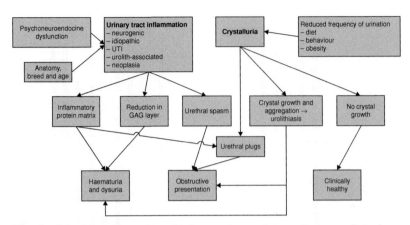

Figure 24 Interrelationship of inflammation and crystalluria on clinical signs in LUTD

4.6.8 Lower urinary tract infection

Bacterial

- Uncommon compared to dogs/man, probably associated with high urine concentration.
  - ○ Increased frequency in older especially female cats and/or low urine SG – UTI reported in 15–20% of cystitis cases in this group.
- Usually secondary.
- Causes:
  - ○ Indwelling urinary catheter.
  - ○ Urolithiasis.
  - ○ iFLUTD.
  - ○ DM.
  - ○ Neoplasia.
- Clinical signs of cystitis.
- Rarely systemically unwell.
- Sediment microscopy showing inflammatory cells.
  - ○ Bacteria reported on sediment examination poorly correlated with positive culture.
- Urine culture is essential to confirm diagnosis.
- $> 10^4$ bacteria/ml cystocentesis.
- $> 10^6$ bacteria/ml catheter or free catch sample.
- Bacterial sensitivity valuable.

Other

- Fungal infection (usually *Candida albicans*) reported after prolonged antimicrobial use.
- FCV and FeSFV have been suggested as being involved in the pathogenesis of iFLUTD.
- *Capillaria feliscati* infects the cat's bladder (in some areas of the world) – usually asymptomatic and responds to benzimidazole parasiticides.

4.6.9 Lower urinary tract neoplasia

- Bladder tumours are uncommon.
- Tumours of the ureters and urethra are very rare.

Transitional cell carcinoma

- Transitional cell carcinoma of the bladder is the most frequent.
  - ○ Older cats (>8 years).
  - ○ Haematuria and dysuria.
  - ○ Secondary bacterial cystitis.
- Diagnosis on ultrasound or contrast radiography.
- Confirmation on biopsy – FNA, catheter or laparotomy.
- Surgery is rarely feasible due to the extent of involvement, as the tumour is usually advanced at presentation.

Other

- A variety of other tumours are described; some, such as leiomyoma, may be surgically amenable.
- Polypoid cystitis may occur but has not been well described in cats.

4.6.10 Incontinence

- Uncommon.

Cause

- Congenital defects:
  - Manx cats (spinal dysraphism).
  - Ectopic ureters.
  - Rare causes – patent urachus, colo-urocystic fistula, ectopic uterine horns.
- Neurogenic.
- Trauma.
- Detrusor atony following severe distension, e.g. obstruction.
- Dysautonomia.
- Urethral incompetence.

Diagnosis

- Dribbling urine may or may not be associated with normal urination.
- Neurogenic:
  - Bladder large and easily expressed indicates LMN damage.
  - Bladder large and difficult to express producing dribbles of urine indicates UMN damage.

Management

- Ectopic ureter – see 4.5.10.

Neurogenic overflow

- Manually emptying needs to be 2–3 times per day.
- Indwelling urinary catheter for 7–10 days will allow the tight junctions to recove if overflow follows severe distension.
- Parasympathomimetics – bethanechol.
  - at 1.25–2.5 mg/cat q12h PO.
  - side effects – lacrimation, salivation, abdominal pain.

Urethral incompetence

- Adrenergic agonists – phenylpro-panolamine at 5 mg/kg PO divided 2–3 times per day.
- Value of testosterone or oestriol equivocal.

Neurogenic disease

- See neurology Section (4.8).

4.7 ENDOCRINE DISEASE

4.7.1 Introduction

Endocrine disease usually presents as a result of the metabolic effects of the increased or decreased secretion of the hormone(s) produced by the gland involved. DM and hyperthyroidism are the most common endocrinopathies reported in cats. HAC, acromegaly, hypoparathyroidism, hyperparathyroidism and hyperaldosteronism are uncommon in cats. Hypoadrenocorticism, hypothyroidism (other than as a consequence of treatment of hyperthyroidism), insulinoma, DI, APUDomas, and phaeochromocytoma have also been reported; all are considered rare or very rare.

4.7.2 Hyperthyroidism

- Hyperthyroidism is recognised as the most common feline endocrine disease, the condition resembles toxic nodular goitre in man.
- 1–3% of cases of hyperthyroidism in cats are due to adenocarcinoma.

Aetiology

Unknown, but a number of risk factors have been identified including indoor living, canned food as the major part of the diet, and exposure to insecticides (e.g. flea control), herbicides, cat litter and flame retardants. Genetic factors are likely to play a role as are abnormal immune and

ORGAN SYSTEMS

hormonal responses. Thyroid growth stimulating immunoglobulins have been demonstrated in cats, but their role is uncertain.

Risk group
- Middle-aged to older cats.
- Youngest documented – 4 years; median age 13 years.
- No sex or breed predisposition although Siamese and Himalayan cats may be under-represented.
- Distinct geographic clusters of disease occur.

History and physical examination
- Gradual onset of weight loss despite an often ravenous appetite.
- Character changes – hyperactivity and irritability.
- Dishevelled appearance.

Clinical signs (Box 6)

Box 6 Frequency of clinical signs in feline hyperthyroidism

Palpable goitre	> 95% cases
Weight loss despite increased appetite	90–95%
Signs of cardiac disease especially tachycardia	60–70%
Hyperactivity	60–70%
Polydipsia/polyuria	50–70%
Diarrhoea	50–60%
Vomiting	30–40%
Skin lesions – alopecia, harsh dry coat, seborrhoea	30–40%
Apathy – probably associated with CHF	5–10%

Other signs
- Neck ventroflexion, hypertensive retinopathy, heat intolerance, excessive panting, dysphonia (change in meow).
- Cardiac abnormalities.
  - Tachycardia, gallop rhythm, heart murmurs, CHF leading to dyspnoea, limb weakness associated with embolus.
- Hypertension.
  - A significant proportion of cats are hypertensive that may be associated with end-organ damage such as ocular haemorrhage, retinal detachment, renal damage, cardiac hypertrophy and cerebrovascular accidents.
- Neuromuscular signs.
  - Secondary to dementia, CVA or thiamine deficiency.

Diagnosis
Usually based on presenting signs, physical examination and biochemical changes.

Radiography
- Enlarged cardiac silhouette on radiography ± pulmonary oedema or pleural effusion.

Ultrasound
- Images of the thyroid gland can be obtained with a high frequency transducer (≥10 MHz).
- Normal gland thin fusiform shape; diseased thyroids are more rounded and nodular.

ECG changes
- Rate >240 bpm, ventricular arrhythmia, widened QRS, tall complexes.

Echocardiography
- Typically – LV hypertrophy, left atrial dilation, hypercontractile ventricle.
- Progression – LV dilation, systolic failure.

ORGAN SYSTEMS

Major differential diagnoses

Causes of weight loss with polyphagia (see sections 2.32 polyphagia and 2.43 weight loss)

- Physiologic/environmental – not meeting caloric need.
- Hyperthyroidism.
- DM – often younger cats, PU/PD usually a prominent sign.
- IBD – younger cats, usually *but not always* GIT signs.
- Lymphocytic cholangitis – usually younger cats, sometimes ascites.
- Drug therapy.
- Exocrine pancreatic insufficiency.
- HAC.
- CKD – cats usually have poor appetites.

Key clinical pathology and imaging changes

- Haematology – about a third of cases show haematological changes, generally leucocytosis, monocytosis and mature neutrophilia.
- Biochemistry – elevation in AST, ALT, ALKP (SAP) and urea occur commonly.

Confirmatory tests

- An elevation in T_4 levels above the laboratory normal.
- Day-to-day fluctuations in T_4 levels do occur.
- Over 95% of cases have a palpable goitre.

NB – *Semi-quantitative in-house tests have a high degree of sensitivity and specificity, i.e. few false positives or negatives, but do not give an absolute value that can be used in monitoring response to treatment.*

Nuclear scintigraphy

Radioactive technetium allows the position of active thyroid tissue to be delineated, with abnormal glands showing increased uptake. The technique can show if both glands are involved, or if the thyroid gland has descended into the thoracic inlet. It will also highlight ectopic thyroid secreting tissue. It is of particular value following the failure of previous thyroid surgery.

Problems with diagnosis

Euthyroid sick cat syndrome

- Concurrent illness can depress thyroid production, and hence T_4 levels may fall to within the normal range. If hyperthyroidism is still suspected other conditions should be treated, and the T_4 level reassessed when the cat appears well.

Borderline hyperthyroid (Figure 25)

- As recognition and awareness of hyperthyroidism has improved, increasing numbers of cats are spotted early in the course of their disease and have borderline increases in thyroid hormone.
- A number of cats will give results at the top end or just above the normal range. Free T_4 and several dynamic tests (feline TSH, T_3 suppression, TRH and TSH

ORGAN SYSTEMS

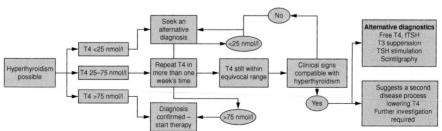

Figure 25 Interpretation of T4 results

stimulation) have been investigated to categorise such cats. Whilst helpful, equivocal results still occur.

- Most borderline cases will, with time, become overtly hyperthyroid. As hyperthyroidism is not a rapidly progressive disease, the best approach is to treat symptomatically if you are confident in your diagnosis, or wait and retest in 1–3 months time.
- Treatment trials are generally not recommended due to the potential risks of medication side effects or causing hypothyroidism.

Treatment (See Figure 26)

- The hypertensive effects of hyperthyroidism can improve renal function in cats with CKD. A number of cats will show a small increase in urea following successful treatment. In a few cases, treatment can precipitate overt signs of renal failure. If this occurs medical treatment should be stopped. If surgery or I[131] has

been used then thyroid supplementation may be required.

- As hyperthyroidism is a chronic slowly progressive disease, rapid reduction in T4 levels is unnecessary and potentially dangerous.
  - Becoming hypothyroid following over-aggressive treatment can result in more rapid progression of renal disease.

Diet

- Recent introduction of a reduced iodine diet for management of hyperthyroid cats.
- Clinical experience to date is limited.

Antithyroid drugs

A variety of drugs have been used in the treatment of hyperthyroidism, the majority being found to be relatively toxic in cats, e.g. propylthiouracil (PTU). Currently two related drugs are used – carbimazole and its metabolite methimazole – these drugs interfere with hormone synthesis preventing organification of iodine in the thyroid gland.

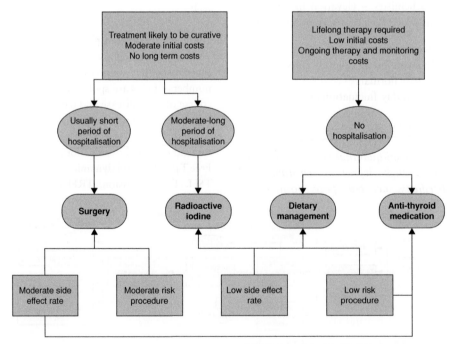

Figure 26   Owner-priority-driven selection of antithyroid therapy

Ipodate

- Inhibits conversion of T_3 to T_4 in the peripheral tissue, and has been used at a dose rate of 15 mg/kg q12h. Experience is limited – reserve for cats where standard medically treatment has been unsuccessful.

Other

- Transdermal methimazole.
- Percutaneous, ultrasound guided intrathyroid ethanol injections.
- Percutaneous radiofrequency ablation.
- Iopanoic acid.

Carbimazole (Vidalta, Neomercazole)

- Licensed product (Vidalta) is a slow release coated 10 and 15 mg tablets.
- Dividing the tablet is not generally recommended as it will alter its pharmacokinetics.
- Dose – 10 mg daily for mild to moderately hyperthyroid cats; 15 mg daily for severely hyperthyroid cats or cat that have not responded to a 10 mg dose rate.
- Side effects with carbimazole
  - Usually occur within 2–3 weeks of beginning treatment, are generally mild (anorexia, vomiting, lethargy, facial excoriation) and relatively common (10–20%). Severe side effects (thrombocytopenia, neutropenia, hepatopathy) are rare (1–5%). All side effects are reversible with withdrawal of carbimazole.
- Monitoring
  - Haematology after 2–3 weeks to check for neutropenia or thrombocytopenia.
    - If a neutropenia develops (<2.5 × 10^9/l) therapy should be stopped for 5 days, and can be re-instituted at a lower dose, so long as the neutrophil count returned to and remains normal.
  - Biochemistry and USG at 2–3 weeks to check renal parameters and liver enzymes and then every 3–6 months.

- T4 level after 2–3 weeks and then every 3–6 weeks until stable; thereafter 3–6 monthly.

Methimazole (Felimazole)

- 2.5 and 5 mg tablets.
- Dosing frequency twice daily.
- Side effects are similar to carbimazole – anecdotally may be more severe/frequently seen.
- Monitoring – as for carbimazole.

Surgical thyroidectomy

Preparation

- Carbimazole/methimazole (diet) – maintain euthyroidism for 1–3 weeks preoperatively (last dose the morning of surgery).
- If resting heart rate is excessive (>200 bpm) then β-blockers should be given – propranolol 2.5–5 mg/cat q8h or atenolol 6.25–12.5 mg/cat q24h (for 7–14 days prior to surgery).

Anaesthesia

- Pre-med – ACP, no atropine. Ketamine or xylazine should be avoided.
- Induction – thiopentone (displays antithyroid activities and does not stimulate catecholamine secretions) propofol or alphaxalone titrated to effect.
- Intraoperative ECG monitoring – arrhythmias are the primary cause of anaesthetic death in hyperthyroid cats.
- Anaesthetic maintenance – gas preferably. Isoflurane/sevoflurane is better than halothane as it causes less sensitisation of the myocardium to arrhythmias.

Complications

Recurrence

- About 15% of cats have bilateral involvement, with one of the glands looking normal at surgery.
- Some cats have ectopic thyroid hormone producing tissue.

ORGAN SYSTEMS

ORGAN SYSTEMS

Hypocalcaemia

- Cats should be monitored for signs of hypocalcaemia over 3–5 days following surgery, hypocalcaemia occurs in around 10% of cases following thyroidectomy.
  - Signs of developing hypocalcaemia – depression, anorexia, agitation, hyperaesthesia.
- Intervene when
  - Calcium <1.5–1.8 mmol/l (iCa^{2+} <0.7–0.9).
  - Cat is showing clinical signs.
- Treat with
  - 50–150 mg/kg of a 10% calcium gluconate solution i/v initially.
  - Then daily calcium supplementation with vitamin D$_3$ analogue.
    - Most require 0.5–1 g calcium carbonate per day.
    - Vitamin D$_3$ analogue
    - One-alpha (0.2 µg/ml solution) – 0.03–0.06 µg/kg q12–24h.
    - Calcitriol (250 mg capsule) – 50 ng q12h.
- Most cats regain normal calcaemic control within 5 weeks.

Radioactive iodine

- Can be used to treat thyroid carcinomas – high dose rates required.

Complications

- Non-response occurs in 2–5% of cases, many will respond to a second dose. Some are adenocarcinomas and require much higher doses.
- Hypothyroidism is common if T$_4$ levels are measured, but rarely (2%) clinically significant signs although the effect on renal function needs to be considered.
- Relapse – 2%

Selection criteria for I^{131} therapy

- Availability and likely hospitalisation period.

- Surgical risk due to intercurrent disease, e.g. severe cardiovascular disease or chronic renal disease.
- No palpable thyroid nodule – ectopic tissue.
- Recurrence following previous thyroidectomy.
- Adenocarcinoma.
- Intolerance/resistance to anti-thyroid drugs.
- Antithyroid drug treatment should be stopped for 1–2 weeks prior to treatment.

Treatment failure

- Has the cat initially responded to therapy – is the cat truly hyperthyroid?
- Has the owner been able to medicate the cat frequently enough and at the correct intervals?
- Could it be an adenocarcinoma?
- Could there be active extrathyroidal tissue?
- Was a bilateral thyroidectomy performed, if not is the other side now involved?
- Has a thyroid remnant regrown at the surgical site – review technique used?
- Are there other diseases which produce similar clinical signs present, e.g. CKD?

Prognosis

- Long-term prognosis is generally good.

2.7.3 Diabetes mellitus

- DM is the second most common endocrinopathy affecting around 1 in 200 cats.

Classification

- Human classification:

Type I – <5% of cases

- Insulin-dependent diabetes mellitus (IDDM).
- Immune-mediated destruction of islet cells.
- Most common form in dogs, relatively rare in cats.

Type II – 80–95% of cases

- Non-insulin-dependent diabetes mellitus (NIDDM).
- Inadequate insulin secretion and impaired insulin action (insulin resistance).
- Can progress to complete failure of insulin secretion.
- Amyloid deposits in islet cells may be significant.
- Most cats, however, require insulin.

Type III – 5–20% of cases

- Secondary DM – other factors having a significant role in the development of DM.
- Diseases leading to impaired pancreatic function – pancreatitis, pancreatic adenocarcinoma.
- Diseases causing insulin resistance, e.g. sepsis, acromegaly, HAC.
- Drug-induced resistance, e.g. progestogens, glucocorticoids.

Glucose toxicity

- Hyperglycaemia suppresses insulin secretion.
- Initially this is reversible and likely accounts for the number of cats reported to have transient diabetes.
- Long-term irreversible structural change occurs in beta cells.

Risk group

- Middle-aged to older cats.
- Burmese cats predisposed.
- Marked sex predisposition with males being affected much more frequently than females.
- Obese cats, physical inactivity, indoor living.
- Neutered cats (irrespective of their sex) compared to entire cats.
- Cats fed on high carbohydrate diets.
- Cats receiving long acting corticosteroids or megoestrol acetate.
- Acromegaly or HAC.

History and physical examination

- Polyuria – due to osmotic diuresis when blood glucose exceeds renal threshold.
- Polydipsia – secondary to polyuria-induced hypovolaemia.
- Weight loss.
- Polyphagia (more variable).
- Lethargy and depression.
- Owners may be unaware of some signs due to the lifestyle of cats, e.g. PU/PD.

Other signs

- May be present, especially with concurrent disease, which may also modify some of the presenting features (e.g. anorexia, etc.).
- Vomiting.
- Plantigrade stance.
- Muscle weakness and wasting.
- Poor hair coat.
- Dehydration.
- Pain.

Diagnosis

Major differential diagnoses (see section 3.11 glucose and 3.16 urinalysis)

NB – *Always check that the case is also hyperglycaemic do not just rely on glycosuria.*

- Stress hyperglycaemia – differentiation of true DM from stress hyperglycaemia can be problematic, and it is essential that the two are not confused before therapy is commenced.
- Hyperthyroidism.
- IBD.
- Intestinal neoplasia.
- CKD.

Key clinical pathology and imaging changes

- Biochemistry – mild to moderate elevation in ALT, ALKP, γ-GT, cholesterol, triglycerides and bilirubin.

ORGAN SYSTEMS

Confirmatory tests

- Persistent, fasting hyperglycaemia.
- In cats, stress hyperglycaemia can be marked, and in excess of 20 mmol/l.
- Glycosuria:
  - Occurs when blood glucose exceeds renal threshold (12–14 mmol/l), and therefore can be seen in stress hyperglycaemia.
  - Can occur in absence of hyperglycaemia, e.g. renal tubular damage.
- Ketonuria.
- Glycosylated proteins – fructosamine >400 μmol/l.
  - Formed primarily by glycosylation of albumin and reflects glycaemic control over the previous 2–3 weeks. Unaffected by short periods of hyperglycaemia (e.g. stress).
    - Some diabetic cats can have fructosamine levels well below 400 μmol/l.
  - Fructosamine levels do not correlate well with the severity of hyperglycaemia, nor do they show evidence of any periods of hypoglycaemia.
  - Serial fructosamine is a relatively poor marker to assess diabetic stability.
  - Glycosylated haemoglobin is measured by some laboratories; it reflects glycaemic control over previous 1–2 months.

Pre-diabetes

- As in man, there is a population of cats that have impaired glucose handling but are not yet overtly diabetic.
- Currently the value in identifying these cats is unknown.
- Diagnosis – fasting hyperglycaemia >9 mmol/l or abnormal glucose tolerance test.

Management of uncomplicated diabetes

- Gradual withdrawal of diabetogenic drugs.
- If obese, dietary manipulation to decrease weight.

- Exogenous insulin therapy.
- Oral hypoglycaemic agents.

Oral hypoglycaemic agents (see Box 7)

- A wide variety of oral agents have been tried in cats, few have undergone significant investigation to establish dose rates, efficacy and safety.
- Reported to give complete or partial control in around 30% of cats, but in many cases control is poor.
- There is a risk that by increasing insulin output the rate of beta cell exhaustion is increased and the opportunity to recover beta cell function lost.

Box 7   Indications and contraindications for the use of oral hypoglycaemic agents in diabetes mellitus

Indications	Contraindications
Obese cats	Diabetic
Mildly affected	ketoacidotic
otherwise healthy	Emaciated/
Recent history of	debilitated cats
diabetogenic drugs	Cats with
Previous response to	concurrent disease
oral hypoglycaemics	

Sulphonylurea

- Increases insulin release from beta cells, mild reduction in peripheral insulin resistance, decreases hepatic glucose production.

Glipizide (Glibenese; Pfizer)

- 2.5–5 mg twice daily with food.
- Most widely investigated and used.
- Initial dose 2.5 mg BID for 2 weeks, check liver enzymes.
- Assess response, if there is no improvement double the dose.
- Cease if no beneficial effect occurs after 12 weeks.

- Side effects – vomiting, hepatotoxicity, jaundice – resolve on withdrawal of treatment.

Transition metals
- Little information on efficacy of vanadium or chromium in cats.

Biguanides
- Decrease hepatic glucose production, reduction in peripheral insulin resistance.

Metformin
- Some studies in cats – may be useful in combination with sulphonylurea.
- GI side effects.

Acarbose
- Delays glucose absorption – may be useful in dogs where post-prandial hyperglycaemia is more marked.
- Adverse effects – diarrhoea and weight loss.

Insulin therapy
- Required for management of most cases of DM in cats.
- 30-iU syringes are available.

NB – *some insulins are in 40 iU/ml concentration not the standard 100 iU/ml of human insulins so it is essential that the correct syringes are used (red top) rather than the standard orange top.*

Diluting insulin
- Improves accuracy of dosing.
- Proprietary diluents from the manufacturer should be used otherwise the pharmacodynamics of the insulin may be altered.

Insulin types
- Potency and duration of action depends on the formulation and individual responses. Cats showed marked variation in sensitivity to insulin, particularly duration of action; hence it is essential to perform a glucose curve to establish dose frequency and peak onset of action.
- Theoretically, as the amino acid sequence of cat insulin is closest to beef insulin compared to pork insulin and least homologous to human insulin, using beef insulin is least likely to result in the formation of anti-insulin antibodies.
- There have been changes in the availability of insulin in the UK currently only one insulin is licensed for use in cats, Caninsulin, which is a porcine insulin containing a mixture of 30% amorphous and 70% crystalline zinc insulin.

Soluble (neutral) insulin
- Rapid onset, short duration, can be given IV.
- Primarily used to stabilise diabetic ketoacidotic cats.

Lente insulin
- Moderate onset of action, peak around 5 hours, duration 8–12 hours; IM or SC use.
- Most cats require twice daily dosing.

Protamine zinc insulin
- Long duration of action (18–20 hours) but can be >24 hours; IM or SC use.
- Contains fish proteins so may be more likely to cause immune response.

Glargine insulin
- Has recently become popular for use in cats and is ultra-long acting.
- It is an insulin analogue.
- Duration of action is >24 hours in many cats (risks of piggy-back effects), peak at around 16 hours.

Initial stabilisation
- Select type of insulin.
- Decide whether to
  - Perform in hospital – stress effects but better observation and accurate dosing more likely.
  - Perform at home – less stress and more likely to reflect effect of insulin give but greater risk of injection issues.
- Start at 0.25–0.5 U/kg.
- Monitor for hypoglycaemia after first injection.
- Give 5–7 days treatment (to allow stabilisation) with minimal interference.
- Monitor to establish glucose nadir.
  - Sampling times will depend on insulin type used.
  - Start 1–2 hours before expected nadir and continue until the glucose level has reached its minimum and begun to rise again.
    - Likely to be of limited benefit if first glucose reading is >20 mmol/l in which case make a dose adjustment and retest 5–7 days after dose adjustment.
- If glucose monitoring is not possible then stabilisation can be attempted based on appetite, body weight, daily water intake and *afternoon* urine glucose levels.

Glucose curves
- When the cat appears to be showing some signs of stabilisation then a 24-hour glucose curve can be performed with samples collected every 1-2 hours.
  - Using hand-held glucometers allow small samples to be taken with a fine needle.
  - Alternatively ear lancing and suck blood into capillary tube.
  - At home curving is possible in some cases and may give more accurate information.
  - Ideally the curve should last a full 24 hours particularly if long-acting preparations are being used.
  - Continuous glucose monitoring is possible and will give more accurate results but can be technically challenging.
- Aim to keep the blood glucose below 14 mmol/l for the majority of the day.
- Glucose level should not fall below 5 mmol/l at any time.
- Do not worry if glucose rises in the early morning – dawn rise phenomenon.
- Assess duration of action and peak activity.
- Alter dose as required – some cats are sensitive to even small increases in insulin.

NB – *Increasing dose will cause a lower nadir* and *increase duration of action.*

Fructosamine and glycosylated haemoglobin
- Fructosamine (primarily glycosylated albumin) is most widely available and reflects glycaemic control over the past 2–3 weeks. It is not affected by short-term stressors such as sampling.
- Results give an impression of how well the cat's diabetes is being controlled.
- Serial evaluation is of limited value as a sole parameter in monitoring response to dose changes.

Diabetic remission
- Transient diabetes is a well-recognised phenomenon in cats, occurring in 20–40% of cases once good glycaemic control is achieved (1–3 months). Hence, initial monitoring needs to be close in order to prevent hypoglycaemia. Remission can be maintained weeks to years.
  - With good dietary management and intensive home monitoring and insulin dose adjustment, resolution of diabetes in as many as 80% of cats has been achieved.

Maintenance therapy
- Good owner education is essential.
- Do not alter dose rate more than once weekly unless intensively monitoring.
- Encourage monitoring by clinical signs – appetite, PU/PD, demeanour.
- Discourage urine glucose monitoring at home, particularly in the morning.
- If urine monitoring is conducted then include ketones and use afternoon sample.
- Periodic (3–6 months) assessments.
- Whilst serum fructosamine will provide useful information about the control of hyperglycaemia over the preceding 2–3 weeks, it will not detect any periods of hypoglycaemia that have occurred.
- 24-hour glucose curve.

What is success?
- Unlike in man, there is no evidence that tight regulation of blood glucose is beneficial and can be difficult to achieve.

Aim to
- Resolve clinical signs.
- Avoid periods of hypoglycaemia.
- Prevent development of complications of diabetes, e.g. diabetic ketoacidosis (DKA), diabetic polyneuropathy.

Role of diet in the management of DM
- Normalise body weight.
- Achieve consistent daily intake – amount and composition.
- Minimise insulin requirement.
- Manage/prevent concurrent disease.

Normalising body weight
- Probably the key nutritional management strategy.
- Usually easiest to achieve with a proprietary diet that restricts energy consumption.
- High fibre diets are poorly tolerated by most cats and can result in malnutrition.
- Malnutrition can lead to insulin resistance and reduced insulin secretion.
- Diabetic cats have increased risk of hepatic lipidosis, so it is essential to ensure that the cat is accepting any new diet.

Timing of feeds
- Can be difficult in cats that catch their own food, or are fed elsewhere.
- Constitutive gluconeogenesis by the liver is high.
- Carbohydrates are not as powerful secretagogues of insulin as protein in cats, so the whole physiology of insulin release may be different.
- Overall, the benefits of closely associated feeding times and insulin injections do not seem to be that great.
- Cats can be stabilised if fed *ad libitum*.

Dietary formulation
- High protein diets with moderate fat content have been shown to improve glycaemic control.

Prognosis
- Dependent on owner commitment.
- Presence of concurrent disorders.
- Reasonably stable cases have a median survival time of 24–36 months.

Diabetic complications

Hypoglycaemia
- Life-threatening event in the management of a diabetic.
- Hypoglycaemic coma results in very rapid onset of irreversible brain damage (faster than hypoxia); hence, every effort should be made to prevent its occurrence.
- Rapid, aggressive treatment is necessary.
- Following an episode, the cause should be investigated, and steps to prevent recurrence should be taken.
- Cats are over-represented (compared to dogs).
  - Predisposed – management factors, concurrent medical problems, high doses (>6 U) of insulin being used.

Cause
- Insulin overdose.
  - Insulin dose miscalculated.
  - Wrong amount drawn into syringe (especially 40 iU/ml syringe used to draw up 100 iU/ml insulin).

○ Accidental IV administration.

○ Incorrect dilution.

- Reduced requirement for insulin.
- Sudden onset anorexia/marked inappetence.
- Transient diabetic.
- Reduced insulin resistance, e.g. management of obesity, resolution of UTI.
- Over-aggressive management of hyperglycaemic episode.

Clinical signs

- All owners should be aware of the signs of hypoglycaemia, and should be advised to have a readily absorbable source of glucose available (Lucozade, honey, glucose solution, Hypostop gel, etc.).
  ○ Lethargy.
  ○ Weakness.
  ○ Head tilting.
  ○ Ataxia.
  ○ Seizures.

Management

- Insulin has a longer duration of action than glucose.
- Half-hourly blood glucose samples following an episode.
- Glucose status unknown – better to give glucose unless ketotic.
- Bolus IV glucose 0.5 g/kg.
- Fluid.
- Monitor – glucose, electrolyte (potassium, phosphorus), blood gas – if available.
- Seizure control – diazepam.
- Glucagon – 0.25–1 mg IM – must be followed by IV glucose.

Failure to respond to therapy

Approach

- What makes you/the owner feel that the cat is not responding?
- The owner's routine should be re-evaluated.
- Is the insulin in date?
- Has it been contaminated?

- Has it been stored correctly?
- Is the owner's injection technique appropriate?
- If the syringes are re-used how are they stored – do they wash them out?
- How consistent is the feeding regime?
- What is the likelihood of the cat feeding elsewhere?
- If the owner's regime seems to be OK then measure fructosamine levels.
  ○ If fructosamine levels are elevated then monitor blood glucose levels – preferably with a 24-hour (or continuous) glucose curve.
  ○ The cat should be injected using a new syringe and a new bottle of insulin by veterinary staff.
  ○ If the cat seems to be responding then the owner's regime should be reconsidered and necessary support in general management, insulin storage and injection techniques given.

24-hour insulin curve abnormal

No/inadequate response

- Insulin problem, injection technique, impaired absorption, e.g. into fat pad (especially ultralente).
- Anti-insulin antibodies (rare).
- Insulin resistance/antagonism.

Inadequate duration of action

- Insufficient dose.
- Rapid metabolism.

Somogyi overswing

- Excessive insulin is being given and the cat is becoming hypoglycaemic. Gluconeogenic mechanisms are switched on (glucagon, glucocorticoids, catecholamines) causing a rise in glucose. The rise is uncontrolled as the cat is diabetic, resulting in a rebound hyperglycaemia.
- Probably a more common cause of insulin curve abnormalities than previously thought.

ORGAN SYSTEMS

NB – *Following an overswing episode a cat can be insulin resistant for 2–3 days.*

Insulin resistance/antagonism

Causes

- Obesity.
- Infection – oral, urinary.
- Diabetogenic drugs.
- Chronic inflammation – especially pancreatitis.
- Hyperthyroidism.
- Neoplasia.
- Renal, cardiac or liver insufficiency (chronic disease).
- Acromegaly.
- Hyperlipidaemia.
- Rarely – phaeochromocytoma, EPI.

Investigation

- Haematology/biochemistry.
- Urine culture.
- Antimicrobial trial therapy.
- Survey radiography.
- Abdominal ultrasound.
- Faecal culture.
- T_4 estimation.
- Insulin-like growth factor 1 measurement.
- Adrenocortical function testing.
- TLI.

Stabilising the diabetic ketoacidotic

- Dehydration, hypovolaemia, thrombosis and shock.

Presentation and clinical signs

- Majority not previously diagnosed as diabetic.
- Middle-aged to older cats.
- Male predominance.
- Cats have usually shown PU/PD, polyphagia, weight loss for up to 6 months or longer.
- Acute deterioration over 1–7 days.
- Anorexia.
- Decreased drinking.
- Vomiting.
- Depression and lethargy.
- Collapse.

Physical examination

- Dehydration.
- Depression.
- Weakness.
- Tachypnoea or deep, slow breathing (severe acidosis).
- GIT signs – vomiting, distension, pain.
- Acetone on breath.
- Concurrent infection, pancreatitis, CHF.

Diagnosis

- History and clinical examination.
- Fasting hyperglycaemia.
- Ketonemia – hand-held ketone monitors are available.
  - Significant numbers of cats are ketonaemic but not acidotic.
- Glycosuria.
- Ketonuria.

NB – *Beta-hydroxybutyrate is not detected by standard dipstick methods.*

- Acidosis.

Therapy

Systemically well

- Give short-acting soluble insulin q8h until ketosis is resolved.
- Encourage cat to eat.
- 0.5 iU/kg/injection and monitor response.
- Lag phase of 2–3 days in resolution of ketonuria.

Sick

- Fluid:
  - Hartmann's or 0.9% sodium chloride fluid of choice given at 2–3 times maintenance, aim to replace deficit over 24–48 hours.
  - Monitor urinary output.
  - Monitor level of dehydration.

ORGAN SYSTEMS

ORGAN SYSTEMS

- Management of hyperglycaemia:
  - Soluble insulin – repeated injection vs. IV infusion.
  - Initially 0.2 U/kg i/m then 0.1 iU/kg hourly i/m until glucose <15 mmol/l.
  - Then 0.5 iU s/c q6–8h.
  - Monitor blood glucose every 1–2 hours initially.
- Acid–base status:
  - Marked and life-threatening acidosis can occur.
  - Ideally measured using blood gas machine.
  - If not, an estimate can be made based on the degree of hypokalaemia (lower potassium ⇒ worse acidosis).
  - Empirical dose 1–2 mmol bicarbonate/kg is safe.
- Hypokalaemia:
  - Can be mildly hyperkalaemic to severely hypokalaemic at presentation.

NB1 – *Correction of the acidosis tends to move potassium out of the cell.*

NB2 – *Insulin causes both glucose and potassium to move into the cell causing profound hypokalaemia.*

  - Potassium supplementation is important, use KCl at 20–80 mmol/l.
  - Overall potassium infusion rate should not exceed 0.5 mmol/kg/hour.
- Hypophosphataemia:
  - Phosphate shifts from intra- to extracellular space with acidosis, and is wasted in the urine.

NB – *Correction of acidosis can cause profound hypophosphataemia leading to haemolytic anaemia, weakness, ataxia and seizures.*

  - Correct by supplementing fluids, e.g. Foston (2.5 mmol/ml phosphate), initially at 20 mmol/l.
  - Aim to keep phosphorus above 0.5 mmol/l.

Monitoring
- Regular monitoring is essential for effective management of the severely ill DKA cat.
- Minimum facilities require the ability to estimate blood glucose.
  - Other parameters can be guestimated by careful patient evaluation.
  - Initially electrolyte and bicarbonate supplementation should be conservative if their values cannot be measured.

Complications
- Concurrent illness and insulin resistance.
- Thromboembolism.
- Hypoglycaemia (see above).
- Cerebral oedema.
- Hypernatraemia and hypochloraemia.
- Severe hypokalaemia.
- Haemolytic anaemia.

Hyperosmolar non-ketotic DM
- Uncommon.
- Severe dehydration and hyperglycaemia without ketosis.
- Usually acidotic and often hyponatraemic.
- Goal to correct dehydration and electrolyte imbalances.
- Prognosis poor.

4.7.4 Hyperdrenocorticism
- HAC is a rare condition in cats being significantly less common than in dogs.
- >80% of HAC cases in cats have concurrent DM.
- PU/PD and polyphagia usually a result of the DM rather than the HAC.

Aetiology
- 75% pituitary dependent and 25% adrenal adenoma/adenocarcinoma.

Risk group
- Mid- to old-aged, mixed breed cats, 70% are female.

History and physical examination
- Signs can be vague but include
- Insulin-resistant DM.
- Skin fragility and bruising.
- Poor coat with alopecia (asymmetric).
- Pot belly and muscle wasting.
- Pigmented skin.

Key clinical pathology
- Glycosuria and hyperglycaemia.
- Urine SG >1.020.
- Proteinuria rare.
- Hypercholesterolaemia.
- Mild increase in ALT.
- Cats do not have an inducible isoenzyme of ALP.
- Hepatomegaly.
- Adrenomegaly on ultrasound useful as a positive finding.

Confirmatory tests
ACTH stimulation
Protocol
- Inject 0.125 mg (½ vial) Synacthen IV or IM.
- Sample at baseline, 1 and 3 or 2 and 3 hours.

Interpretation
- Values over 600 nmol/l supported by clinical signs are supportive of HAC.
- False positive and negative results occur.

Low-dose dexamethasone suppression
Protocol
- 0.1 mg/kg IV (low dose volume so dilute 1:10 with sterile water for accuracy).
- Sample at baseline, 3 and 8 hours.

Interpretation
- HAC supported by a failure to suppress.
  - 95% of HAC cats fail to suppress.
- Care should be taken in the interpretation of results in cats, as the endogenous cortisol production during the test is likely to be high.

Urine cortisol:creatinine ratio
- Not been fully evaluated in cats.
- Reference range $2-36 \times 10^{-6}$.
- Likely to be of similar interpretation as in dogs, i.e. a normal ratio makes HAC unlikely and an elevated ratio indicates the need for confirmatory tests.

High dose dexamethasone suppression test
- Failure to suppress indicates HAC, but does not discriminate pituitary from adrenal dependent causes.

Endogenous ACTH
- Undetectable levels indicate adrenal dependence.
- Normal to high levels supports pituitary dependent.
- Validation of assay for use in cats and sample handling should be checked with the clinical pathology laboratory to be used.

MRI or CT
- Adrenal glands not always identified, but can be valuable to detect spread and metastasis.
- Pituitary gland can also be imaged.

Treatment
Medical
- Trilostane has been shown to be effective in small numbers of cases.
  - Suggested dose 30 mg/cat q24h.
  - Monitoring as for dogs using ACTH stimulation test.
  - Continued management of diabetes usually required.
- Op'DDD (mitotane) poor results in early trials.
  - May require higher doses and/or longer course.
- Ketoconazole, metapyrone and L-deprenyl have not been shown to be effective.

ORGAN SYSTEMS

Radiation
- Limited success – speak to radiation oncologist.

Surgery
Adrenalectomy
- The best option at this present time; bilateral for pituitary dependent.
- Surgical complications are common; facilities for intensive post-operative management should be available.
- Adrenal adenocarcinomas tend to be locally invasive and commonly involve the vena cava or aorta, making full surgical resection difficult. The extent of invasion is difficult to assess with pre-operative imaging.

NB – *Despite the histopathological appearance, adrenal neoplasms exhibit a malignant behaviour.*

Hypophysectomy
- Available at a few centres, surgical risks are relatively high.

Prognosis
- Poor without treatment.
- Short-medium term reasonable with treatment.

4.7.5 Acromegaly
- Rare in cats although some evidence may be undiagnosed.

Aetiology
- Pituitary neoplasia.

Risk group
- Mid- to old-aged cats.
- Male.

History and physical examination
- Insulin-resistant diabetes:
  - Incidence of non-diabetic acromegalic cats is unknown.
- Weight gain despite poorly controlled DM.
- Change in body shape:
  - Increased body size.
  - Enlarged abdomen and head.
  - Prognathia.
- Arthropathies.
- Organomegaly.
- Heart – murmur, cardiac hypertrophy and CHF.
- Liver, kidney, spleen.
- Tongue – stridor and upper airway obstruction.

Key clinical pathology changes
- Poorly controlled DM.
- Hyperphosphataemia without azotaemia.
- Comparison of photographs over time.

Confirmatory tests
- Insulin-like growth factor 1 (IGF-1) estimation.
  - False-positive and false-negative results.
  - Many cats with DM without acromegaly have raised IGF-1.
- CT/MRI of pituitary.

Treatment
Cobalt irradiation of pituitary
- Good success reported, treatment of choice.

Octreotide
- A long-acting somatostatin analogue not shown to be effective in cats.

Surgery
- See hyperadrenocorticism.

Management of DM
- Reasonable to good quality of life can be provided by treating the secondary diabetes, as acromegaly is generally a slowly progressive disease.

- Very large doses of insulin may be required – 10–15 iU/kg.
  - Severity of insulin resistance fluctuates – repeated 12–15 iU injections through the day safer than single larger doses.

Prognosis
- Survival times of 4–42 months reported.
- Many acromegalic cats die from hypoglycaemic episodes.

4.7.6 Parathyroid disease

Hypoparathyroidism
- Rare as primary disease, relatively common following bilateral thyroidectomy.

History and physical examination
- Primary disease – young-middle aged cats.
- Abrupt to gradual onset of intermittent neurologic signs.
- Tremor.
- Seizure.
- Ataxia.
- Stilted gait.
- Disorientation.
- Weakness.
- Nictitating prominence.
- Lethargy and anorexia.
- Panting.
- Fever.
- Hypothermia.
- Bradycardia.
- Mild to severe dehydration.
- Posterior lenticular cataracts.

Key clinical pathology changes
- Hypocalcaemia.
- Hyperphosphataemia without azotaemia.
- ST and QT prolongation on ECG, bradycardia.
- Magnesium levels should be checked, as severe hypomagnesaemia can mimic the effects of hypoparathyroidism.

Confirmatory tests
- Primary disease – low PTH in the face of hypocalcaemia.

Treatment

Emergency
- IV calcium gluconate (10%) 1.0–1.5 ml/kg over 10–30 minutes (see Table 56).
- SC 2.5% calcium gluconate can also be given for less critical cases.
- Monitor cardiac rhythm during administration.

Maintenance therapy (Tables 54 and 55)
- Vitamin D analogues and calcium – in the majority of iatrogenic cases calcium regulation will recover over time.
- Dose rate of calcium for hypocalcaemic cats usually elemental calcium 50–100 mg/kg/day initially but some cats will require as much as 500 mg/kg/day. Longer term most cats require 0.3–0.5 g /cat/day.
- It is important to check the product label of calcium supplements as many are combined with other minerals notably phosphorus and magnesium. Some are mixed salts, e.g. calcium gluconate and lactate, making it difficult to calculate the elemental concentration. Some are combined with vitamin D or cod liver oil.

Hyperparathyroidism
Hyperparathyroidism can occur as a result of primary disease of the parathyroid gland, or secondary to inappropriate nutrition or CKD. In the latter two cases serum calcium is low or low/normal, whereas in primary disease the calcium is high (see 3.8 for differential diagnosis of hypercalcaemia). Primary hyperparathyroidism will be discussed below; it is very rarely diagnosed in cats.

Table 54 Vitamin D supplements

Generic	Forms	Manufacturers	Daily dose rate	Time to maximal effect	Duration of toxicity
Vitamin D_2 (ergocalciferol)	Capsules – 25 000 and 50 000 U Oral syrup – 8000 U/ml Injectable 50 000 U/ml	Not recommended	4000–6000 U/kg/day	5–21 days	1–18 weeks
Dihydrotachysterol	Oral solution – 0.25 mg/ml	AT 10	Initially – 0.02–0.03 mg/kg/day Maintenance – 0.01–0.02 mg/kg q24–48h	1–7 days	1–3 weeks
Alfacalciferol (Alfacalcidol)	Capsules – 0.25–1 mg Solution – 2 mg/ml Injectable – 2 mg/ml	One–alpha One–alpha One–alpha	0.05 mg/kg q24h for 3–4 days then 0.01–0.025 mg/kg q24h	1–4 days	1–14 days
Vitamin D_3 (calcitriol)	Capsules – 0.25, 0.5 mg Injectable – 1.0 mg/ml	Rocaltrol Calcijex	10–15 ng/kg/q12h for 3–4 days then 2.5–7.5 ng/kg q12h	1–4 days	1–14 days

Table 55 Calcium supplementation

Compound	Amount of elemental calcium	Forms	Initial dose rate (divided into 3–4 doses)	Other
Calcium carbonate	40%	Most are available as tablets, chewable tablets or capsules. Some liquid forms are available.	125–250 mg/kg/day	
Calcium citrate	21%		250–500 mg/kg/day	
Calcium gluconate	9%		500–1000 mg/kg/day	
Calcium lactate	13%		350–700 mg/kg/day	
Calcium oleate	7%		N/A	Collocal D contains 0.52 mg/ml calcium and 70 U vitamin D_2
Calcium gluconate	9.3 mg/ml	(Injectable 10%)	10–15 mg/kg as initial dose (1–1.5 ml/kg 10% solution) 60–90 mg/kg/day as a CRI	Usually diluted to 2.5% solution for use in cats. Can be given IV, IM (care regarding muscle necrosis and volume) or SC

Risk group for primary disease
- Older female and Siamese cats predisposed.

Clinical signs of hypercalcaemia
- PU/PD, lethargy and anorexia.
- Ectopic calcification causing significant organ dysfunction (renal failure, urolithiasis, gastric dysfunction).
- Parathyroid masses are usually small and not palpable.

Key clinical pathology and imaging changes of hypercalcaemia
- Hypophosphataemia.
- Renal, and rugal fold calcification on radiography.
- Calcium oxalate crystals or uroliths.

Confirmatory tests
- Increased serum PTH concentrations in the face of hypercalcaemia.
- Ultrasound.

Treatment
- Parathyroidectomy is a relatively straightforward procedure; post-operative calcium regulation however can be a major problem (see Hypoparathyroidism).
- Cases should be diuresed and given furosemide prior to surgery, to reduce serum calcium.

Prognosis
- Appears good > 1.5 years, in case series reported.

4.7.7 Hyperaldosteronism

Excess aldosterone production can be primary or secondary in origin. Secondary hyperaldosteronism results from increased stimulation of RAAS usually as a compensatory mechanism to hyponatraemic hypovolaemia, such as chronic use of diuretics. Reduced renal perfusion secondary to CKD can also increase aldosterone levels.

Primary hyperaldosteronism (PHA) uncommon associated with adrenal adenoma/carcinoma, MEN and hyperplasia. Bilateral neoplasia is reported.

Signalment
Middle-aged to older cats.

Presentation
- Hypokalaemic polymyopathy – muscle weakness and head ventroflexion.
  - Less commonly limb stiffness, dysphagia and collapse.
  - Mild and episodic → sudden and acute onset.
- Hypertensive retinal detachment and acute onset blindness.
  - Other signs of severe hypertensive disease are possible but not, as yet, reported.
- Occasional additional signs of hyperprogesteronism – similar signs to hypercortisolemia.

Diagnosis
- Hypokalaemia often present but degree is variable and persists despite supplementation.
- Elevated creatine kinase.
- Elevated FE of potassium.
- Hypertension.
- Elevated basal aldosteronism in the face of a low-normal plasma renin activity.
- An aldosterone to renin ratio (ARR) in healthy cats of 0.3–3.8 has been published.
- Adrenal mass on radiography, ultrasound or advanced imaging.

NB1 – *pulmonary metastasis are reported so the thorax should be evaluated.*

NB2 – *Diagnosis of PHA in the face of chronic renal disease can be difficult* *as aldosterone levels can be significantly elevated and incidental adrenal masses do occur.*

Treatment
- Immediate treatment with potassium may be necessary with some cats requiring very high doses up to 6 mmol PO q12h.
- Treatment of hypertension with amlodipine may also be required (0.625 mg PO q24h → 1.25 mg q12h).
- Spironolactone (as a competitive inhibitor of aldosterone) – 2–4 mg/kg PO q24h.
- Adrenalectomy for unilateral masses – specialist surgical procedure:
  - Medical stabilisation prior to surgery.
  - High perioperative mortality of around one-third of cases is reported.
  - Invasion of the vena cava is common.

Prognosis
- Medically managed – reported 7–30 months.
- Surgically treated – 8/17 alive at 1 year 2/17 alive at 3 years.

4.7.8 Other endocrine disease (Table 56)

Hypothyroidism
Naturally occurring disease is rare, and only primary hypothyroidism has been documented in cats. Both congenital and acquired forms have been described. The most common form of hypothyroidism is iatrogenic following I^{131} treatment or bilateral thyroidectomy. Although T_4 levels are often very low following these procedures, clinically significant hypothyroidism requiring supplementation is rare.

Hypothyroidism following treatment for hyperthyroidism has been associated with more rapid progression of renal disease.

Amine precursor and uptake decarboxylation (APUD) omas
- In the CNS and GIT are groups of Peptide secreting cells in CNS and GIT. Clinical signs are dependent on the peptide produced. Include insulinomas (see Table 53) and phaeochromocytoma (very rare in cats). Other APUDomas reported in small animals include gastrinoma (Zollinger–Ellison syndrome), glucagonoma (superficial necrolytic dermatitis [hepatocutaneous syndrome]), pancreatic polypeptide-producing tumour, carcinoids.

Multiple endocrine neoplasias
- Rare.

Polyendocrinopathies
- Relatively common, particularly in association with DM.

4.8 NEUROLOGIC DISEASE

4.8.1 Introduction
Neurologic signs are a common part of the presentation in many cats. Much information can be gained by performing a full neurologic examination. Cats are not ideal subjects for neurologic examination as many will not tolerate a complete examination conducted in a single session, and responses can be inconsistent between examinations without necessarily meaning there has been a change in the neurologic status.

4.8.2 Neurologic examination

Objectives
- Confirmation of neurological abnormalities.
- Localisation of the disease.
- Assessment of severity.
- Construction of a differential list.
- Formulation of a diagnostic and therapeutic plan.

ORGAN SYSTEMS

Table 56 Rare endocrinopathies in cats

Endocrinopathy	Congenital hypothyroidism	Acquired hypothyroidism	Hypoadrenocorticism	Insulinoma	Diabetes insipidus
Presentation and history	From 6–8 weeks old Disproportionate dwarf – Large head & short limbs	Lethargy, inappetence, obesity	Idiopathic, trauma, chronic glucocorticoid use	? Siamese predisposition	Idiopathic, trauma, neoplasia, cystic, inflammatory. Young cats
Clinical signs	Lethargy, mental dullness, constipation, bradycardia, hypothermia, retained deciduous teeth	Seborrhoea, hair loss, thick skin, pale mucous membranes	Lethargy, depression, weight loss, anorexia. Waxing and waning course. Dehydration and poor CO	Hypoglycaemia (see 4.7.3)	PU/PD (see 2.33) Variable CNS signs
Diagnosis	Low T_4 with elevated fTSH		ACTH stimulation test	Elevated insulin in face of low blood glucose	Rule out other causes PU/PD ADH response test Water deprivation test – not recommended
Treatment	Thyroid supplementation at 10–20 µg/kg q24h – aim for T_4 of 20–40 nmol/l		Crisis – 0.9% saline IVFT, dexamethasone 0.2 mg/kg q12h Chronic therapy Fludrocortisone – 0.05–0.1 mg/cat Prednisolone – 0.1–0.2 mg/kg/day	Surgery Hyperglycaemic agents	CDI – ADH replacement with DDAVP drops or tablets
Prognosis	Very good Clinical signs should resolve over 4–6 weeks, but bone and joint abnormalities may persist in kittens causing chronic problems		Good	Tumours are malignant and micrometastasis usually occurred by the time of presentation.	Good if responds to treatment

DDAVP, desmopressin acetate; fTSH, feline thyroid stimulating hormone;

Approach

- Full history – likelihood of trauma, access to toxins, use of medication, onset, duration and progression of signs.
- General clinical examination, including ophthalmic.
- Observation – mental status, posture, gait.

Clinical examination

Initial assessment

- Mentation – how alert and responsive is the cat?
- Pupillary light response
- Blink reflex.
- Head position.
- Ability to stand, position adopted when standing.
- Movement – lameness, ataxia, ability to negotiate obstacles.
- Weakness – single, fore, hind or all four limbs.
- UMN – involving the CNS or LMN – involving the PNS (Table 57).

Table 57 Comparison of clinical signs associated with upper and lower motor neuron damage

LMN damage	UMN damage
Loss of voluntary motor activity	Limited voluntary movement
Loss of reflex motor activity	Increased tone
Loss of resistance to passive movement (tone) resulting in flaccidity	Intact local reflexes which may be hyperactive (due to loss of higher control)
Atrophy of muscles	Occurrence of abnormal reflexes
Loss of sensation	Loss of conscious sensation
Loss of proprioception (limb position sense)	

Cranial nerves

CN I – olfactory

- Olfactory defects are rare.
- Assess with noxious or irritating substance, e.g. surgical spirit

CN II – optic

- Not ruled out by normal ophthalmic examination and PLR.
- Assess with following or menace response (also involves CN VII, avoid touching the cornea or the blink can be mediated by sensory CN V), obstacle test and visual placing responses, owner history.

CN III – oculomotor

- Pupillary constriction and extraocular muscles.

Deficit

- Mydriasis (inability to contract pupil) and ventrolateral (down and out) strabismus.

CN IV and VI – trochlear and abducens

- Extraocular muscles and retractor bulbi (VI).

Deficit

- Mild dorsolateral rotation (IV).
- Medial strabismus.
- Inability to retract globe in response to touching cornea (sensory via V) (VI).

CN V – trigeminal

- Facial sensation and motor to muscle of mastication.

Deficit

- Motor.
  - Atrophy of temporal muscles.
  - Inability to close mouth.
- Sensory.
- Ophthalmic branch:
  - Loss of corneal sensation resulting in a negative palpebral (with VII) and corneal (with VI) reflex.

ORGAN SYSTEMS

- Maxillary:
  - Loss of twitching in response to touching whiskers (with VII).
  - Loss of response to noxious stimuli to oral or nasal mucosa.
- Mandibular:
  - Lack of response to noxious stimuli, e.g. pin-prick to skin of mandible or oral mucosa.

CN VII – facial

- Motor function to facial muscles.
- Taste sensation to rostral two-thirds of tongue.

Deficit

- Facial paralysis.
- Drooping lip.
- Lack of response to pin prick.
- Loss of palpebral and menace reflex.
- Facial asymmetry (if unilateral).
- Lack of aversion response to atropine-soaked swab placed on the rostral tongue.

CN VII – auditory (vestibulocochlear)

- Hearing.
- Postural responses – see Table 58.

Deficit

- Deafness:
  - Lack of response to loud noise (startle).
  - Difficult if unilateral – absence of auditory evoked brain stem potential.
- Nystagmus:
  - Horizontal – fast phase away from lesion site that can be central or peripheral.
  - Vertical implies lesion is central in origin.
  - Rotatory or positional nystagmus is associated with peripheral or central (vestibular nucleus) disease.

NB – *Hereditary horizontal (physiologic) nystagmus occurs in some Siamese cats without other signs of vestibular dysfunction.*

Table 58   Comparison of clinical signs associated with central and peripheral vestibular disease

Clinical signs of vestibular disease	Central	Peripheral
Head tilt	Yes	Yes
Asymmetrical ataxia	Yes	Yes
Nystagmus	Yes	Yes
Positional nystagmus	Yes	No
Conscious proprioceptive deficits	Yes	No
Paresis	Yes	No

- Head tilt.
- Mild/unapparent tilt can be exaggerated if the cat is suspended from the pelvic limbs, normally thoracic limbs reach forward and the head is held approximately 45° to the ground.
- Circling.
- Hyperflexed head implies bilateral disease.

CN IX (glossopharyngeal) and X (vagus)

- Sensory and motor function to the larynx.
- Negative chronotrope to the heart (X).
- Sensory and motor function to the abdominal viscera.

Deficit

- Lack of gag response.
- Dysphagia.
- Dysphonia.

CN XI (accessory)

- Motor input to neck and shoulder muscles.

Deficit

- Rare.
- Wasting of muscles.
- Torticollis and inability to flex neck.

CN XII (hypoglossal)

- Motor function to tongue.

Deficit

- Inability to lick muzzle on the affected side.
- Contracture and deviation to the affected side.

Postural reactions

- Coordination of a complex series of sensory and motor functions.
- Highlights subtle defects.
- Poor at providing localisation.

Postural tests

- Wheel barrowing.
- Extensor postural thrust – cat suspended around thorax, pelvic limbs lowered to touch the surface; this should be associated with limb extension and a short backward pace.
- Hemi-standing and hemi-walking – detects incoordination and paresis.
- Hopping – detects single limb defects.
- Proprioception.
- Righting response of all four paws to knuckling.
- Return of limb to normal position after foot placed on piece of card and slowly slid laterally.
- Visual and tactile placing – step up as fore or hind legs meet table top.

Spinal reflexes

- Can be difficult in cats and vary day-to-day.
- Reduced or absence suggests LMN lesion, complete cord dysfunction, coma.
- Increased responses in UMN disease or unopposed action.
- Limb tested with cat in lateral recumbency, limb relaxed and slightly flexed.

Thoracic limb

- Biceps – proximal to insertion on elbow (C6–C8).
- Triceps – proximal to insertion on olecranon (C7–T2).
- Flexor withdrawal (C6–T2).
- Crossed extensor response (opposite limb extends) suggest UMN or central lack of suppression.

NB – *The presence of flexor withdrawal without central recognition of the stimulus does not reflect an intact spinal cord.*

- Extensor carpi radialis – muscle belly distal to elbow should elicit carpal extension (C7–T2).

Pelvic limb

- Patellar reflex (L4–L6).
- Gastrocnemius reflex – proximal to hock (L6–S2).
- Cranial tibial – just distal to the lateral tibial tuberosity should cause hock flexion (L6–S2).
- Flexor withdrawal (L6–S2).

Other

- Perineal (anal) reflex – stimulation causes anal contraction (S1–S3).
- Panniculus – twitch of truncal muscle as the spinal segmented is stimulated by a needle prick.
  - Afferent (sensory) T3–L1.
  - Efferent (motor) C8–T1.

Muscle tone

- LMN integrity is necessary to cause muscle cell contraction and maintain tone.
- The UMN has both a facilitatory and an inhibitory effect on the LMN. Loss of the UMN control has an overall hypertonic/spastic effect.
- Neurogenic atrophy is much more rapid than atrophy of disuse.

Nocioception

- If superficial sensation is present then no need to assess deep pain.
- Deep pain assessed by central response to progressively increasing stimulation.

ORGAN SYSTEMS

4.8.3 Approach to the neurologic case

See also section 2.5 ataxia, 2.6 behavioural change, 2.9 weakness, 2.31 paresis and paralysis, 2.37 seizures, 2.39 stiffness, 2.40 stupor and altered states of consciousness and 2.41 tremor.

Is the lesion
- Intracranial or extracranial?
- Primarily neurologic or secondary to another systemic disease?
- Unifocal or multifocal?

What is
- The location of the lesion?
- The nature of the lesion – i.e. malformation, inflammation, degeneration, trauma, neoplasia, infarction?
- Degenerative lesions usually in older cats, except specific abiotrophies.

Multifocal disease
- Inflammatory until proven otherwise.
- FIP meningoencephalomyelitis.
- Meningoencephalitis, e.g. granulomatous meningoencephalitis – perivascular proliferation of reticulohistiocytic cells.
- Toxoplasmosis.
- Cryptococcosis.
- Thiamine deficiency encephalopathy.
- Rabies.
- (Aujesky's).
- Feline spongiform encephalopathy.
- Meningitis (bacterial meningitis is very rare).
- Encephalitis.
- Aberrant parasitic migration/*Coenurus* cysts.

Occasionally
- Neoplastic if multiple metastases.
- Multiple injuries.
- Multiple malformations.

Differential diagnosis

Extracranial

Metabolic
- Hepatic encephalopathy – especially associated with PSSs.

- Hypoglycaemic – insulinomas, insulin overdose, xylitol.
- Azotaemia.
- Hypocalcaemia – primary hypoparathyroidism, post hyperthyroid surgery, pregnancy, toxaemia.
- Hypophosphataemia (rare), ketoacidotic diabetic cat.

Toxins
- Alpha-chloralose.
- Bromethalin.
- Cannabis.
- Dieldrin (wood preservative).
- Ethylene glycol.
- Lead.
- Metaldehyde.
- Organochlorides.
- Organophosphates/carbamates.
- Strychnine.
- Thallium.
- Theobromide (in chocolates).

Medications
- ACP.
- Enrofloxacin.
- Flea sprays (Fenvalerate, permethrins and DEET).
- Metoclopramide.
- Metronidazole.
- Piperazine.
- Theophylline.

Hyperviscosity
- Polycythaemia (primary or secondary, e.g. erythropoietin therapy).
- Multiple myeloma.
- Chronic leukaemia.

Others
- Acromegaly.
- Acute pancreatitis.
- Feline precursor porphyria.

Intracranial

Idiopathic epilepsy
- Comparatively rare in cats.
- No breed association has been documented, though it is thought to

occur more commonly in pedigree cats.

- Onset in mid-adulthood.
- Seizures frequently occur when the cat is asleep.

Neoplasia
- Relatively common.
- Meningioma, lymphoma and gliomas most frequent.

Infectious/inflammatory disease
- See Section 5 for staggering disease (Borna virus).
- Rabies.

Ischaemic encephalopathy (see Section 4.8.7).
  Lysosomal storage diseases (see Section 4.8.7).

Trauma
- Can potentially cause any number of signs.
- Seizures following cranial trauma (usually RTAs) are not uncommon.
- Majority of cats do not progress to epilepsy.

Thiamine deficiency
- Rare.
- Associated with
  ○ Feeding raw fish (thiaminase).
  ○ Cooked meat diets (thiamine destroyed by heat).
  ○ Sodium metabisulfite preservatives (destroys thiamine).
  ○ May be precipitated in anorexic cats with PU/PD or on fluid diuresis.
- Clinical signs include
  ○ Seizuring.
  ○ Cranial nerve deficits.
  ○ Ataxia.
  ○ Neck weakness.
- Treatment
  ○ Injectable 10–20 mg i/m.
  ○ Oral 5–30 mg/cat/day.

Hydrocephalus
- Congenital.
- Secondary to CSF obstruction, common in FIP.

4.8.4 Diagnostic approach to neurologic case

Rule out extracranial disease
- Haematology.
- Biochemistry including pre- and post-prandial bile acids (or ammonia).
- FeLV/FIV serology.
- Cryptococcus antigen.
- Toxoplasma serology.

Lesion localisation (Figure 27)

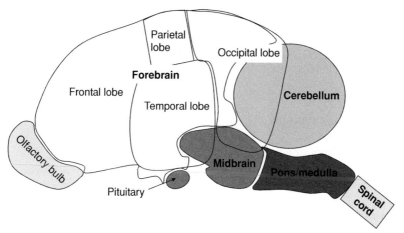

Figure 27 Sagittal section of a cat brain showing major anatomic regions

ORGAN SYSTEMS

Cerebellum

Dysmetria (high-stepping forelimb gait, wide base stance, truncal swaying), generalised or intention tremors, and vestibular signs.

Pons and Medulla

Weakness or proprioceptive deficits similar to cervical spinal cord disease, deficits CN V–XII, autonomic dysfunction including respiratory centres.

Midbrain

CN III and IV, changes in consciousness, rigidity, postural deficits.

Forebrain

Changes in mentation, seizures, circling or pacing, central visual loss.

Spinal cord

C1–C5 – UMN signs in thoracic and pelvic limbs.

C6–T2 – LMN signs thoracic, UMN pelvic.

T3–L3 – UMN signs pelvic limbs, Schiff-Sherrington signs if lesion severe (forelimb rigidity despite voluntary movement).

L4–S3 – LMN signs pelvic limbs, tail and perineum.

Coccygeal – LMN signs tail.

- LMN in all four limbs suggests diffuse PNS or neuromuscular disease.
- If there is cranial nerve involvement – brain is affected too.
- Common causes of lesions at each location are listed in Table 59.

Imaging

Radiography

- Of non-neurologic structure.
- Vertebral column:
  ○ Disc abnormalities are not uncommon.
  ○ Clinically significant disease is rare and requires myelography or MRI.
- Skull:
  ○ Generally provides limited diagnostic information other than in trauma cases.

Magnetic resonance imaging (MRI) and computer assisted tomography (CT)

- Powerful techniques available for the diagnosis of intracranial disorders:
  ○ Image quality can be an issue with some systems due to the size of the cat's head.
  ○ Gadolinium – IV contrast medium which has enhanced electromagnetic properties, demonstrates damage to blood–brain barrier on MRI.
- Expensive.
- General anaesthesia required.
- Sensitive for the detection of lesions.
- Non-specific for pathogenesis.
- Can be used to examine spinal cord for disc herniation.

MRI or CT?

- MRI has superior contrast resolution hence is preferred for imaging the CNS.
- MRI has an extensive range of sequences allowing differentiation of fluid and CSF, and potentially haemorrhages and mass lesions within the CNS.
- Combination of good contrast and spatial resolution enables quite subtle pathology to be identified.
- CT is quicker and less expensive but has poorer resolution that may miss smaller lesions
- CT will show mineralised disc extrusions but the spinal cord can only be assessed using myelography.
- Brain CT may demonstrate a mass effect, severe haemorrhage, mass, or meningeal lesions, but is not useful to assess herniation of the cerebellum through the foramen magnum.
- CT valuable if skull or vertebral pathology especially trauma.

CSF sampling

Technique

- General anaesthesia.
- Intubation to protect airway, uncuffed, one tube size smaller (reduces risk of kinking).

Table 59 Differential diagnosis of CNS lesions in cats according to site, chronicity and pain

Site of lesion	Acute, painful	Acute, non-painful	Chronic, painful	Chronic non-painful
C1–C5	Disc disease[a] Atlantoaxial subluxation[b] Neoplasia Inflammatory CNS disease[b] Discospondylitis[b] Trauma[b]	Ischaemic myelopathy (due to fibrocartilaginous emboli)	Disc disease[a] Atlantoaxial subluxation[a,b] Neoplasia Inflammatory CNS disease[b] Discospondylitis[b]	Storage diseases[b] Congenital vertebral malformations
C6–T2	Disc disease[a] Neoplasia Inflammatory CNS disease[b] Discospondylitis[b] Trauma[b]	Ischaemic myelopathy	Disc disease[a] Neoplasia Inflammatory CNS disease[b] Discospondylitis[b] Trauma[b]	Congenital vertebral malformations
T3–L3	Disc disease Neoplasia Inflammatory CNS disease[b] Discospondylitis[b] Trauma[b]	Ischaemic myelopathy	Disc disease Neoplasia Inflammatory CNS disease[b] Discospondylitis[b]	Degenerative myelopathy Hereditary myelopathy[b] Spinal dysraphism[b] Syringomyelia Congenital vertebral malformations[b] Neoplasia
L4–S3	Disc disease Neoplasia Inflammatory CNS disease[b] Discospondylitis[b] Trauma[b] Sacrocaudal injuries	Ischaemic myelopathy	Disc disease Lumbosacral disease Neoplasia Inflammatory CNS disease[b] Discospondylitis[b]	Spina bifida[b] Spinal dysraphism[b] Sacrocaudal dysgenesis Syringomyelia Congenital vertebral malformations[b] Neoplasia

[a]Rarely significant in cats. [b]Common in young animals

ORGAN SYSTEMS

- Lateral recumbency.
- Head is flexed to create a 90° angle with the vertebral column.
- Nose should be raised to maintain the sagittal plane parallel to the table top.
- Occipital crest and wings of the axis are palpated; the needle is placed in the midline, midway between the intersection of the two lines, and the occipital crest perpendicular to the neck.
- 40 mm/22 gauge spinal needle is ideal, but a hypodermic needle (25 mm/23g) of a similar size can be used.
- The needle is slowly advanced until there is a popping sensation and sudden loss of resistance as the needle enters the subarachnoid space.
- CSF should ideally be allowed to flow passively.
- If flow is very slow then gentle positive pressure with a 1-ml syringe can be applied.
- If there is blood contamination, from passage through a small vessel, the first 1–2 drops of fluid should be discarded.
- Gross contamination renders the sample non-diagnostic and needle should be removed.
- CSF should be placed in an EDTA and a plain tube.
- If the lesion is caudal to the foramen a lumbar puncture may be more diagnostically valuable; but this is technically difficult and usually only produces a few drops of CSF.
- Following CSF collection, myelography can be performed if indicated.
- Use non-ionic water soluble contrast medium (0.25–0.5 ml/kg).

Analysis
- Record gross appearance.
- Cytology of the CSF should be as rapid as is practical.
- If rapid analysis is not possible contact the diagnostic laboratory for preferred preservative, e.g. paraformaldehyde, ethanol or nothing.
- Protein levels are stable for around 4 hours.
- Other parameters that are sometimes measured include.
  - Glucose (reduced relative to blood in bacterial meningitis).
  - ALT or CPK (indicate non-specific neuronal damage).
- The diagnostic value of viral titres, e.g. coronavirus, in the CSF is unclear.

Interpretation of changes
- General rather than specific diseases.
- Increases in cell count and proteins indicating inflammatory or neoplastic disease.
- Neoplastic cells in the CSF are rare.

NB – *A normal CSF analysis does not exclude inflammatory or neoplastic disease.*

Reference range
- Gross appearance – clear and watery.
- Cells <6 white cells/ml.
- Protein <30 mg/dl.
- Glucose >60–80% of serum value.

Complications and contraindications to CSF sampling
- Small but appreciable risk of brain stem herniation or spinal cord laceration accompanies attempts at CSF collection.
  - Risk increased if there is raised ICP or intracranial masses causing distortion of the brain architecture, e.g. neoplasia.
  - Raised ICP leading to herniation can be difficult to appreciate (papilloedema is often not present) and distortion of intracranial anatomy on clinical examination.
- Fracture/luxation of bone in the sample area.
- Post-anaesthetic complications including seizures can also occur.

Electroencephalogram (EEG)

- May be useful in revealing focal disease, generalised cortical damage in encephalitis, hydrocephalus, and cortical depression in hepatic and toxic syndromes or post-traumatic scarring.
- Not widely used in cats.
- Criteria for normality are poorly defined.

4.8.5 Management of neurologic disease

Oxygen

- Many cases with reduced cerebral function following trauma or seizure activity will be suffering from hypoxia.
- O_2 enriched environment can reduce further hypoxic damage and cerebral oedema.

Fluids

- Maintenance of perfusion of the nervous system is essential to ensure adequate oxygenation.
- Reduces the build-up of neurotoxic metabolites.
- Overhydration can worsen cerebral oedema.

Acid–base balance

- Acidosis is more frequently encountered following injury.
- Alkalosis can occur due to inappropriate hyperventilation caused by pain or damage to the respiratory control centres.
- Brain and CSF pH are more profoundly affected by respiratory rather than metabolic disturbances in acid–base balance.
- Care must be taken if bicarbonate is used to correct an acidosis, as CO_2 readily diffuses across the CSF producing paradoxical *CSF acidosis*.
- CSF acidosis is usually associated with coma.
- Alkalosis causes hyperexcitability and potentially seizures.

Glucose

- All seizuring cats should have their blood glucose level assessed.
- Hypoglycaemia may cause seizures, but can also be the result of prolonged seizure activity.
- Hypoglycaemic seizures are difficult to control with anticonvulsant therapy, unless glucose levels are restored.

Nutrition

- Total parenteral nutrition may be necessary in comatose animals.
- Other injuries can lead to an inability or reluctance to eat; in such cases nutritional support is important to aid recovery (see section 4.13 – nutrition).

Pain relief

- Pain can be severe, associated with spinal or cranial injuries
- Acute phase pain is probably best managed using opiates either alone or in combination e.g. methadone, lidocaine and ketamine (MLK) or fentanyl, lidocaine and ketamine (FLK) (see section 1.5 – analgesia).
- Longer term pain relief can be provided by NSAIDs, but they should not be used concurrently with corticosteroids.
- Pain relief can be contraindicated in head injuries as it can mask the state of alertness making it difficult to assess clinical trends

Nervous system oedema

- Can be extremely difficult to diagnose without advanced imaging.
- Fundoscopy can be of value if papilloedema is present.
- Oedema can occur secondary to infection, trauma, neoplasia, hypoxia, and other metabolic disturbances.
- Oedema should be suspected in cats whose neurological status is deteriorating without other obvious cause, particularly if they are becoming progressively less alert and responsive.

ORGAN SYSTEMS

Management
- Hypertonic saline if hypovolaemic
- Mannitol
- Elevate head and neck by 15–30°
- Hyperventilation (short term)
- Surgery
- Methylprednisolone succinate – 30 mg/ kg slow IV then 15 mg/kg at 2 and 6 hours has shown limited efficacy

Mannitol
- Most widely used in the treatment of nervous system oedema, being more effective than furosemide.
- Dose – 0.5–2.0 g/kg of a 20% mannitol solution is given *very* slowly over a 10–15 minute period
- Mannitol dose can be repeated in 30–60 minutes.
- Contraindications of mannitol therapy.
  ○ Dehydration – correct prior to administration
  ○ CHF
  ○ Suspected ongoing cerebral/spinal haemorrhage
  ○ Acute spinal cord injury from trauma (or disc herniation)
- If urine has not been produced within 1 hour of mannitol administration furosemide should be given to induce diuresis.

Infection
- Few antimicrobials will cross the intact blood–brain barrier; however, in many cases there will be sufficient inflammation to allow therapeutic concentrations to be achieved.
- Toxoplasmosis – clindamycin.
- *Cryptococcus* – fluconazole has good penetration into the CSF.

Glucocorticoids
- For acute (within the first 24 hours) or severe nervous system inflammation methylprednisolone sodium succinate can be given at 30 mg/kg and repeated at 15 mg/kg every 6–8 hours for the first 24 hours or as a CRI at 2.5 mg/kg/hour.
  ○ Evidence for the value of corticosteroids in most forms of CNS disease remains poor and use more than 24 hours post injury is generally considered contraindicated.
- Dexamethasone at 2 mg/kg given i/v may be less effective acutely than methylprednisolone but it has a longer duration of action, a second dose of 1 mg/kg can be given after 12 hours.
- Use of high doses of steroid *is* associated with side effects including haemorrhagic gastroenteritis, pancreatitis and hepatopathy.
- GIT side effects can be reduced by using H_2 blocker, proton-pump inhibitor and/ or sucralfate.
- A number of rare steroid responsive non-suppurative inflammatory conditions of the CNS have been reported, such as GME and meningoencephalitis.
- Chronic glucocorticoid usage can be of value in cats showing multifocal CNS disease, or in palliation of CNS neoplasia.

4.8.6 Prognosis in neurologic disease
- For many owners the most important consideration in neurological cases is
  ○ Likelihood of recovery.
  ○ Time that recovery may take.
  ○ Likelihood of residual deficit.
  ○ Nursing care required.

Modified Glasgow coma scale (Box 8–10)
- Subject to personal interpretation.
- General trends rather than absolute values are often the most helpful particularly with client management.
- 3–8 represents a grave prognosis.
- 9–12, a poor to guarded prognosis.
- Above 12, a reasonable to good prognosis.
- A rising score on repeated examinations also represents a more favourable prognosis.

Box 8 Modified Glasgow coma scale – motor activity

Motor activity

Normal gait, normal spinal reflexes	6
Hemiparesis, tetraparesis or decerebrate activity	5
Recumbent, intermittent extensor rigidity	4
Recumbent, constant extensor rigidity	3
Recumbent, constant extensor rigidity and opisthotonus	2
Recumbent, hypotonia of muscles, depressed or absent spinal reflexes	1

Box 9 Modified Glasgow coma scale – brain stem reflexes

Brain stem reflexes

Normal pupillary light response and oculocephalic reflexes	6
Slow PLR and normal to reduced oculocephalic reflexes	5
Bilateral unresponsive miosis with normal to reduced oculocephalic reflexes	4
Pinpoint pupils with reduced to absent oculocephalic reflexes	3
Unilateral, unresponsive mydriasis with reduced/absent oculocephalic reflexes	2
Bilateral, unresponsive mydriasis with reduced/absent oculocephalic reflexes	1

Box 10 Modified Glasgow coma scale – level of consciousness

Level of consciousness

occasional periods of alertness and responsive to environment	6
depression or delirium, capable of responding to environment but may be inappropriate	5
semicomatose, responsive to visual stimuli	4
semicomatose, responsive to auditory stimuli	3
semicomatose, responsive to noxious stimuli	2
comatose, unresponsive to repeated noxious stimuli	1

ORGAN SYSTEMS

Oculocephalic reflex – eyes should track with the head movement as the cat's head is turned from side to side.

Peripheral nerve injury
- Generally resistant to stretch injuries, as both the nerve bundle and nerve itself are semicoiled to allow for stretch.
- Most common cause of monoplegia is injury to the nerve plexus or peripheral nerve.
- Other diagnoses do have to be considered, e.g. neoplasia (primary, secondary or compressive) or space-occupying lesions causing external pressure on the nerve or nerve root.

- Occasionally polyneuropathies, e.g. endocrine, can initially appear as a monoparesis.

Neurapraxia
- A transient loss of nerve function following injury with no resultant nerve degeneration.
- Prognosis is good, function usually returns rapidly, but can take up to 3 months.

Axonotmesis
- Rupture or severance of an axon with the supporting structures left intact.

- Most nerve injuries caused by stretching, direct blow or excessive pressure are a combination of neurapraxia and axonotmesis.
- Axon distal to the point of injury degenerate.
- Regeneration begins after 1 week and proceeds at around 1 mm per day.
- Can be complicated by neurogenic atrophy and fibrosis of the muscles, so passive physiotherapy is essential.

Neurotmesis
- Complete severance of a nerve.
- Recovery of function is unlikely unless the cut ends are closely apposed.
- Neuroma formation may occur.

Spinal cord paraparesis and paraplegia

Acute paralysis
- Trauma
- Aortic embolism
- Neoplasia

Chronic progressive disease
- Neoplasia
- Discospondylitis
- Rarely disc disease

Prognosis
- Guarded – aortic thromboembolism, neoplasia
- Variable – trauma depending on degree of damage
- Variable to good – discospondylitis, disc disease

Trauma
- Most common cause of spinal injury in the cat. Acute cases may be treated with methylprednisolone.
- Early decision on surgical intervention should be made if there is myelographic evidence of compression.
- Many cats respond well to conservative management with strict cage rest.

- Prognosticating in such cases is best based on repeated neurological examinations. Although the initial status is important any sustained improvements carry an improved prognosis.

Good prognostic signs
- Normal anal reflex.
- Urinary control.
- Conscious perception of pain.
- Tail movement (conscious).
- Paraparesis (weakness) rather than paralysis.
- Normal spinal reflexes.

Intermediate prognostic signs
- Lack of urinary control.
- Hyperactive spinal reflexes.
- Only conscious of deep pain.
- Paralysis.

Poor prognostic signs
- Schiff-Sherrington syndrome (pelvic limb paralysis with forelimb rigidity).
  - Better outlook if normal or hyperactive spinal reflexes.
- Loss of spinal reflexes.
- Primitive spinal reflexes, e.g. crossed extensor.
- Loss of anal tone.
- Ascending loss of panniculus.
- Absence of deep pain.

NB – *Some of the above features may be due to spinal shock and considerable improvement may occur over the first 24–72 hours. Any prognostic decisions on cases of spinal trauma should be delayed for this 72-hour period. Combinations of features representing poor prognosis also worsen the outlook, e.g. paralysis with loss of bladder control and loss of deep pain sensation.*

4.8.7 Specific disease states

Cognitive dysfunction
See Section 1.4 – Gerontology.

ORGAN SYSTEMS

Seizures

See Section 2.37 for differential diagnosis.

Pathophysiology

- Change in balance of excitatory and inhibitory neurones.
- Increased excitatory or decreased inhibitory neurotransmitters.
- Changes in proportions of receptor sites.
- Denervation hypersensitivity.
- The result of these changes is to increase the rate of firing of a group or groups of neurones, and increase the susceptibility of other neurones to be captured by them.
- Repeated exposure of normal neurones to spontaneous discharge will increase their inherent excitability leading to the expansion of the focus = *kindling*.
- Seizures often occur at times of changing brain activity, e.g. during phases of sleep, at waking, excitement, feeding.

Systemic changes

- Initially increased then decreased blood glucose
- Increased temperature and lactic acidosis
- Ventricular arrhythmias
- Neurogenic pulmonary oedema

Diagnostic approach

- As for other neurologic disease.
- Initial approach is to differentiate intracranial from extracranial causes.

Therapy

- Phenobarbital (phenobarbitone) remains the first choice drug for chronic treatment at 1.5–3 mg/kg q8–12h.

When to treat?

- Kindling means that it is important to begin treatment of epilepsy early.
- Guidelines – cat seizes more than once every 6 weeks or has clusters of fits more frequently than every 2 months.

Phenobarbital

- Acts to decrease the excitability of ALL tissues including the myocardium, fortunately CNS depression occurs at lower doses.
- Absorption can be variable between patients.
- Half-life of phenobarbitone in cats is approximately 40 hours; steady state is achieved after 5 half-lives, hence assessment of the effect of therapy is difficult to make until 8 days after therapy has been instituted.
- In cases where the cat is fitting severely a loading dose of 1.5× the daily maintenance dose can be given.

Side effects
- Sedation.
- Behavioural changes.
- Polydipsia.
- Tolerance.
- Paradoxical hyperactivity.
- Anaemia (rare).
- Induction of hepatic microenzymes – this will result in more rapid metabolism of the drug so steady state levels will decrease over a number of weeks, which can lead to destabilisation of the patient.

Drug interactions
- Antimicrobials.
- Antacids and H_2 antagonists.
- Cardiac medication.
- Theophylline.
- NSAIDs.
- Corticosteroids.
- ACP.
- Metoclopramide.
- Anthelmintics.

Diazepam

- Second choice therapy.
- Tends to give less reliable control as its half-life is only 7 hours.
  - Tolerance tends to develop.

ORGAN SYSTEMS

- Acts to limit the spread of seizure activity and elevates the seizure threshold.
- Idiopathic hepatotoxicity is reported.
- Frequent and regular dosing is required 1–2 mg q6–8h.

Side effects
- Sedation.
- Polyphagia (temporary).

Taurine
- Acts as an inhibitory neurotransmitter in cats.
- Few reports of successful use but no widespread trials have been performed.

Other agents
- Potassium bromide should be avoided as it causes allergic pneumonitis in around one third of cats and is only efficacious in around one third of cases.
- Relatively less information is available about the pharmacokinetics and toxicity of other antiseizure agents in cats.
  - Specialist advice should be sought before using agents such as levetiracetam, zonisamide, gabapentin or pregabalin in cats.

Treatment failure
- Owner non-compliance.
- Drug interaction.
- Precipitating causes, e.g. additional medication, other disease processes, physical/psychological stress.
- Failure of diagnosis.
- Seizures have an extracranial cause.
- The disease process is progressive.
- Medication failure.
- Inappropriate drug.
- Insufficient drug.
- Rapid changes in dose rates.
- Excessive serum fluctuations (timing).
- Inappropriate combination.

Response to apparent therapeutic failure
- Measure serum levels.
- Peak and trough levels should be assessed.
- Therapeutic range (for barbiturates) being 15–45 µg/ml.

Idiopathic epilepsy
- Uncommon in cats compared to dogs.
- Usually seizure start when cat is a young adult (6 months–5 years).
- Initial seizure frequency is usually low.
- Diagnosis is by exclusion of other causes of seizuring.
- Treatment is with anti-epileptic medication.

Treatment of status epilepticus
- Prompt, aggressive management is required.
- Place a cephalic catheter as early on as possible, makes subsequent treatment considerably easier.
- Diazepam 0.25–0.5 mg/kg IV, wait 2–5 minutes for effect.
  - Repeat dose up to three times until effect – maximum 20 mg diazepam/cat.
  - If diazepam effective consider CRI at 0.5 mg/kg/hour
    - Diazepam is substantially absorbed by some plastics used in syringes/giving sets – non-absorbent materials include glass, polyolefin, polypropylene and polyethylene.
- If seizuring is not controlled then 3–6 mg/kg pentobarbital IV.

NB – *Can cause respiratory depression especially in combination with diazepam.*

- Repeat dose after 30 minutes to maximum 20 mg/kg.
- If still seizuring then anaesthetise with propofol and try and maintain on propofol CRI.
  - Note it can be difficult to distinguish anaesthetic recovery from seizuring in some cases as they are weaned off propofol CRI.

ORGAN SYSTEMS

- Supply oxygen enriched environment to reduce CNS hypoxia.
- Monitor blood glucose.
- IV fluids preferably lactated Ringer's solution.
- Elevation of the head – controversial as reduces cerebral perfusion pressure.

Brain diseases

- Increased ICP.
  - Clinical signs of ICP – altered mental state, paresis, seizures, CN deficits, altered respiratory pattern – also see section 4.8.4 cerebral oedema.
- Hydrocephalus.
- Mentation change and seizures.
- Corticosteroids and diuretics, surgical shunt.
- Neoplastic.
- Inflammatory.
- Idiopathic.
- Narcolepsy.
- Vascular disease.

Brain tumours

- Less frequent in cats than dogs – 3.5/100 000 cats.
- No apparent breed predisposition.
- Meningioma most commonly seen and can be amenable to surgical removal.
- Aged cats.
- Most common intracranial tumour in cats.
- Malignancy rates are low.
- Tumour is slow growing.
- Sometimes multiple.
- Good candidates for surgery as they are usually accessible.
- Variety of other primary tumours reported.
- Secondary tumours include lymphoma, pituitary adenoma, and metastatic carcinoma.
- Local extension can also occur from middle ear, nasal and skull tumours.

Presentation

- Often long history of vague signs e.g. behavioural change.
- Seizuring most frequently recognised sign – generalised or focal.
  - Associated with altered consciousness and circling.
- Other reported signs
  - Altered posture, ataxia, head tilt, behaviour change, depression, incontinence and cervical spinal hyperaesthesia.

Diagnosis

- Exclude extracranial causes.
- CSF changes often non-specific and associated risk of herniation.
- Advanced imaging – MRI most sensitive for intracranial soft tissue mass lesions.

Spinal cord and disc disease

Differential diagnosis for spinal disease

- Bilateral orthopaedic disease – cruciate rupture, tibial crest avulsion, fractures, coxofemoral degenerative joint disease.
- Generalised orthopaedic disease – polyarthritis.
- Muscle disease.
- Thromboembolic disease.

Localisation of lesions

See Section 4.8.4 and Table 60.

Diagnosis

- Lumbar CSF aspiration.
- Radiography usually requiring myelography.
- CT +/– myelographic CT.
- MRI.

Causes of myelographic changes

Extradural

- Disc herniation.
- Congenital abnormality.
- Neoplasia – vertebral, metastatic soft tissue, lymphoma.

ORGAN SYSTEMS

ORGAN SYSTEMS

- Discospondylitis.
- Vertebral osteomyelitis.
- Trauma – disc, bone fragment, haematoma.

Intradural/extramedullary
- Neoplasia – lymphoma, meningioma, other.

Intramedullary
- Acute stage ischaemic myelopathy.
- Inflammatory CNS disease.
- Neoplasia.
- Haematoma.

Single limb deficits
Common injuries
- Brachial plexus – most common, causes complete loss of sensation ± Horner's syndrome and loss panniculus.
- Radial nerve – following humeral fracture, causes dropped elbow and knuckled carpus.
  - Treatment – tendon relocation, carpal arthrodesis.
  - Complications – contracture of joints, abrasions on foot, trophic ulcers (as denervated skin has less resistance to pressure) and poor vascular tone.
- Lumbosacral trunk deficits:
  - Inability to extend hip and flex stifle or flex/extend hock.
  - Often bear weight as fix stifle.
  - Analgesia distal to stifle except medially.
- Sciatic nerve:
  - Preserve gluteal function ± hamstrings.
  - Injuries are most commonly iatrogenic, associated with intramedullary pin, ischial or acetabular fractures.

Peripheral neuropathies
- Associated with multisystemic disease, e.g. DM, hyperchylomicronaemia.

Polyneuropathy
- Paresis.
- Ataxia.
- Muscle atrophy.
- Hyporeflexia.
- Hypotonia.

Diagnosis
- EMG.
- Nerve biopsy.

Ischaemic neuropathy
- Secondary to thromboembolism.
- Paresis/paralysis.
- Painful hard muscles.
- Cold extremities.

Polyneuropathy associated with coccidiostat toxicity
- Mild paresis to severe tetraparesis.
- Respiratory and autonomic signs.
- Secondary to peripheral neuropathy (axonopathy).
- Contamination of food with salinomycin (ionophore coccidiostat).
- Outcome dependent on severity of signs and veterinary support.

Diabetic polyneuropathy
- Associated with poor glycaemic control.
- Many diabetic cats show electrophysiological evidence, relatively few have clinical signs.
- The majority of distal polyneuropathy especially of hind limbs.
- Plantigrade stance, progressive paresis, hyporeflexia and muscle atrophy.
- Significant improvement in early cases if diabetic control is good.

Neoplasia
- Primary neoplasia – neurofibroma, schwannoma.
- Compression from secondary neoplasm, e.g. xanthoma.
- Infiltration, e.g. lymphoma.
- Sensory (paraesthesia, excessive licking) and motor signs.

Chronic inflammatory polyneuropathies

Idiopathic laryngeal paralysis

- Reported in cats, although the majority of cases are secondary to another disease.

Trauma

- Peripheral nerve dysfunction. Recovery will depend on the degree of axonal disruption and if there is axonal die- back the distance for regrowth (1–2 mm/day).
- Nerve root avulsion carries the worst prognosis.
- Stretch and compression injuries can cause temporary interruption of axonal flow (recovery in days) or may lead to die-back.
- Demyelination is rapidly repaired.

Feline hyperaesthesia syndrome

- Varying irritation of dorsal thoracolumbar area.
- Rippling skin.
- Chew hair/skin.
- Scream when touched.
- Frantic meowing, growling, hissing, swishing tail and apparent hallucination.
- Varying success with phenobarbital, gabapentin, corticosteroids, megoestrol acetate, amitriptyline, clomipramine.

Aujesky's disease (pseudorabies, mad itch)

- Herpes virus.
- Cat is dead-end host, and although they can shed virus – it is usually fatal.
- Contact with pigs or pork.
- Currently no Aujesky's disease in pigs in the UK.
- Notifiable disease.

Clinical signs

- Behavioural change – restless, hypersalivate, isolate.
- Intense pruritus – self-mutilate.
- Rarely aggressive.
- Not all animals are pruritic.
- Terminal within 48 hours – paralysis and coma.
- Peracute death can occur.

Diagnosis

- At PM.
- Usually antibody negative.

Horner's syndrome

Signs

- Miosis, 3rd eyelid prolapse, enopthalmia and ptosis.
  - Not all components need to be present but there is always miosis.

Localisation

- Varies from midbrain through spinal cord to T1–T3 up the vagosympathetic trunk and cranial cervical ganglion next to the tympanic bulla.
- Classified as 1st, 2nd or 3rd order.
- Most cases are 3rd order and idiopathic but if necessary, pharmacologic testing with phenylephrine.

Ischaemic encephalopathy

- Peracute onset of unilateral forebrain signs ± seizures.
  - Mental depression, confusion, circling, hemiparesis.
  - Sudden onset blindness.
- Suspected to be secondary to vasospasm.
  - May occur as a complication of anaesthesia.
- Young to middle-aged adults.
- Usually show rapid neurologic improvement over 24–72 hours.
- Residual signs tend to be minimal.
  - Persistent personality changes or post-ischaemic epilepsy.

ORGAN SYSTEMS

- Diagnosis requires MRI.
  - CSF cytology and proteins often unremarkable.
- Treatment is symptomatic and supportive aimed at reducing cerebral oedema.
- Prognosis is usually very good.
  - A few cats die/are euthanised in first 24 hours due to deteriorating neurologic status.

Idiopathic vestibular syndrome
See section 2.5.8.

Inherited neuropathies

Adult-onset motor neurone disease
- Chronic progressive generalised weakness associated with tremor, neck weakness, dysphagia and muscle atrophy.
- Spinal reflexes initially present are gradually lost.
- 4 years of age and older.

Diagnosis
- Denervation and fibrillatory potentials, normal nerve conduction.
- Postmortem changes in spinal cord.

Treatment
- None available but progression is slow, so good period of survival with supportive care.

Table 60 Inherited neuropathies

Disease	Pathology and inheritance	Breed and prognosis	Clinical presentation	Diagnosis
Hyperoxaluric neuropathy	Suspected autosomal recessive axonopathy	DSH	Oxalate crystals/ uroliths, CKD develops by 1 year of age. Profound LMN weakness begins at 5–9 months	Biochemistry, urinalysis, electrophysiology
Hyperchylo-micronaemia	Formation of lipid granuloma		Monoparesis – particularly Horner's syndrome, facial/ masticatory muscle paralysis	Low lipoprotein lipase activity, elevated triglyceride + cholesterol
Sphingomyelinase deficiency (feline Niemann–Pick disease)	Autosomal recessive lysosomal storage disease – demyelinating polyneuropathy	Siamese	2–5 month old Progressive LMN signs – paresis, tremor Hepatospleno-megaly	Nerve conduction velocity – slow. Nerve biopsy, skin fibroblast culture, urinalysis
Distal axonopathy	Degenerative neuropathy – sciatic nerve and areas of spinal cord and brain	Birman Poor	6–10 week male – progressive hind limb ataxia	

Lysosomal storage diseases
- A group of inherited, progressive and lethal multisystemic degenerative disorders (see Table 61).
- Initial clinical signs are often neurologic:
  - Usually single gene mutation/deletion with a recessive or X-linked inheritance.
  - Cerebellar signs are frequently seen.
- Diagnosis is based on
  - Familial patterns.
  - Evaluation of serum, white blood cells or various biopsies to establish enzyme levels.
  - Urinalysis.

4.8.8 Autonomic nervous system

Diarrhoea – nictitating membrane prominence
- See GIT disease.

Dysautonomia (Key–Gaskells syndrome)
- Usually young adults.
- Incidence has been low, but prevalence may be increasing.

Clinical signs
- Autonomic dysfunction.
- Anorexia, constipation.
- Dry mouth (xerostomia) and nasal passages.
- Third eyelid prolapse.
- Vomiting, regurgitation and megaoesophagus.
- Bradycardia.
- Urinary/faecal incontinence.
- Anal areflexia.

Diagnosis
- Thoracic and abdominal radiographs.
- Schirmer tear test.
- Absence of inflammation to intradermal histamine.
- Abnormal pupillary response to 0.1% pilocarpine.

Treatment
- Palliative – feeding (gastrostomy tube may be required), artificial tears, laxatives (lactulose).
- Bethanechol.
- Cisapride or metoclopramide.

Prognosis
- Depends on severity of signs.
- Severely affected cats 20–30% survival.

Table 61 Lysosomal storage diseases in cats

Condition	Enzyme deficiency	Breed
Mucopolysaccharidosis I	Alpha-L-iduronidase	DSH, Siamese, Korat
Mucopolysaccharidosis VI	Arylsulphatase B	Siamese
Metachromatic leucodystrophy	Arylsulphatase	DSH
GM₁ gangliosidosis	Beta-galactosidase	Siamese, Korat, DSH
GM₂ gangliosidosis	Beta-hexosaminidase	DSH, Korat
Globoid leucodystrophy	Beta-galactocerebrosidase	DSH
Glycogenosis	Alpha-glucosidase	DSH, Norwegian forest cat
Mannosidosis	Alpha-mannosidase	DSH, Persian
Sphingomyelinosis	Sphingomyelinase	DSH, Balinese
Ceroid lipofuscinosis	Unknown	Siamese

ORGAN SYSTEMS

4.9 NEUROMUSCULAR AND MUSCULAR DISEASE

4.9.1 Introduction and general approach

Neuromuscular disease – weakness on exercise (myasthenia), complete, flaccid paralysis (botulism) or rigidity (tetanus).
Myopathies – muscle weakness or pain, reduced exercise tolerance and abnormal (stiff) gait. Neck ventroflexion. Sensation is normal; reflexes may be slow due to decreased motor ability.

- Neuromuscular and muscular disease is rarely diagnosed in cats.
- Cats with muscular or neuromuscular disease present with a variety of clinical signs depending on the muscles that are involved.
  - Weakness.
  - Stiffness and pain.
  - Collapse, inability to stand.
  - Regurgitation, constipation and dysuria.
    See sections 2.9, 2.31, 2.36 and 2.39

General approach
- Physical examination.
- Observation of walking.
- Neurological.
- Video evidence if intermittent signs.
- Routine haematology and biochemistry – include cholesterol, triglycerides, AST, CK and potassium.
- Retrovirus and Toxoplasma serology.
- Serum acetylcholine receptor antibodies, acetylcholine esterase activity.
- EMG and nerve conduction velocities.
- Nerve and muscle biopsy.
  - Muscle biopsies are best if taken from affected but not end-stage muscle. Specialist staining is often required. Sample numbers, preservation and preservatives, postal conditions should be discussed with the

diagnostic laboratory *prior* to samples being taken.

4.9.2 Neuromuscular disease

Myasthenia gravis
- Relatively rare in cats, associated with an immune-mediated destruction of acetylcholine receptors.
- Abyssinian and Somalis breeds may be over-represented.
- Trigger for antibody production is unknown but can occur following a variety of diseases, e.g. URT viral infection. It has also been associated with thymomas (20% of cases).
- Generalised muscle weakness following exercise or stress exhibiting as crouching gait progressing to lateral recumbency.
- Focal myasthenia not reported in cats.
- Collapse may occur very rapidly and the most severely affected cats are unable to stand.
- Dysphonia and dyspnoea are common.
- Megaoesophagus is rare, compared to dogs.
- Toxic side effect of methimazole therapy.

Diagnosis
- Fatigable blink response.
- Edrophonium test (IV 0.05–0.1 mg/kg).
- Repetitive nerve stimulation.
- Anti-acetylcholine receptor antibody assay.

Treatment
- Thymectomy if mass.
- Pyridostigmine 0.5–3 mg/kg daily:
  - Depending on severity of signs start at low dose and gradually increase.
  - Can be difficult to distinguish signs of under and over dosage.
  - In cats unable to take oral medication neostigmine can be used initially.

- Prednisolone started 2–3 days after pyridostigmine, increasing the dose every few days from 0.5 mg/kg to 2–4 mg/kg. Once signs are resolved prednisolone can be gradually withdrawn.

Chronic organophosphate poisoning

- Neurotoxicity after prolonged exposure causing neuromuscular weakness.
- Some cats are particularly sensitive as they have naturally low acetylcholine esterase levels.

Diagnosis

- Whole blood acetylcholine esterase levels.
- Signs worsen after edrophonium.

Treatment

- Remove from source and most will recover in 3–6 weeks.
- Diphenhydramine 4 mg/kg q8h if severely affected.

Botulism

- Uncommon in cats.
- Progressive flaccid paralysis.

Differential diagnosis depending on local flora and fauna.

- Snake envenomation.
- Tick paralysis.
- Ciguatera and tetrodotoxin toxicity.
- Red-back spider bite.
- Acute onset sepsis.

Tetanus

- Cats seem very resistant to disease.
- Often develop localised signs.
- Diagnosis is based on clinical signs – spastic paralysis.
- Treatment is symptomatic and supportive.
- Debride and clean wound.
- Antitoxin is of limited value in established disease.

4.9.3 Muscular disease

Myopathies

Inherited myopathies (Table 62)

Hypokalaemic polymyopathy

- Secondary to any cause of severe hypokalaemia (see Section 3.10).
- Generalised weakness characterised by neck ventroflexion – signs are variable and wax and wane.
- Severe hypokalaemia may impair renal function and cause weight loss and lethargy.
- CK is markedly elevated, potassium usually <3 mmol/l.
- Rapid response to oral supplementation (potassium gluconate 2–4 mmol/kg [= 2–4 mEq/kg]).
- Similar signs can occur with hypernatraemia.

Hypocalcaemic myopathy

- Secondary to any cause of hypocalcaemia (see section 3.8).
- Calcium usually <1 mmol/l (total) or 0.5 mmol/l (ionised).
- Present with weakness, tetany and tremors.
- Peripaturient queens – anorexia, lethargy, muscle twitching.
- Treatment (see section 4.7.6).
- 50–150 mg/kg of a 10% calcium gluconate solution IV initially.
- Then daily calcium supplementation with vitamin D_3 analogue.

Polymyositis and polymyopathy

Toxoplasma gondii (see section 5.10)

- Associated with myositis as well as other systemic signs, particularly neurologic and respiratory.

Neospora

- As yet unreported as a natural infection in cats. Experimental infection causes clinical disease.

Table 62 Inherited myopathies

Disease	Pathology and inheritance	Breed and prognosis	Clinical presentation	Diagnosis
Feline X-linked muscular dystrophy	Absence of dystrophin	Male (<2 year old) Poor	Bunny hopping gait, difficulty in walking/jumping, cervical rigidity, symmetric muscle hypertrophy (including heart), tongue enlargement and dyspnoea	CPK, EMG, muscle biopsy
Laminin alpha-2 (merosin) dystrophy			Weakness, hind limb atrophy and contracture	Immunohistochemistry on muscle biopsy
Nemaline myopathy	? inherited		6–18 months – reluctant to walk, hypermetric gait, muscle atrophy and tremors, hyporeflexia	EMG/CK unhelpful Muscle biopsy
Generalised ossifying myositis	Extensive calcification – skeletal muscles and connective tissue	Young Poor	Weakness, stiffness, decreased limb movement, muscle pain	Radiography and biopsy
Myotonia	Muscle spasm/ stiffness persisting after a voluntary effort	DSH Depends on degree	Stiff gait, abducted limbs, unable to open mouth fully, ± dysphagia Startling causes spasm of facial muscle, fall into lateral recumbency with extended limbs	Dimpling of tongue/skeletal muscle after percussion UGA, 'dive bomber' potentials on EMG, muscle biopsy
Hereditary myopathy	Muscle weakness and tremor especially of head, cause unknown	Devon Rex Reasonable	1–4 months – high stepping gait and ventroflexion of neck. Poor exercise tolerance, adopt a 'dog-begging' posture. Problems prehending and swallowing food	Biopsy Quality of life reasonable with management
Hypokalaemic polymyopathy	Muscle weakness	See page 305		

Immune-mediated polymyopathy
- Has been suspected in cats.
- Muscular, especially neck weakness.
- Muscle pain and exercise intolerance.
- Waxing and waning course in some cats.
- CK elevated, EMG abnormal.
- Biopsy shows lymphocytic infiltrate and myonecrosis.
- Spontaneous recovery in some cases, otherwise corticosteroids therapy.

Hyperthyroid myopathy (also see Section 4.7.2)
- May present with generalised weakness, neck ventroflexion, muscle tremor, gait disturbance and collapse associated with thyrotoxicosis.
- Reflexes normal to exaggerated.
- Signs usually reversed following management of the hyperthyroidism.

4.10 SKELETAL DISEASE

4.10.1 Introduction
This section is not intended to cover all aspects of orthopaedic disease in the cat, but will focus on non-traumatic, non-surgical skeletal disease.
- Bone disease.
- Joint disease.
- Disc disease.

Skeletal disease is particularly common in older cats with >65% of cats over 12 years old having evidence of osteo-arthritis.

Obvious clinical signs of skeletal disease are less frequently observed than in dogs, due to the cats' small body frame, ability to adapt to disease and the fact that cats are rarely taken for walks. Indications that there may be underlying skeletal disease include sleeping more and going outside less often with a reduced activity.

4.10.2 Presentation and physical examination

Presentation
Major more specific, presenting signs that suggest skeletal disease are
- Pain ± fever.
- Lameness.
- Collapse.
- Weakness.
- Inability to move normally – particularly seen as a reduced ability to jump up/down from surfaces in the home.
- Skeletal deformity.
- Joint swelling (often difficult to appreciate in cats).

Physical examination
- General physical.
- Neurologic/spinal examination (see section 4.8.2).
- Limb position, symmetry and muscle mass.
- Gait analysis can be difficult as cats are often reluctant to walk around a consulting room.
  - Encourage owner to video cat at home.
  - Forelimb lameness:
    - Head nodding – head up on painful limb.
  - Hind limb lameness:
    - Hock higher to reduce weight bearing.
    - Leg may be held away from body.
    - Pelvis rotated towards sound side during the swing phase of movement reducing joint excursion.
  - Bilateral forelimb disease – can be difficult to detect, tend to
    - Shift weight backwards and have a hunched back.
    - Crouched hind limb stance and a very upright neck position especially on rough surfaces.
  - Bilateral hind limb disease tends to
    - Wobbling gait and a shift of weight forward.

Table 63 Normal range of movement

	Flexion (°)	Extension (°)
Shoulder (relative to scapular spine)	60–70	180
Elbow	50–60	80–90
Carpus	130–140	30–40
Hip relative to axis of pelvis	50–60	190–200
Stifle	50–60	90
Tarsus	50–60	90–110

- Assess joints for pain, swelling and range of movement (Table 63).
  - Include paws, pads, claws and phalangeal joints.

4.10.3 Investigation

Imaging

Radiograph acquisition

- Generally requires heavy sedation or anaesthesia to acquire radiographs.
- Fine detail film/screen combination or computed setting.
- At least two orthogonal views; may require flexed, extended and oblique views as well.
- Exposures appropriate for bone and surrounding soft tissue.
- Radiographs of contralateral limb may be helpful.
- Myelography may be required for spinal cord disease.
  - Cisternal puncture (see Section 4.8.4).

Radiograph assessment

- How many lesions are there – do they all look the same?
- What's going on in the bone?
  - Generalised increase in bone density (osteopetrosis).
  - Generalised decrease in bone density (osteopenia).
  - Focal increase in bone density (proliferation).
  - Single or multiple.

- Focal decrease in bone density (lysis).
- Single or multiple.
- Mixture of increase and decrease.
- Periosteal reaction.
- Solid, lamellated, spiculated, amorphous, Codman's triangle.
- Does the process cross the joint (rare in neoplasia)?
- What's going on in the overlying soft tissue?
  - Loss of fascial planes.
  - Gas in the soft tissue.
  - Mineralisation of the soft tissue.
  - Enlargement of the soft tissue.
- More detail can be obtained in some cases using CT especially for skull lesions.
  - CT is poor for imaging of bone around teeth.
- Ultrasound of the soft tissues around joints may add information.

Arthrocentesis

- Figure 28 for needle placement.
- In many cases it is difficult to obtain more than one or two drops of synovial fluid from a cat joint.
  - Make direct smears for cytology and Gram staining if indicated.
    - Occasional extracellular bacteria may represent contamination during collection.
    - Blood contamination during collection can make interpretation difficult – comparing the red and white cell counts to those of a peripheral blood smear.
- More fluid is recovered then nucleated cell counts and culture can be performed.
  - Isolation rates are improved by placing the sample in blood culture bottles – 1 part joint fluid to 9 parts blood culture medium.

Arthroscopy

- Appropriate experience and arthroscopes required.
- Not all joints can be examined.

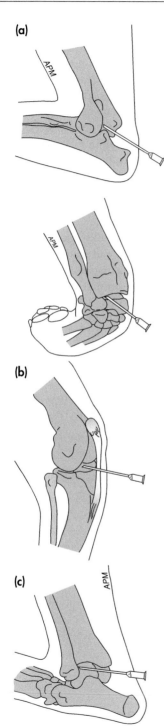

(a)

(b)

(c)

Figure 28 Needle placement for arthrocentesis. Reproduced by kind permission of Andy Moores.

Scintigraphy
- Specialist technique to look for 'hot spots' indicative of inflammation.

Biopsy
- Standard surgical approach to joint with biopsy of synovium.
- Bone biopsy using a Jamshidi needle – obtain several samples.

4.10.4 Bone disease

Congenital bone disease
- A variety of congenital disorders have been reported in cats, some of which appear breed related. Others appear sporadically or are inherited and not breed related.
- Pelger-Huet anomaly.
- Osteogenesis imperfecta – an inherited collagen defect causing excessive bone fragility. A much more common cause of osteopenia in kittens, however, would be nutritional secondary hyperparathyroidism.
- Osteopetrosis – a rare condition resulting in thickened cortical bone due to defective osteoclastic activity. It can also be seen as an acquired disorder and can be associated with FeLV infection
- Polydactyly (autosomal dominant inheritance); extra toe(s).
- Syndactyly – rare; fusion or absence of toe(s)
- Radial agenesis – most common absence of a bone portion in cats.
- Amelia – absence of limb(s) – reported in kittens.
- Hypochondrodysplasia – 'Kangaroo' and 'Munchkin' cats have been bred with foreshortened front limbs or all limbs respectively.
- Osteochondrodysplasia – Scottish fold ear cats also have thickened, inflexible tails, shortened and malformed distal limbs and caudal vertebrae. It is an autosomal dominant trait.
- Mucopolysaccharidosis (Table 61) associated with abnormal skeletal development (face shape and limb length), joint disease and generalised osteopenia.

ORGAN SYSTEMS

- Dwarfism – congenital dwarfism is most commonly endocrine related – thyroid (see section 4.7.8) or pituitary.
- Multiple cartilaginous exostoses – rare in cats, characterised by protuberances of cancellous bone. Clinical signs are associated with a mass effect and therefore depend on location. Rarely malignant transformation will occur.
- Abnormalities of the vertebra.
  - Wedge-shaped, butterfly and transitional vertebrae causing deviation of the vertebral column.
  - Spinal dysraphism – failure of normal neural tube closure can affect the vertebral column or spinal cord.
    - Spina bifida – incomplete fusion of vertebral arches (usually lumbar) – common in Manx cats especially 'rumpies'.
- Abnormalities of the ribs and sternum.
  - Pectus excavatum – inward deviation of the xiphisternum.
  - Flat chestedness – dorsoventral flattening of the rib cage – common in Burmese and Bengal cats.

Acquired bone disease

- Osteopetrosis.
- Secondary hypertrophic osteopathy (Marie Bamberger's disease) – rare in cats.
  - Lateral pallisading new bone on distal limbs associated with intrathoracic disease (usually neoplastic).
  - Limbs are swollen and painful.
  - Treat underlying disease, as this results in rapid resolution of pain and gradual remodelling of bone.
  - Vagotomy has also provided temporary relief.
- Aneurismal bone cysts – rare, non-neoplastic locally destructive lesions.
- Fibrous dysplasia – expansile fibrous lesions within one or several bones in young cats. Successful surgical resection has been reported.

Metabolic and nutritional bone disease

A variety of conditions resulting in a reduction in bone mass – *osteopenia*. Osteopenia can be subdivided into diseases leading to excessive resorption (*osteolysis*) – e.g. nutritional secondary hyperparathyroidism, and defective bone formation. Defective bone formation can be as a result of insufficient osteoid production (*osteoporosis*) or defective mineralisation (*osteomalacia*).

Nutritional secondary hyperparathyroidism

- Associated with diets providing excessive phosphate and inadequate calcium (all meat) resulting in marked osteopenia due to resorption of bone calcium in an attempt to maintain serum calcium.
- Calcium:phosphorus ratio < 1:16.

NB – *Adding milk to an all-meat diet will not redress the balance.*

- Kittens are at greater risk than adult cats due to their increased calcium requirement.

Key history
- Current and recent diet.

Clinical signs
- Lameness.
- Reluctance to stand.
- Pain.
- Enlargement of costochondral junction and metaphyses.
- Pathological fractures leading to angular limb deformities or neurologic signs associated with vertebral fractures.
- Constipation.
- Hypocalcaemic cataracts.

Diagnosis
- Biochemistry:
  - Low serum calcium and phosphorus *may* be present.

- ○ Increased alkaline phosphatase.
- ○ Increased PTH.
- Radiography:
  - ○ Area of relative osteopenia in metaphyses especially distal radius and ulna.
  - ○ Osteopenia – best appreciated in the dorsal spinous processes of the thoracic vertebrae.
  - ○ Thin cortices.
  - ○ Bowed diaphysis.
  - ○ Pathological fractures.

Management
- Severe cases – parenteral calcium gluconate (1–2 ml of 10% solution/kg/day for 3 days).
- Diet.
- NSAID pain relief.
- Calcium:phosphorus ratio of 2:1 for the first 2–3 months (may require calcium supplementation).
- Confined for the first 2–3 weeks whilst remineralisation occurs to reduce the risk of folding fractures as the cat becomes more active.

Prognosis
- Good unless there is severe skeletal, especially spinal, deformity.

Rickets
- Rare disease of kittens (acquired disease in adults = osteomalacia) due to insufficient calcium and/or phosphorus for adequate mineralisation of newly formed osteoid. Cats are unable to synthesise cholecalciferol in skin exposed to UV light.
- Usually associated with
  - ○ Vitamin D deficiency.
  - ○ Dietary deficiency.
  - ○ Inborn error of vitamin D metabolism.
  - ○ Low availability of minerals.
  - ○ Impaired absorption.

Key history
- Current and recent diet.

Clinical signs
- Lethargic.
- Weak.
- Lame.
- Reluctant/unable to walk.
- Folding fractures or bending of long bones.
- Enlargement of costochondral junction and metaphyses.
- Neurologic signs associated with hypocalcaemia.

Diagnosis
- Biochemistry:
  - ○ Low serum calcium and phosphorus *may* be present.
  - ○ Increased alkaline phosphatase.
  - ○ Increased PTH.
  - ○ (Low 25-hydroxycholecalciferol).
- Radiography:
  - ○ Axial and radial thickening of growth plates.
  - ○ Cupping of adjacent metaphyses.
  - ○ Distal radial growth plates most affected.
  - ○ Osteopenia.
  - ○ Thin cortices.
  - ○ Bowed diaphysis.
- Management:
  - ○ Feed a balanced diet.
  - ○ Improve mineral absorption – management of GIT disease.
  - ○ Vitamin D supplementation if inborn error of metabolism.
- Prognosis:
  - ○ Good unless severe skeletal, especially spinal, deformity.

Renal secondary hyperparathyroidism
- See Section 4.5.

Primary hyper and hypoparathyroidism
- See Section 4.7.6

ORGAN SYSTEMS

Hypovitaminosis A

- Cats require a preformed source of vitamin A – daily requirement 1600–2000 iU.
- Vitamin A is involved in growth, maturation and remodelling of bone.
- Lack of vitamin A decreases osteoclast activity resulting in long bone and spinal deformity with bones becoming bulky reducing the size of the vertebral canal, cranial vault and foramina.
- Affected cats are lame or show neurologic signs.
- Corneal vascularisation and ulceration, retinal degeneration, infertility, weight loss and muscular weakness are also reported.
- Diagnosis is radiographic.
- Management by dietary correction.
- Rare.

Hypervitaminosis A

- Usually associated with feeding excessive liver.
- Effects depend on age and chronicity.
- Young cats – suppression of osteoblasts and degeneration in the cartilaginous epiphyseal plate with reduced long bone growth.
- Mature cats – exostoses in ligaments and tendons resulting in bony proliferation especially around the cervical and thoracic spine and limb joints.
- Changes are not reversible on correction of the diet.

Other conditions

- Osteochondrosis dissecans – forelimb, cats <1 year old.
- Femoral neck metaphyseal osteopathy.

Neoplastic bone disease

Bone neoplasia is relatively rare in cats compared to dogs. It can be primary, e.g. osteosarcoma, secondary due to local invasion, e.g. SCC, or metastases from a distant neoplasm and often multiple, e.g. bronchial carcinoma.

Osteosarcoma

- Commonest bone neoplasia in cats (70–80% of cases).
- Aged cats.

- Females over-represented.
- Humerus, femur and tibia most common sites.
- Can affect skull and vertebral column.

Key history

- Previous fracture sites.

Clinical signs

- Lameness.
- Swelling.
- Pain.

Diagnosis

- Radiographic features.
  - Destructive lesion – radiolucent areas within bone, thinning and loss or cortices.
  - Joints preserved.
  - Periosteal new bone ('sunburst' appearance) classical, but may not be present.
  - Codman's triangle.
  - Pathological fracture.
  - Changes not pathognomonic – confirmation based on biopsy

Management

- Survey imaging.
- Evaluation of major organ function.
- Generally metastasise slowly.
- Surgical excision has been curative in non-metastatic disease.

Other bone neoplasms

- A variety of other primary bone tumours have been described in cats, they are generally rare.
- Fibrosarcoma – second most common primary neoplasm, primary bone involvement, osteolytic.
- Osteoma – rare, benign masses of variable mineral density, firm, non-painful and slow growing extraskeletal, parosteal and osteoid forms described.
- Chondrosarcoma – rare, firm, fixed mass involving bone.
- Multilobular chondromas – rare, invasive, usually arising from skull, can be malignant.

- Osteoclastoma (giant cell tumour) – lameness and swelling, osteolytic, slow growing, variably malignant.
- Giant cell sarcoma – rare, periosteal, destructive.
- Spindle cell sarcoma – rare, densely calcified mass.

Metastatic bone neoplasia
- Rare in cats.
- Mammary gland carcinoma, bronchial carcinoma, pulmonary carcinoma.
- Pulmonary carcinoma has been reported to affect multiple digits.

Direct extension of neoplasms to bone

Fibrosarcoma
Some cases will invade bone causing lysis. Local surgical resection, e.g. mandibulectomy, has been successful. Multiple, invasive, s/c fibrosarcomas involving bone have been reported in young cats. Prognosis in these cases is poor.

Squamous cell carcinoma
Invasion of skull bones and digits from cutaneous or mucosal SCCs is relatively common. Bone appears moth-eaten with mineralisation erosion and, sometimes, periosteal new bone. Soft tissue swelling associated with these changes can be seen. Prognosis is guarded unless radical resection is possible. Survival times of cats with oral SCCs involving bone are slightly better than those without bone involvement.

Other
A variety of other tumours including lymphoma reported.

Bone infection
Primarily bacterial, associated with haematogenous spread, local extension or direct implantation (e.g. cat bite, RTA). The severity depends on the site, number, type and strain of the bacterium involved, degree of local soft tissue damage and the host's immune response (age, intercurrent disease). Where the infection is poorly contained, vascular thrombosis can occur resulting in the formation of a sequestrum. In most cases there will be an attempt to wall off the infection producing a localised lesion with proliferative and destructive features. Such changes can be difficult to distinguish from neoplastic bone disease.

Bacterial osteomyelitis

Common pathogens
- *Staphylococcus*.
- *Streptococcus* spp.
- *Pseudomonas* spp.
- Mixed infection.
- Anaerobes.

Clinical signs
- Usually localised.
- Lameness.
- Pain.
- Swelling.
- Pyrexia.

Diagnosis
- Clinical signs.
- Radiography.
  ○ Lysis and/or increased bone density (usually at the edge of the lesion).
  ○ Periosteal new bone may extend a considerable distance, can cross joint space.
  ○ Sequestra may be present.
  ○ Local soft tissue swelling and loss of fascial plane architecture.

Clinical pathology
- Haematological changes are uncommon.
- Culture of bacterial species is helpful.

Treatment
- Medical
  ○ Antibacterials preferably based on culture and sensitivity. Empirical choices include potentiated amoxicillin, clindamycin, cephalosporin and fluoroquinolone; combination therapy may include metronidazole. Therapy should be continued for a minimum of 4–6 weeks.

ORGAN SYSTEMS

- Surgical
  - Removal of any surgical implants.
  - In acute cases drainage of purulent material (including intramedullary) accompanied by external support.
  - Curettage of sequestra.
  - Local resection of diseased bone or amputation.
  - Fracture fixation is usually best achieved using remote methods, e.g. external fixation.

Non-bacterial osteomyelitis

Fungal osteomyelitis is reported, its frequency is variable according to the area of the world. In the UK cryptococcosis is most common. Less commonly *Aspergillus fumigatus* is involved. Outside the UK coccidiomycosis and histoplasmosis are encountered. Diagnosis is based on the presence of lytic lesions and the demonstration of fungal elements preferably in tissue biopsies. Cases are treated in a similar fashion to bacterial osteomyelitis; imidazoles, such as fluconazole are first choice drugs.

Spondylosis, spondylitis and discospondylitis (see Table 64)

4.10.5 Joint disease

Arthritis in cats can be divided into two broad groups: degenerative (traumatic and osteoarthritis) and inflammatory (infective and immune-mediated). Degenerative joint fluid tends to be clear, and contain relatively few white cells, most of which are lymphocytes and macrophages. Inflammatory fluids tend to be more turbid with higher white cell counts, predominantly neutrophils. Although haemophilia has been reported in cats, degenerative haemophilic arthropathy has not.

Degenerative arthritis

Trauma

Usually follows an acute injury – falls, RTA or catfight. In many cases only one joint is affected presenting as pain and swelling. Systemic signs may be present, but may not be primarily related to the joint damage. Severity can be very variable from mild inflammation 'sprain' to more severe injury involving ligamentous, joint capsule or articular cartilage damage.

Table 64 Differentiating spondylosis, spondylitis and discospondylitis

Spondylosis (Spondylosis deformans)	Spondylitis (= vertebral osteomyelitis)	Discospondylitis
Common	Infection within the body of the vertebra particular lumbar	Involves disc and vertebral end-plate
New bone on the ventral aspect of vertebrae in the region of the end-plate	Bone destruction	Disc space narrowing
Early stages hook-like projections that become more pronounced and adopt a ventrocaudal/cranial course eventually bridging	Periosteal reaction and bone formation	Destruction ± collapse of end-plates with sclerosis as the end-plate joins the body causing shortening of the body.
Bone surface is smooth	Sclerosis of the surrounding bone	Periosteal new bone on ventral & lateral aspect of vertebra(e).
		Healing usually results in fusion of adjacent vertebrae

Clinical examination
- Lameness.
- Pain.
- Swelling.

NB – *Patient should be checked for signs of damage to other organs that may be life threatening if significant trauma involved.*

Diagnosis
- History of trauma.
- Physical examination.
- Radiography – increased soft tissue density, fractures, and ligamentous damage. New bone is not present unless the injury is long standing (greater than 10–14 days).
- Synovial fluid – viscous with normal to increased white cells, mainly mononuclear. Blood may be present.

Management
The joint should be carefully assessed; however, the majority of cases will recover with supportive treatment – rest and NSAIDs if not infected. Further investigation should be considered if there is evidence of ligamentous damage resulting in joint instability or there is a penetrating wound with the possibility of infection.

Osteoarthritis
- Primary common in aged cats – no obvious underlying cause.
- Secondary – more common young cats, occurs as a result of another joint disorder.

Clinical examination
- Primary disease usually multiple joints.
- Secondary disease usually single joints (but can be bilateral, e.g. hip dysplasia).
- Cat systemically well.
- Intermittent to persistent lameness, usually chronic.
- Reduced range of joint movement, activity and ability to jump.

- Joint manipulation may be resented.
- Joint swelling usually not palpable.
- Slowly progressive.

Diagnosis
- Radiography:
  - Bone changes present.
  - New bone present around the joint.
  - Osteophytes, spurs, exostoses, lipping.
  - ± Calcification of articular soft tissue.
  - Sclerosis of the subchondral bone in long-standing cases.
  - Narrowing of the joint space.
  - Marked changes can be associated with relatively low grade clinical signs.
  - Underlying cause of osteoarthritis, e.g. hip dysplasia, may be evident.
- Synovial fluid:
  - Increased in quantity.
  - Reduced viscosity.
  - Cell count low mainly macrophages and some lymphocytes.

Management
- Dependent on the severity of clinical signs.
- Physiotherapy/encouraging the cat to exercise, though difficult are worthwhile.
- NSAIDs usually treatment of choice, e.g. meloxicam.
- Weight loss if BCS 6/9 or greater.
- Nutraceuticals – a variety of products are available either as nutritional supplements or incorporated in specialist diets.
  - Antioxidants (PUFA).
  - Glucosamine.
  - Sodium hyaluronate.
  - Chondroitin.
  - Green-lipped mussel.
  - Others – lysine, carnitine, methionine, turmeric and Boswellia extract.
- Corticosteroids – should be reserved for resistant cases or for short-term

ORGAN SYSTEMS

management of flare-ups; corticosteroids may promote cartilage degeneration in the long term.
- Surgery
  - E.g. excisional arthroplasty, arthrodesis.
- Other modalities of unproven benefit, e.g. acupuncture, homeopathy, magnets.

Inflammatory arthritis

Infection

Septic (bacterial) arthritis
- Entry to the joint is usually by penetrating wound, especially cat bites; haematogenous spread is uncommon, except in kittens where it is associated with spread from the umbilicus.

Clinical signs
- Usually a single joint.
- Swelling, heat, pain.
- Loss of movement.
- Crepitus suggests extensive bony and cartilage damage.

Diagnosis
- Radiography:
  - Soft tissue swelling.
  - Distension ± thickening and displacement of facial planes.
  - Loss of intra-articular fat pad lucency.
  - Widened and deformed joint space → loss of articular cartilage and joint collapse.
  - Long-standing disease can lead to extensive periosteal new bone.
  - Secondary osteoarthritic changes.
  - Bone sclerosis adjacent to infection.
  - Ankylosis.
- Laboratory changes:
  - Leucocytosis and mild anaemia.
  - Synovial fluid changes.
    - Increased quantity.
    - Turbid.
    - Watery.
    - Sometimes blood contamination.
    - Increased white cells predominantly toxic polymorphs.
    - Culture results variable, increased success using synovial membrane.

Management
- Systemic antibacterials based on culture and sensitivity for 4–6 weeks.
- Joint lavage.
- Pain relief – NSAID.
- Surgical intervention.
- Debridement.
- Arthrodesis
- Excision arthroplasty
- Amputation
- Corticosteroids may be required in some cats that have an immune-mediated component to microbial antigens that can persist within the joint

Other infectious agents
L-forms
- Cell-wall-deficient bacterial haematogenous infection associated with joint destruction. Organisms are difficult to culture but responsive to tetracycline.

Mycoplasma
- *M. gateae* has been associated with polyarthritis. Synovial changes similar to bacterial septic arthritis, but the neutrophils are not degenerative.

Mycobacterium
- Can cause a septic arthritis

Coronavirus
- Has been associated with polyarthritis.

Calicivirus
- Associated with certain field and vaccine strains of FCV – 'transient limping syndrome', usually in kittens.
- Clinical signs:
  - Lame, stiff and sore.
  - Muscle and joint pain.
  - Fever, lethargy and inappetence.
  - Self-limiting within 2–4 days.

- Management:
  - Supportive care.
  - NSAID.
  - Corticosteroids contraindicated.

Lyme disease
- Serological evidence of exposure is relatively high in the UK (around 15%); there is, however, no clear evidence of disease association.

Immune-based arthritis
- Immune-based disease can be associated with polyarthropathy; they are rare causes of joint disease in cats.
- Broadly they can be divided into erosive and non-erosive forms.
- Clinical signs associated with joint pain and swelling. May be concomitant joint laxity and deformation.
- Other non-joint associated clinical signs may be present with SLE and idiopathic forms.
- Synovial fluid is watery with increased volume, and contains large numbers of non-degenerate polymorphonuclear cells.

Erosive arthritis
- Radiographic destruction of the joint.

Rheumatoid arthritis
- Multiple hot, swollen, painful joints.
- Serological evidence of rheumatoid factor.
- Characteristic synovial changes.
- Management with immunosuppressive doses of corticosteroids.

Periosteal proliferative arthritis
- Male cats over-represented.
- Extensive new bone around joints including enthesophytes, especially hocks and carpi.
- Suggested to be retrovirus associated (FeLV, FeSFV), but this is unsupported.

Idiopathic arthritis (see Box 10)
- Four forms are described; radiographic changes may be minimal, associated with limited periosteal new bone and soft tissue changes (periarticular thickening, distension of the joint capsule, loss of intra-articular fat shadow).

Box 10 Classification of idiopathic arthritis

Type I	Uncomplicated
Type II	Associated with remote infections
Type III	Associated with GIT disease
Type IV	Paraneoplastic syndrome

Synovial neoplasia
- Synovioma – rare, usually distal limbs, relatively benign.
- Synovial sarcoma – very rare, destructive rapidly metastatic, poor prognosis.

4.10.6 Intervertebral disc disease
Discospondylitis
See Section 4.10.4.

Disc degeneration, prolapse and herniation
- Radiographic evidence of disc disease is not uncommon in cats, but it is rarely associated with clinical signs.

Clinical signs
- Dependent on site, severity, lateralisation and speed of onset.
- Cervical discs slightly more common.

Diagnosis
- Plain radiographs can be unhelpful, calcification is uncommon.
- Disease can be associated with normal to narrowed disc space.

- Normal discs can have apparently narrowed disc spaces.
- Myelography, MRI or CT is required to demonstrate compression.

Management
- Depends on severity and speed of onset of signs.
- Decompressive surgery not usually indicated.
- Rest and pain relief usually sufficient.
- Corticosteroids within the first few hours following an acute disc protrusion may be helpful.

4.11 DISORDERS OF THE BLOOD, HAEMOPOIETIC AND IMMUNE SYSTEM

4.11.1 Introduction
Morphologic changes in red cells
- Poikilocytes – abnormal shape
- Acanthocytes – surface projections found in liver disease/splenic tumours
- Crenation – occur relatively rapidly in cats, artefactual spur found in old sample, excess EDTA
- Spherocytes – common in normal cats, can suggest membrane damage, e.g. immune-mediated haemolytic anaemia
- Leptocytes – thin flat cells seen in anaemia of chronic disease, shunts
- Target cells – leptocytes with dark-staining centre
- Howell-Jolly bodies – nuclear remnants seen as basophilic spheres – <1% of red cells in normal cats.
- Heinz bodies – small, irregular, refractile areas of denatured haemoglobin indicate oxidant damage – <10% cells in normal cat.

Toxic changes in neutrophils
- Purple-black cytoplasmic granules.
- Diffuse cytoplasmic basophilia.

- Angular cytoplasmic inclusions – Döhle bodies.
- Giant neutrophils with bizarre nuclei.

4.11.2 Anaemia
See section 3.1.
- Anaemia is associated with many diseases in the cat.
- Mild (>22%) or moderate (>18%) non-regenerative anaemia is common in chronic disease.
- Initial investigation should be directed towards confirmation of the clinical suspicion and classification of the anaemia as regenerative vs. non-regenerative.
  - There is a poor correlation between mucosal pallor and anaemia in cats (see Section 2.30).
- Non-regenerative anaemias, other than deficiency diseases and reversible drug toxicities, generally carry a guarded prognosis.

History and clinical signs
Presentation
- Anaemic cats often present with non-specific signs such as lethargy, malaise, inappetence or inability to jump onto surfaces.
- Access to toxins, medication, e.g. NSAIDs.
- Lifestyle (FeLV/FIV risk).
- Diet.
- External evidence of bleeding.
  - Melaena/haematochezia.
  - Haematemesis.
  - Epistaxis.
  - Haematuria.
- Abdominal distension.
- Dyspnoea.
- Weight loss.
- Pica – eat soil/cat litter, lick concrete.
- Heat seeking.

Major clinical signs
- Pallor.
- Tachypnoea.

- Tachycardia (> 200 bpm), cardiomegaly, haemic murmur (decreased viscosity).
- Lethargy – usually goes unnoticed until anaemia is profound.
- Pain – due to chronic hypoxia.
- Lymphadenopathy.
- Splenomegaly – extra-marrow haematopoiesis.
- Hepatomegaly.
- Jaundice – rare except in acute haemolytic anaemia.
- Evidence of haemorrhage – petechiae, ecchymoses, blood in faeces/urine/nasal/oral.

Diagnostic aids

- Haematology including reticulocyte count and FIA (Haemoplasma) screen.
- Serology – FeLV, FIV, Coombs' test.
- Biochemistry and urinalysis.
- Iron and iron binding protein levels.
- Faecal occult blood.
- Survey imaging.
- Bone marrow biopsy.
- Erythropoietin.

Haematology

- Feline red blood cells clump easily as do their platelets (which can then be misinterpreted as RBCs by automated machines).
- Crenation is also a common occurrence.
- For these reasons RBC counts and their derived indices (MCV, MCHC, MCH) need to be interpreted with care.
- PCV (not HCT) and haemoglobin concentrations are of most reliable.
- Blood smear interpretation for anisocytosis, polychromasia, erythrocyte fragmentation, parasites and autoagglutination is vital.
- Chronic loss can lead to a non-regenerative (microcytic, hypochromic) anaemia due to iron deficiency.
- Haemolysis is associated with only red cell loss, so protein levels, etc. will be normal.

Feline reticulocytes

Two forms of reticulocytes are present in feline blood. Punctate erythrocytes (small clumps and specks of ribosomes) are common in normal cats (up to 10%). Aggregate reticulocytes (clumped reticular material), however, are rare (<0.5%). Aggregate reticulocyte counts peak 4–7 days after the initiation of a regenerative response. Reticulocyte counts are less valuable in mild or chronic anaemias or in cats with concurrent inflammatory illness.

Bone marrow aspirate biopsy

Indicated if

- The anaemia appears non-regenerative and unassociated with chronic disease.
- Pyrexia of unknown (POU) origin.
- And/or if peripheral blood changes suggest.
  - Leukaemia.
  - Myeloproliferative, myelodysplastic or myelophthisic disease.
  - Dyshaematopoiesis.
  - Pancytopenia.
  - Unexplained, marked neutrophilia.
  - Suspected hypereosinophilic syndrome.

Erythropoietin assay

- Appropriate in non-regenerative anaemia.
- Supraphysiologic levels of EPO replacement may still be helpful if endogenous level high.
- High EPO levels are associated with renal tumours (in which case PCV is high) or primary bone marrow failure.

Use of erythropoietin

- 30% of cats develop antibodies to recombinant human erythropoietin.
- 50 iU of alpha/beta erythropoietin SC or IV three times weekly until PCV normalised.

ORGAN SYSTEMS

- Darbopoietin (modified human erythropoietin) with prolonged half-life.
  - 0.25–0.5 μg/kg s/c weekly.
  - Antibody development appears less common.

Diagnosis of anaemia
See Figure 29

Specific causes

Haemoplasma (Feline infectious anaemia, Haemobartonellosis)
See section 5.5.

Neonatal isoerythrolysis
See section 1.3.6.

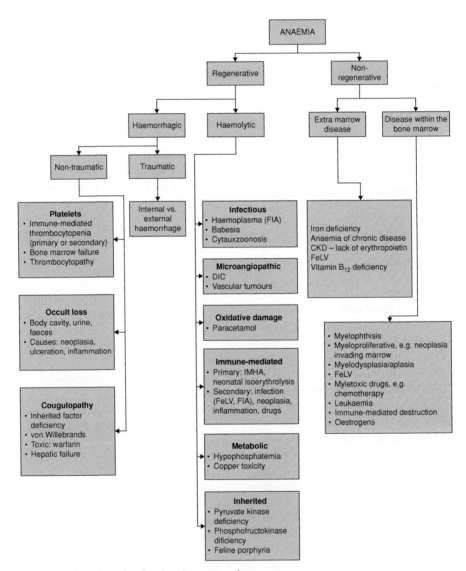

Figure 29 Algorithm for the diagnosis of anaemia

Immune-mediated haemolytic anaemia (IMHA)

- Relatively uncommon in cats compared to dogs.
- Primary or secondary causes.
- More often extravascular.
- Jaundice and intravascular haemolysis is rare.

Clinical signs

- Pyrexia.
- Lethargy.
- Tachycardia.
- Tachypnoea.
- Pallor.
- Hepatosplenomegaly.
- Lymphadenopathy.

Diagnosis

- Look for causes of secondary IMHA.
- Exclude haemorrhagic causes – coagulation profile, imaging, iron levels, faecal occult blood.
- Positive Coombs' test.
- Smear changes suggestive of immune-mediated disease – agglutination, spherocytes.
- Regenerative response – appropriately elevated reticulocytes.

NB – *Positive Coombs' test can occur with other diseases, e.g. Haemoplasma, lympho- and myeloproliferative disease.*

Management of primary IMHA

- Acute symptomatic support and transfusion if necessary.
- Immunosuppressive prednisolone at 1–2 mg/kg q12h.
- Withdraw therapy slowly over months monitoring PCV and reticulocyte count.
- Non-responsive case may require further immunosuppression consider chlorambucil, ciclosporin or cyclophosphamide.

Immune-mediated bone marrow disease

- Bone marrow aspirate/biopsy shows maturation arrest of red cells only.
  - This condition may be referred to as pure red cell aplasia.
- Considered to be immune-mediated destruction of red cell precursors in most cases.
- Response to immunosuppression variable.
  - More difficult to balance effects on immune system and those that will suppress the bone marrow itself.

General approach to the management of anaemia

- Diagnosis and treatment of underlying cause.
  - Cases where a clear diagnosis is made generally carry better prognosis.
- Acute management of the anaemia – transfusion (Section 4.11.6), colloids, haemostasis.
- If underlying cause not diagnosed or untreatable consider.
  - Repeat blood transfusion.
  - Haematinics – iron, sufficient protein in diet.
  - Erythropoietin.
  - Anabolic steroids – nandrolone dodecanoate at high dose (5 mg/kg) weekly.
  - Immunosuppression.

4.11.3 Polycythaemia

See Section 3.2

Clinical signs

- All cases:
  - Congested mucous membranes.
- Some cases depending on severity or cause:
  - Lethargy and depression.
  - Neurologic signs – confusion, seizures.
  - Systolic ejection murmur.
  - History of bleeding diatheses.
- PU/PD

ORGAN SYSTEMS

Diagnosis
- Increased red cell count in a normally hydrated individual.
- Stressed cats can increase red cell counts to some extent, but PCV >50% is abnormal.
- Arterial blood gas analysis.
- Erythropoietin level.
- Investigate causes of hypoxemia – cardiorespiratory disease, haemoglobinopathy
- Bone marrow biopsy is of limited value as regardless of cause erythroid precursors will be increased and abnormal cells, suggesting erythroid neoplasia, are unusual.

Erythropoietin level
- Elevated suggests hypoxemia, renal tumour.
- Low/normal erythropoietin in the absence of anoxic disease suggests primary polycythaemia (polycythaemia vera).

Management
- Treat underlying disease where possible.
- Reduce red cell count PCV < 60%.
  - Phlebotomy
  - Hydroxycarbamide (hydroxyurea) at 10–25 mg/kg q12h.
    - Start at low dose and assess response after 2–3 weeks, increase dose if there is no response.
    - Once PCV is normalised reduce dose frequency to maintain PCV at high end of reference range
  - Surgical leeches.

4.11.4 White blood cell disorders

Lymphoma
See section 4.11.7.

Many cats with lymphoma will have no evidence of abnormal lymphocytes in the circulation.

Hypereosinophilic syndromes
- More common in female cats.
- Can be difficult to distinguish from eosinophilic leukaemia.

Clinical signs
- Related to organ involvement.
- GIT signs are common.
- Usually accompanying weight loss, lethargy and inappetence.

Diagnosis
- Circulating eosinophilia.
- Eosinophilic infiltrate in multiple organs.
- Commonly – spleen, lymph node and GIT.
- Less commonly – liver, kidney, skin and heart.
- Bone marrow involved in all cases.
- Can present as mass-like lesions or diffuse infiltration.

Differential diagnosis of eosinophil count >1.5 × 10^9/l
See Section 3.4.

Treatment
- Prednisolone at 1–2 mg/kg q12h.
- Hydroxycarbamide (hydroxyurea) at 10–15 mg/kg q12h.
- Routine monitoring of haematology for excessive bone marrow suppression.

Leukaemias

Eosinophilic leukaemia
- Can be difficult to distinguish from hypereosinophilic syndromes.
- Tend to have
  - Higher myeloid:erythroid ratio.
  - More frequent immature eosinophils.
  - Lower red cell counts.
  - Higher peripheral eosinophil counts.

Myeloproliferative disorders
- Myelogenous leukaemia – granulocytes lines affected.
- Myelomonocytic leukaemia.
- Erythroleukaemia – red and white cell series affected.
- Lymphocytic leukaemia – may be associated with lymphoma.
- Megakaryocytic myelosis.

- Myelodysplastic syndromes – refractory anaemias and chronic leukaemia, polycythaemia.
  - Poorly characterised group of conditions associated with bone marrow failure of all or some lineages.
  - Some cases may have an immune-mediated basis.

Myelofibrosis
- Fibroblast proliferation within bone marrow.
- Associated with acute leukaemias, myelodysplastic disease, FeLV and drug reactions.

Clinical findings
- Associated with loss of functional bone marrow components.
- Anaemia.
- Haemorrhage.
- Infection.

Acute leukaemias
- Very rare.
- >30% of cells are blastic.
- Clinical signs are usually severe on presentation.
- Response to treatment is very poor.
- Euthanasia should be considered on diagnosis.

Chronic leukaemia
- Rare.
- Lymphocytic or granulocytic.
- Very high circulating white cell counts.
- Clinical signs often mild and associated with debilitation of chronic disease and hyperviscosity.

Management
- May be unnecessary.
- Ensure body weight is maintained.
- Chlorambucil may control rate of increase.

Mastocytosis
- Two forms recognised in cats.

Diagnosis
- Fine needle aspirate biopsy (FNAB) of mass lesions.
- Disseminated disease.
- Splenic aspirate.
- Buffy coat smear.
- Bone marrow aspirate.
- Survey imaging.

Systemic mastocytosis
- Splenomegaly and vomiting.
- Anaemia and mastocytaemia.
- Usually FeLV negative.
- Splenectomy may prolong survival.
- Medium-term prognosis poor.
  - Consider using tyrosine kinase receptor inhibitors (masitinib, toceranib).

Cutaneous mastocytosis (histiocytic mast cells)
- All ages but usually <4 years.
  - Particularly young Siamese cats.
- Generally cutaneous swelling.
- Low grade.
- Some cases spread to local lymph nodes.
- Some cases spontaneously resolve in young cats.
- Surgical excision is advisable.

4.11.5 Clotting disorders

Clotting mechanism (see Figure 30)
See also section 2.7, 2.19, 2.20 and 3.3
- Clotting is initiated in response to vascular injury and involves
  - Reflex vasoconstriction.
  - Adhesion of platelets to the exposed subendothelium mediated by proteins, e.g. VWF (primary haemostatic plug) – primary plug.
  - Initiation of coagulation cascade with fibrin forming the secondary haemostatic plug.
  - Coincident activation of the fibrinolytic and kinin pathways and other anticoagulant factors, e.g. ATIII to prevent excessive thrombus formation.

ORGAN SYSTEMS

ORGAN SYSTEMS

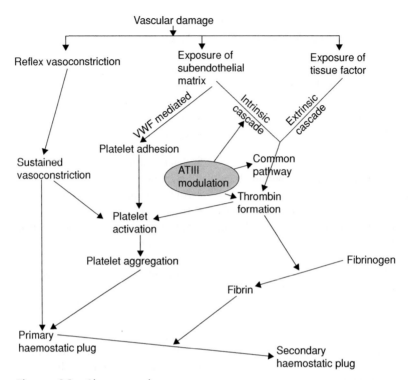

Figure 30 Clotting mechanism

- Recent studies have emphasised the importance of cells bearing tissue factor in the process.
- Rather than a cascade clotting occurs as a series of overlapping processes.

Laboratory assessment of haemostasis
- Tests are poor predictors of tendency to haemorrhage which is heavily influenced by the underlying disease process.
- Excitement causes increased platelet count, activation and increase factor V (FV), FVII, VWF, fibrinogen.
- Clotting mechanisms activated by catheter.
- Use sodium citrate tubes – accurate filling and good mixing is important.

Disorders of primary plug
- Platelet count, but will not evaluate platelet function.

NB – *Machine counts (especially in-house) can be very unreliable, if there is doubt then smear assessment and manual counts should be performed.*

Von Willebrand's factor deficiency
- Rare → very rare in cats.
- Requires specific measurement of factor levels AND state of polymerisation.

Vascular disorders
- Difficult to diagnose.

Buccal mucosal bleeding time
- Global evaluation of clotting.
- Method:
  - Sedation usually required.
  - Evert upper lip and tie.
  - Standardised incision made in buccal mucosa.

○ Careful blotting of blood from site without disturbing clot.

○ Time to stop bleeding.

• Prolonged in platelet disorders, von Willebrand's disease, vascular abnormalities.

• Normal cats 1–3.25 minutes.

Whole blood clotting time and clot retraction

• Whole blood placed in glass tube and time to clot formation measured.

• Quality of clot and clot retraction subjectively assessed.

• Unreliable test – some normal cats appear not to clot.

• Does not assess vascular effect or von Willebrand's factor.

Activated clotting time

• Intrinsic pathway.

• Diatomaceous earth in glass tube at 37°C.

• Mixed by inverting five times.

• Look for first evidence of clotting.

• Whole sample should clot as one.

• Abnormal samples – often tiny clots.

• Interpretation:

○ <90 seconds normal.

○ 90–165 seconds equivocal depending on collection method.

• Also available as cassette-based test.

Activated partial thromboplastin time (APTT)

• Intrinsic pathway.

• Greater than twofold increase is significant.

• Prolonged with factor deficiencies (XI, X, IX, XII, prothrombin), DIC.

One-stage prothrombin time (OSPT)

• Extrinsic system.

• Greater than twofold increase is significant.

• Factor X, VII and prothrombin deficiency.

• Liver disease.

• Coumarin intoxication.

• Vitamin K deficiency.

• Consumptive coagulopathies.

Proteins induced by vitamin K antagonists (PIVKAs)

• Diagnosis of suspected coumarin toxicity.

• Reference ranges are being developed for cats.

Coagulation activation

Fibrinogen assays

• Low levels are associated with decreased production or consumption:

○ Hereditary.

○ DIC.

○ Liver disease.

○ Chronic DIC may be high/normal.

Fibrin(ogen) degradation products (FDPs) assay

• Indicate accelerated fibrinolysis.

• Increased in DIC.

• D-Dimers may be more sensitive than FDPs.

Platelet disorders

See Section 3.3.

Thrombocytopenia

• Usually acquired due to decreased production, increased consumption, increased destruction or sequestration.

• Platelet count is usually only mildly to moderately decreased in haemorrhagic disease.

• Spontaneous haemorrhage becomes likely if count falls below $40 \times 10^9/l$.

Primary thrombocytopenia

• Very rare single lineage bone marrow disorder.

Immune-mediated thrombocytopenia
- Uncommon compared to dogs.
- Primary or secondary.

Management
- Identify and treat underlying disease.
- Immunosuppression if primary disease:
  - Prednisolone at 1–2 mg/kg BID.
  - Gradual reduction every 3 weeks, if platelet count is within reference range.
  - Severe cases may require other agents, e.g. cyclophosphamide.
- Splenectomy may become necessary.
- A single injection of vincristine (0.03 mg/kg) will temporarily raise platelet count if there are functional megakaryocytes in bone marrow.
- Transfusion BUT
  - Platelet-rich plasma not generally available.
  - Platelet survival is short (half-life <24 hours).

Thrombocytopathy
- Normal or increased platelet numbers.
- Platelets dysfunctional.

Cause
- Von Willebrand's disease.
- Uraemia.
- NSAID.
- Platelets coated with proteins – myeloma, excessive use of colloids.
- Chédiak–Higashi syndrome.

Thrombocytosis
- Not usually of clinical significance.
- May reflect recent haemorrhage.
- Can be a bystander reaction to intense marrow stimulation, e.g. in anaemia.
- Rarely as a paraneoplastic syndrome or primary myeloproliferative disorder.
- Mild increase in inflammatory and infectious disease.
- Iron deficiency.

Coagulation abnormalities

Haemophilia
- Congenital, breed-associated diseases:
  - Haemophilia A – FVIII deficiency.
  - Haemophilia B (Christmas disease) – FIX.
  - Haemophilia C – FXI deficiency.
- Severity of signs related to factor level.
- Spontaneous bleeding is rare.
- Bleeding usually occurs following trauma or surgery.
- Diagnosis based on
- Abnormal APTT and bleeding times.
- Specific factor measurement relative to normal controls.

Management
- Avoid drugs that interfere with coagulation, especially NSAIDs.
- Blood transfusion should be available if surgery is required.
- Blood transfusion should be given if there is active haemorrhage following trauma.
- Desmopressin has been used in dogs prior to surgery.

Coumarin intoxication
- Ingestion of poisoned bait or vermin.
- Coumarins antagonise the vitamin K-dependent hepatic production of factors II, VII, IX and X.
- Affects intrinsic and extrinsic pathways but OSPT increases first as factor VII has the shortest half-life.

Clinical signs
- Pallor.
- Tachycardia.
- Epistaxis.
- Associated with the site of haemorrhage.
- Dyspnoea is common due to pulmonary or pleural haemorrhage.

Diagnosis
- Likely access.
- Elevated OSPT, APTT.
- Increased PIVKAs.

Management

- Induce vomiting and use absorbent and cathartics if ingested within last 12 hours.
- Control of haemorrhage with pressure.
- Avoid jugular venipuncture or SC injections in suspected cases.
- Fluids and blood transfusion.
- Haemorrhage around catheter sites and injection points can be a problem.
  - Catheters should be inserted with minimum trauma and mild pressure applied for several minutes.
- Vitamin K_1:
  - 2–5 mg/kg by injection only if the cat is vomiting or oral administration not possible.
  - IV administration potentially dangerous.
  - Alternative is SC or IM injection using a fine needle at several sites.
- Once OSPT is normal – oral therapy 2–5 mg/kg daily – absorption is improved if given with food especially fatty food.
- Duration of treatment is dependent on coumarin involved, most recent products have very prolonged effects (months).

Disseminated intravascular coagulation (DIC)

- Generalised activation of haemostatic and fibrinolytic system.
- Eventually results in a consumptive coagulopathy.
- Common as a subclinical problem in many disease states.
- Precipitated by septicaemia, endotoxaemia, viraemia (particularly FIP), immune complex production, red cell haemolysis, major organ failure, trauma, burns or post-surgical.

Diagnosis

- Increased whole blood clotting time, APTT, PT and ACT in later stages.
- Thrombocytopenia.
- Increased FDPs.
- Elevated D-dimer levels.

Management

- Value of heparinisation of cats at risk is unclear.
  - Unfractionated heparin (70–300 iU/kg s/c q8h).
  - Low molecular weight heparin – 80–150 iU/kg s/c q4–8h.
- Management of underlying disease.
- Aggressive and intensive supportive care:
  - Fluids.
  - Blood or blood products.
  - IV antimicrobial.

Prognosis

- Guarded to poor associated with the underlying cause of the DIC.

4.11.6 Blood transfusion

NB – *Blood for diagnostic testing should be taken prior to any form of transfusion as this will severely affect the haematology results as well as the protein levels.*

- Blood products are likely to be required in
  - Severe anaemia (PCV<12–15%).
  - Severe hypoalbuminaemia.
  - On-going haemorrhage associated with a lack of coagulation factors or platelets.
- Whole blood transfusions provides three critical factors:
  - Oxygen-carrying capacity.
  - Clotting factors if petechiation or ecchymotic haemorrhage, cavity bleeding, etc. is caused by clotting factor deficient.
  - Proteins – whole blood provides both albumin and globulins; some of the globulins such as α_1-macroglobulin have important roles in regulating the levels of inflammatory mediators for example in pancreatitis.

ORGAN SYSTEMS

ORGAN SYSTEMS

Indications

- Haemorrhagic shock:
  - Usually still sufficient oxygen-carrying capacity to support life but inadequate distribution. Initially, volume replacement is sufficient. Chronic haemorrhage requires transfusion as these cats are rarely hypovolaemic.
- Non-regenerative non-haemolytic anaemia:
  - Provides critical support allowing time for a diagnosis to be made and treatment (where possible) to be implemented.
- Coagulopathies:
  - Halt active bleeding.
  - As clotting factors and platelets are labile, freshly collected blood should be used.
- Haemolytic anaemias.
- Hypoproteinaemia.
- DIC.
- Septic shock.
- Acute pancreatitis.

Volume

Anaemia

- Post-transfusion PCV of 20% should be aimed for but is rarely achievable unless the patient is a kitten or multiple donors are available:

$$\text{amount ml} = \frac{\text{bodyweight of recipient kg} \times [20 - \text{PCV of recipient}]}{\text{PCV of donor}}$$

- 2.5 ml/kg will raise the PCV by approximately 1%.

Hypoproteinaemia/coagulopathy, etc.

- More difficult to calculate. 30–50 ml of blood can be given and the response in terms of raising the protein levels or the effect on clotting monitored.

Compatibility

This is a crucial issue in feline blood transfusion as cats have three blood groups, A (70–80%), B (20–30%) and AB (1–2%).

- Cats with blood group B frequently have high levels of naturally occurring anti-A alloantibodies which can cause fatal reactions without prior transfusions having to be given.
- Blood group distribution varies with breeds (see Box 11).
- Cross matching better than blood grouping before transfusion.

In-house cross matching

- Rapid slide method.
- Important to distinguish rouleaux formations from agglutination.
- Collect EDTA and serum samples from donor and recipients.
  - Minimise sample volume from recipient.
- Centrifuge samples.
  - If no centrifuge allow red cells to precipitate (takes one to several hours).
- Label four glass slides:
  - Donor control – donor red cells + donor serum.
  - Major crossmatch – donor red cells and recipient serum.
  - Minor crossmatch – recipient red cell and donor serum.
  - Recipient control – recipient red cells and recipient serum.

Box 11   Distribution of blood groups amongst cat breeds in the UK

Breeds with no type B cats	Siamese, Burmese, Tonkinese, Oriental short hair, Ocicat
Breeds with <5% type B cats	DSH, DLH, Maine Coon, Norwegian Forest Cat
Breeds with 10–20% type B cats	Abyssinian, Birman, Himalayan/Persians, Scottish fold ear, Somali, Sphinx
Breeds with >20% type B cats	British and exotic short hairs, Cornish and Devon rex

- Place one drop of undiluted red cells and two drops of serum on slide and mix.
- Gently rock the slides from side-side and observe for 2 minutes.
- Examine for agglutination within 5 minutes of mixing.
- Dilute red cells 0.1 ml of packed red cells + 2.4 ml of saline to distinguish rouleaux from agglutination.

Emergency administration

- Extreme situations – no alternatives are available.
- Administer 1 ml of blood to the recipient.
- Observe closely for 5–10 minutes for the development of a transfusion reaction.
  - If no reaction occurs the transfusion can continue with close monitoring.
  - If transfusion reaction, treat as below.

Collection and storage

Donor cats

- Large (not fat) FIV, FeLV and haemo-plasma-negative cat less than 8 years old.
  - Regularly vaccinated and periodically given a general health check and in particular routine haematology, FeLV and FIV tests.
- Full physical examination prior to each donation.
- If sedation of donor requires use IM sedatives that cause minimal hypotension:
  - ACP at 0.02 mg/kg + buprenorphine at 0.01 mg/kg. If this is insufficient then 10 μg/kg of medetomidine can be added.
  - Midazolam at 0.25 mg/kg + ketamine at 5 mg/kg – can be mixed in the same syringe and given as a single injection.

Collection

- Via jugular puncture using an 18/19 g needle; site surgically prepared.

- Use 20 ml syringes + anticoagulant or 70 ml bags with coagulant for the amount of blood to be collected (need sensitive weighing scales to measure amount collected).

Anticoagulants

- Acid citrate dextrose – 15% of collected volume (not suitable for storage).
- Citrate phosphate dextrose ± adenine – 12.5% of collected volume.
- Adsol, Nutrisol, or Optisol – contained in human blood collection bags – 16% of collected volume.
- Emergency situation where heparin can be used at 5–12.5 iU/ml.

Administration

- Directly from the syringe via a 21 g catheter with extension tube or a 20 g butterfly needle.
- Syringe driver is available this is ideal + small volume inline filter such as Haemo-nate.
- Given at the rate of about 1 ml/kg/hour for the first 30 minutes:
  - Temperature, pulse and respiration (TPR) at the start of the transfusion and then at 15 and 30 minutes.
  - TPR stable at 30 minutes increase transfusion rate can be increased – aim of giving the whole volume over 3–4 hours.
  - Periodic monitoring should continue throughout the transfusion.
- In an emergency situation blood can be given at a rate of 0.5 ml/kg/minute.
- Measure PCV 6–12 hours post transfusion.

Synthetic blood

- Haemoglobin glutamer available:
  - Good oxygen carrying capacity and colloidal effects.
  - Remains in circulation for 24–48hrs.
  - Can cause pulmonary oedema – maximum dose rate 7ml/kg given slowly.

Transfusion reactions

- Clinical signs see Table 65.

Table 65 Clinical signs of acute and chronic transfusion reactions

Acute transfusion reaction	Delayed transfusion reaction
Rise in temperature	Patient lethargic and depressed, inappetent, nauseated and has not improved as expected post transfusion
Tachycardia, arrhythmia	
Increased respiratory rate	
Tremors, vocalisation	Jaundice
Ptyalism and/or vomiting	Haemoglobinuria and bilirubinuria
Angioedema (usually noticed as head swelling)	Haemoglobinaemia and hyperbilirubinaemia
Urticaria	Raised liver enzymes
Collapse, seizure, coma, cardiopulmonary arrest	Falling PCV, as the transfusion is haemolysed

Management
- Depends on severity of reaction:
  - Stop transfusion.
  - Start monitoring ECG, BP and get crash trolley ready.
  - Administer crystalloids to maintain BP.
  - Chlorphenamine 2–5 mg/cat slow IV.
  - Dexamethasone sodium phosphate 0.5–1.0 mg/kg *not until normotensive*.
  - Adrenaline 1:100 000 – 0.5–1 ml/kg IV can repeat every 2–30 minutes.
  - Give omeprazole or H_2 blocker, antiemetic.
  - Start colloids if vascular leakage (oedema) and BP not being maintained.
  - Give dobutamine if severe, non fluid-responsive hypotension.
  - CPCR is not hopeless if arrest occurs depending on underlying disease.
- Mild, once reaction subsided the transfusion can be restarted at 10–25% of the rate.

4.11.7 Lymphoma
- Most common neoplasm in cats.
- Incidence of FeLV-positive lymphomas is declining, currently around 10–20% of cases but there is local and country–country variation.
- Median age is increasing (now 9–10 years) but is bimodal, with mediastinal lymphoma still presenting primarily in young cats.

Classification
- Based on
  - Anatomic site:
    - Multicentric (nodal) – uncommon to solely involve lymph nodes; may involve solitary nodes of especially of the head and neck.
    - Alimentary – most commonly small intestine. Low-grade smouldering, diffuse small cell lymphoma carries a reasonable – good survival or high grade focal blastic lymphoma that has a worse prognosis.
    - Mediastinal – thymus or lymph nodes, pleural effusion common.
    - Extra nodal – nasal, renal, ocular/retrobulbar, CNS and skin most common sites.
  - Immunophenotype.
  - FeLV result.
  - WHO classification (see Box 12).

Presentation

Signalment
- No clear breed or sex predilection.
- Male cats and Siamese may be over-represented.
- Chronic inflammation may increase risk.

Box 12 WHO classification of lymphoma

Stage I	Single lymph node
Stage II	Multiple regional lymph nodes
Stage III	Generalised lymphadenopathy
Stage IV	Liver and/or splenic involvement
Stage V	Bone marrow or blood involvement and/or any non-lymphoid organ
Substage a	Asymptomatic
Substage b	Clinical signs of disease

Clinical signs

- Tend to be organ specific.
- Diverse group of neoplasms can be present in any organ and differential diagnosis for most presenting clinical signs.
- Usually accompanying weight loss, lethargy and inappetence.

Diagnosis

- Lymphomegaly or diffuse organomegaly on physical examination or imaging.
- Paraneoplastic hypercalcaemia is rare in cats.
- Histopathology of FNA or biopsy.
  - Ideally immunohistochemistry should be performed.
    - Confirms it is lymphoma and not another type of round cell tumour.
    - Subtypes tumour B vs. T cell.
  - Diagnosis is relatively simple when cells are blastic or morphologically abnormal.
  - Problems differentiating benign hyperplastic lymph node syndromes, especially on FNA.
    - Submandibular lymph nodes can be especially problematic.
- In cases where there are high numbers of mature, morphologically normal lymphocytes infiltrating solid organ the differentiation from severe lymphocytic inflammatory disease can be difficult.
- L-Asparaginase test – where access to biopsy is not possible or desirable a single injection of 400 U/kg of L-asparaginase will cause marked reduction in the size of the mass in 2–3 days if it is a lymphoma.

Therapy

- There remains a lack of clear evidence as to which is the 'best' protocol.
- Cats are not always ideal patients for IV protocols.
- Whatever protocol is used, monitoring should be undertaken, initially weekly for most therapies.
- Wherever possible breaks in therapy should be avoided.
- WBCC $<3 \times 10^9/l$ or neutrophil count $<2 \times 10^9/l$ is an indication to delay therapy.
- Pre-treatment for more than 3–4 days with prednisolone should be avoided, as it will reduce the response rate to other agents significantly.
- Efficacy of rescue therapies largely unknown.
- In patients that are difficult to catheterise a long-term injection port can be considered.
- Adjunctive antibacterial therapy is NOT recommended unless there is evidence of infection or to cover short periods of neutropenia ($<2 \times 10^9/l$).

Single agent therapy

Prednisolone

- 2–4 mg/kg q12h.
- Has a palliative action increasing survival times by 1–2 months.

Chlorambucil
- Valuable in the management of low grade, smouldering mature cell intestinal lymphoma.
- Associated with few side effects – intermittent monitoring of haematology required.
- Needs to be stored in the fridge.

Dose rate – various described but tablets should not be split.
- 15 mg/m^2 for 4 days every 3 weeks.
- 20 mg/m^2 q14 days.

Doxorubicin/epirubicin
- Not shown to have significant efficacy as a single agent in cats.

Combination chemotherapy
- Complete response rates of 50–70% expected.
- Duration of treatment is difficult to determine but 6–9 months is the general recommendation.
- Pre-medication with IV glucocorticoids and antihistamine may reduce the incidence of acute side effects.

COP protocol
- Remission rates of above 80% are reported in some studies.
- Median remission of 5 months.

Prednisolone
- 2 mg/kg q12h week 1 then reducing by 50% for the next 3 weeks.
  - Some protocols use 2 mg/kg weekly throughout treatment period.

Vincristine
- 0.75 mg/m^2 IV every 3 weeks.

Cyclophosphamide
- 200–300 mg/m^2 every 3 weeks (preferably IV to decrease the need for owners to handle cytotoxic drugs).

- Following induction (8 weeks) maintenance with doxorubicin (25 mg/kg IV every 3 weeks) as a single agent may be more effective.

COAP protocol
- L-*Asparaginase* can be added into the initial treatment (day 1) at 400 iU/kg by SC injection and can result in rapid reduction of lymphoma size.
  - Not been shown to improve survival times.

Modified Madison-Wisconsin protocol
- Reported remission rates lower than COP at 50–70%.
- Median remission rates longer at 9 months.
- Can be continued biweekly sequence weeks 11 → 25 for 12 months.
- Then triweekly 6 months and monthly thereafter.

Prednisolone
- 2 mg/kg q24h weeks 1 and 2, then 1 mg/kg weekly.

Vincristine
- 0.5–0.75 mg/m^2 IV.
- Weeks 1, 3, 6, 8, 11, 12, 15, 19 and 23.

Cyclophosphamide
- 250 mg/m^2 IV – weeks 2, 7, 13 and 21.

Methotrexate
- 0.8 mg/kg IV – week 7.

Doxorubicin
- 20 mg/m^2 IV – weeks 4, 9 and 25.

Rescue
- Variety of other agents can be considered depending on original protocol – vinblastine, methotrexate, doxorubicin.

Radiation
- Consider for extra-nodal lymphoma especially nasal.

NB – *Most cats have spread outside of the primary site at the point of diagnosis.*

Response to myelosuppression
- Delaying treatment.
- Reducing dose or substituting agent that caused myelosuppression:
  - Chlorambucil instead of cyclophosphamide may be necessary 2–4 mg/m^2 PO q48h.
- Use of granulocyte colony stimulating factor.
- Supportive therapy as indicated.
- Substitution or reducing dose of vincristine.

Prognosis
- Depends on stage at diagnosis and morphology of lymphocytes.
- Overall remission rates and survival times seem shorter than dogs.
  - Subpopulation that achieve complete remission have greater chance of long term (>1 year survival).
  - Low grade alimentary lymphoma median survival time 19–29 months.
- *No* clear association with
  - Organ involvement/site.
  - Bone marrow involvement.
  - Phenotype B vs. T cell.
  - Retrovirus status.

4.11.8 Diseases of the immune system
Immune-mediated disease
- Common underlying pathology in many chronic disease states:
  - Gingivitis-stomatitis.
  - IBD.
  - Idiopathic lower urinary tract disease.
  - Polyarthritis.
  - Immune-mediated haemolytic anaemia uncommon.

Use of immunosuppressive drugs
- Corticosteroids:
  - Prednisolone – 2–4 mg/kg.
  - Dexamethasone – 0.35–0.7 mg/kg.
- Ciclosporin – 5 mg/kg q24h (25 mg/cat).
- Cyclophosphamide – 2.5 mg/kg q24h (usually 1 × 50 mg tablet every 4–5 days).
- Chlorambucil:
  - 1–2 mg/m^2 q24h (usually 2 mg tablet every 4–5 days).
  - 15 mg/m^2 for 4 days every 3 weeks.
  - 20 mg/m^2 q14 days.
- Azathioprine – cats lack the enzyme systems necessary for metabolism hence toxicity is significantly increased, a dose rate of 0.3 mg/kg daily has been suggested. Haematological parameters should be regularly monitored.

Systemic lupus erythematosus
- Rare multisystemic disease.
- Can be drug induced.
- Variety of clinical signs dependent on the organs involved.
- Pyrexia, lethargy and inappetence.
- Anaemia, skin lesions, polyarthritis, oral and renal involvement.

Diagnosis
- Poorly defined in cats.
- At least two separate manifestations of autoimmune disease.
- Positive anti-nuclear antibody titre.
- Positive lupus erythromatosus (LE) cells.

Cold agglutinin disease
- Anti-erythrocyte IgM antibodies.
- Haemolysis with minimal anaemi.
- Erythrocyte aggregation in peripheral vessels causes necrosis and sloughing of extremities in cold weather.
- Pinnae, tail and digits most commonly affected.
- Rarely eyelids and rostral nose.

ORGAN SYSTEMS

Myeloma
- Relatively rare.
- Non-specific presentation – depression, anorexia, weight loss.

Diagnosis
- Plasma cells – rarely seen in blood.
- Multiple erosive lesions of bone cortices.
- Hypergammaglobulinaemia with a monoclonal spike on serum electrophoresis.

NB – *Other diseases can cause monoclonal gammopathies, e.g. FIP, ehrlichiosis.*

- Granulocytopenia and thrombocytopenia secondary to marrow infiltration.
- Flame cells in bone marrow, spleen or peripheral masses.

Management
- Therapy is less successful in cats than in dogs.
- Prednisolone at 1–2 g/kg q12h and reducing.
- Melphalan at 0.1 mg/kg orally for 10 days then reduce to 0.05 mg/kg orally continuously.

Thymoma
- Uncommon.
- Middle-aged to older cats.
- Differentiate from thymic cysts and thymic lymphoma.

Clinical signs
- Dyspnoea.
- Vomiting.
- Dysphagia, anorexia.
- Coughing.
- Lethargy.
- Dysphonia.

Paraneoplastic syndromes
- Myasthenia gravis.
- Polymyositis.
- Myocarditis.
- Dermatitis.

Physical examination
- Bilaterally muffled heart and lung sounds.
- Poor compressibility of cranial thorax.

Diagnosis
- Imaging cranial mediastinal mass ± fluid.
- FNA:
  - Mixed population of thymic epithelial cells.
  - Immunohistochemistry advisable.

Treatment
- Surgical via median sternotomy.

Prognosis
- Post-surgical complications are common.
- Median survival time is 21 months.

Splenic disease
- Mild splenic changes in cats on ultrasound are common.
- Significant splenic disease is uncommon.
- Splenic bleeding as a cause of haemoabdomen even following RTA is rare.

Splenic masses
- Rare in cats.
- Primary neoplasia (haemangioma/haemangiosarcoma).
- Metastatic neoplasia.
- Haematoma.
- Splenic abscess.
- Nodular change.

Splenomegaly
- Uncommon.
- Seen more frequently than masses.

Investigation
- Spleen is often not seen on abdominal radiographs.
- Haematological changes are variable and may often be unremarkable.

- Presence of a splenic shadow on radiography may be normal or can indicate splenomegaly, but is also associated with splenic displacement by other abdominal organs.
- Ultrasound is sensitive in demonstrating focal changes, but it can be difficult to interpret a generalised increase or decrease in echogenicity.
- Ultrasound changes are non-specific.

Biopsy
- FNA:
  - Easy to perform.
  - Relatively safe.
  - Low diagnostic yield.
  - Most valuable in diffuse, infiltrative disease.
- Tru-cut biopsy:
  - Not recommended unless a large, localisable avascular mass.
- Biopsy at laparotomy/laparoscopy.

Causes of splenomegaly
- Suppurative – penetrating wound, migrating foreign body, *Toxoplasma*, mycobacteria (can also be granulomatous), secondary to endocarditis.
- Necrotising – salmonellosis.
- Eosinophilic – hypereosinophilic syndrome.
- Lymphoplasmacytic – pyometra, haemoplasma.
- Pyogranulomatous – FIP.
- Hyperplasia – haemolytic or bone marrow disorders.
- Congestion – drugs, portal hypertension.
- Diffuse neoplasia – lymphoma, mastocytosis, myeloma, leukaemia.

4.11.9 Inherited disorders of the coagulation, haematopoietic and immune system

Inherited coagulopathies
- Increased bleeding tendency, variation of severity between individuals.

- Clinical signs:
  - Excessive bleeding from umbilical cord.
  - Gingival bleeding during tooth eruption.
  - Spontaneous haematoma/haemarthrosis.
  - Haematoma following vaccination.
  - Excessive haemorrhage at neutering.

Factor VII
- DSH.

Factor VIIIC – haemophilia A
- Most common, relatively mild.
- DSH.
- Havana Brown.
- Siamese.
- Persian.

Factor IX – haemophilia B
- Sex-linked.
- DSH.
- British shorthair.
- Himalayan.
- British Shorthair (BSH).

Factor X
- DSH.

Factor XII (Hageman trait)
- DSH.

Von Willebrand's factor
- Himalayan.
- Devon Rex.
- Other breeds.

Vitamin K-responsive coagulopathy
- Devon Rex.

Inherited anaemia
Pyruvate kinase deficiency
- Chronic intermittent haemolytic anaemia associated with a deletional mutation.

ORGAN SYSTEMS

ORGAN SYSTEMS

- Somali.
- Abyssinian.
- DSH.

Inherited white cell abnormalities
Neutrophil granulation anomaly
- Functionally silent, fine eosinophilic granules present.
- Birman.

Chédiak–Higashi syndrome
- Associated with colour dilution gene, e.g. blue smoke. Enlarged granules present in leucocytes and melanocytes, early cataract development, bleeding tendency.
- Persian.
- Other breeds.

4.12 ONCOLOGY AND CHEMOTHERAPY

4.12.1 Introduction
- Three principal treatment modalities exist – surgery, chemotherapy and radiation.
- Other modalities that are applicable to certain tumours include immunotherapy with antitumour vaccines, use of biological response modifiers such as acemannan or bacillus of Calmette and Guerin (BCG), cytokine therapy, cryotherapy, hyperthermia, specific receptor inhibitors and photodynamic therapy.
- Method chosen in each case should be appropriate to the tumour, location, patient and owner.
- In many cases a combination of modalities will provide the best long-term outcome.
- It is essential that the owners appreciate that the majority of treatments are not curative but palliative.

4.12.2 Approach to neoplasia
Diagnosis
- Many cats that have neoplasia do not present with a palpable mass – approximately one-third of cases

referred to internal medicine services will have neoplasia as the underlying diagnosis.
- Routine blood tests tend to have low sensitivity for neoplasia.
- Imaging has high sensitivity but lacks specificity and other causes of mass lesions should always be considered.
- Histologic/cytologic diagnosis is usually required to confirm the presence and type of neoplasm.

NB – *Histological grading does not always correlate with biological response, e.g. most adrenal neoplasms appear histologically benign but will metastasise.*

- If treatment is considered staging is important.
  - Tumour Node Metastasis system is appropriate for most cases.

Surgery
- First surgery has the highest chance of success.
- Pre-surgical biopsy to define type and aggressiveness of tumour allows better surgical planning.
- Removing masses without FNA or biopsy may lead to choosing inappropriate margins of resection.
- Imaging.
  - Define extent of tumour, invasion and relations – may require advanced imaging.
  - Excludes distance metastasis.
- Plan the extent of resection to remove the palpable tumour and a surrounding area of normal tissue to remove all tumour cells.
- Higher grade tumours require a wider area of resection.
- A lateral skin margin of 1–5 cm (depending on tumour type and grade) and a deep fascial layer is mandatory.
- The deep margin is the most common margin for incomplete excision.

- 'Shelling out' will only remove the grossly visible tumour tissue and recurrence is likely.
- Wound reconstruction after tumour resection may require advanced surgical techniques.
- Early referral for definitive treatment is likely to have a better outcome than referral after resection with dirty margins.

Chemotherapy

- As with other drugs, dose rates and toxicities can be unpredictable in cats, safety in other species is not necessarily transferable to cats.
- Safe handling of drugs is of paramount importance.
  - Each chemotherapy agent in the practice should have an individual risk assessment.
  - Designated personnel should be trained to dispense and administer chemotherapy.
  - Appropriate accompanying literature should be given to clients regarding handling of medication, urine and faeces.
  - For IV drugs, gowns, masks and gloves are required.
  - Drugs should be reconstituted in a fume cupboard or using an appropriate sealed system, e.g. PhaSeal.
  - Closed systems should be used for administering the drugs and patients should be actively monitored at all times during administration.
  - Hospitalised patients should have their kennels clearly marked.

Commonly used drugs

Prednisolone

- Lymphocytolytic to neoplastic lymphocytes, initial dose rate 2 mg/kg or 40 mg/m^2
- Also have some effect to reduce tumour-associated inflammation and therefore effective tumour size

Vincristine

- Interferes with microtubule assembly.
- Used primarily to treat lymphoproliferative disorders.
- Value in thrombocytopenia questionable.
- Always give via IV catheter; very irritant perivascularly.

Side effects
- Bone marrow suppression usually mild.
- Peripheral neuropathy.
- Constipation.

Cyclophosphamide

- Cross-links DNA preventing synthesis and function.
- Used to treat lymphoproliferative, myeloproliferative and immune-mediated disease.
- Some sarcomas and carcinomas also responsive.

Dose
- Varies with protocol.

Side effects
- Bone marrow suppression – nadir 7–14 days.
- GIT upset.
- Hepato- and nephrotoxicity.
- Reduced hair growth.

Chlorambucil

- Similar to and a substitute for cyclophosphamide, less myelosuppressive.
- Used as an immunosuppressive agent, management of small cell lymphoma in cats, chronic lymphocytic leukaemia.

Dose
- Varies with protocol.

Side effects
- Anorexia.
- Nausea and vomiting.

Doxorubicin

- Antibiotics.
- Inhibits DNA synthesis and function.
- Used in treatment of lymphoma and sarcomas.

ORGAN SYSTEMS

Dose
Usually 20 mg/m^2 IV every 3–4 weeks.

Side effects
• Anaphylaxis reported.
• Severe bone marrow suppression.
• Nephrotoxicity.
• Anorexia and vomiting.
• Cardiotoxicity not documented.

Radiation
• Effective for a number of tumour types alone or in combination.
• Use is generally limited by availability and the need for repeated anaesthesia as treatment requires fractionation:
  ○ Side effects include mucositis, skin changes, ocular damage.
  ○ Radioactive iodine is highly effective for the treatment of hyperthyroidism only requiring a single dose in most cases.
• Commonly treated tumours include
  ○ Oral tumours.
  ○ Nasal tumours.
  ○ Pituitary macroadenoma.
  ○ Tumours extremities – vaccine-associated sarcomas, lymphoma.
• Advice of a radiation oncologist should be sort if radiation therapy is considered.

4.12.3 Dose calculation for chemotherapy agents
• Due to their potential toxicity, many chemotherapeutic agents are given on a body surface area (BSA) basis to allow more accurate dosing (see Table 66).
• Tablet sizes are usually inappropriate for cats but recompounding should only be undertaken by a compounding pharmacy.
• In most cases, dosing interval has to be extended to accommodation tablet size.

4.12.4 Nutritional management of neoplasia
• Maintaining body weight improves survival times in patients with neoplasia.

Table 66 Relationship between weight and body surface area in cats

Weight (kg)	BSA (m^2)
2	0.16
2.5	0.18
3	0.21
3.5	0.23
4	0.25
4.5	0.27
5	0.29
5.5	0.32
6	0.33

• Omega-3 polyunsaturated fatty acids reduce tumour necrosis factor-α that can be associated with weight loss.
• Inappetence can be a major factor, hence highly palatable energy-dense diets are recommended.
• Energy is best provided as fats.
  ○ Energy requirements can be twice that of a similar sized animal without neoplasia.
• Protein levels should be increased at 30–45% of metabolisable energy High dose arginine supplementation (>2% on dry matter basis) may be helpful.
• A wide variety of other food ingredients and nutraceuticals have been recommended for cancer patients; evidence of efficacy is lacking.

4.12.5 Paraneoplastic syndromes
• Disease states that occur secondary to the metabolic, endocrine or haematologic effects of a tumour.
• Can be distant from the tumour itself and be responsible for the clinical presentation, e.g. hypercalcaemia associated with lymphoma causing a presentation for PU/PD.

Haematologic

- Anaemia due to chronic disease, bone marrow invasion, immune-mediated or microangiopathic haemolysis, GI and external loss, hypersplenism.
- Thrombocytopenia and altered coagulation (DIC).
- Hyperviscosity due to monoclonal gammopathy, polycythaemia.
- Leucocytosis and eosinophilia – rare.

Metabolic and endocrine

- Cancer cachexia – anorexia, weight loss, fatigue and immune dysfunction – MER can double in cancer cases. Caused by alterations in carbohydrate, protein and lipid metabolism. Cancer cachexia decreases survival times.
- Fever – induced by cytokines about 10% of PUO cases.
- Hypercalcaemia due to release of parathyroid-related peptide.
- Hypoglycaemia – insulinomas but also liver, pulmonary and muscle tumours. Secondary to sepsis, e.g. GI tumour rupture.
- Hyperhistaminaemia – release from mast cells causing local oedema, erythema and pruritus and distant GI ulceration.

Neuromuscular

- Demyelination and axonal degeneration – likely underlying autoimmune mechanism.
- Myasthenia gravis – usually secondary to thymoma.
- Hypertrophic pulmonary osteopathy (Marie's disease).

Dermatologic

- Alopecia (cats).
- Exfoliative dermatitis (cats with thymoma).
- Small hyperplastic dermal collaginous nodules.

4.13 NUTRITION

4.13.1 Introduction – nutritional requirements of cats

- Cats have major nutritional idiosyncrasies which need to be addressed when considering nutritional management of disease.
- Cats have
  - A higher protein requirement; arginine-deficient diets such as some baby foods can rapidly cause hepatic encephalopathy.
  - Significantly lower (about one-third the level) amylase activity than dogs as well as lower levels of disaccharidases making the feeding of a low-fat diet more difficult in terms of an alternate source of calories.
  - More selective eating habits and therefore dietary manipulation that results in reduced palatability, such as the addition of fibre, can have low acceptance rates.
  - An essential requirement for taurine. Taurine deficiency is usually associated with attempts to feed a vegetarian/vegan diet. Taurine deficiency can lead to central retinal degeneration, DCM and reproductive failure. In the early stages these changes are reversible.
  - A requirement for a source of pre-formed vitamin A.
  - An essential requirement for arachidonic acid in their diet.
  - Stronger insulin secretion in response to amino acids than carbohydrates.
  - A greater sensitivity to oxidants in their food which can cause Heinz body anaemia. Such changes have been associated with feeding some baby foods which use onion powder as a base.

Vegetarian/vegan diets for cats

- It is not possible to formulate vegetarian/vegan diets for cats without careful addition of essential ingredients that are usually animal derived.

ORGAN SYSTEMS

- Even when produced, balanced vegetarian/vegan diets do not seem to have the same health benefits as meat-based diets.

Fibre

- Dietary fibres are forms of carbohydrates and can be classified as soluble or insoluble.
- Non-fermentable fibre has little value in most veterinary diets other than to reduce nutrient density and produce a bulky stool.
- Fermentable fibre could be a conditionally dependent nutrient; the short-chain fatty acids that are produced may have a role in promoting restoration of normal intestinal function.
- Preferentially metabolised by the indigenous bacterial flora of the GIT which may inhibit overgrowth of potentially pathogenic bacteria.
- Increasing dietary fibre has a number of potential benefits, but high-fibre diets are not readily accepted by cats.
- Daily recommendation for fibre intake is 0.28 g crude fibre/100 kcal of ME.
- Change onto a high-fibre diet can lead to flatulence, increased borborygmi and increased faecal output particularly when the changeover is rapid.

Effects of fibre

- Lowers the nutrient density of the diet.
- Binds water increasing faecal bulk and frequency of defaecation, soluble fibre has a greater capacity for this than insoluble fibre.
- Decreases the digestibility of protein, fat and carbohydrates.
- Slows the release of carbohydrates from the food.
- Decreases the absorption of calcium and zinc.
- Increases the undigested residue and microbial content of the faeces.

- It may influence the bacterial flora of the intestinal system.
- Increased fermentable fibre can act to
  - Trap nitrogen in bacterial cells reducing the amount of nitrogen that is converted into urea.
  - Short-chain fatty acid production has an osmotic effect increasing the amount of urea moving from the blood into the colon.
  - Helps to maintain the structural integrity of the intestine.
  - Affects intestinal transit time tending to increase transit in hypermotile states such as diarrhoea and decrease transit time in constipation.

Fibre supplementation

- Psyllium – 1–2 teaspoon mixed with each meal.
- Wheat bran – 1 tsp per meal.
- Canned pumpkin or creamed corn – 1–4 tsp per meal – sweeter and more palatable.

4.13.2 Life stage nutrition and energy requirements

Energy

- Energy requirement is dependent on life stage and to a smaller extent on lifestyle (Table 67).
  - Where energy demand is high e.g. when kittens, during gestation or lactation, cats are usually best fed *ad libitum*.
- Dietary energy is the prime regulator of food consumption in cats.
- The most useful measurement for comparing the energy contents of a diet is the metabolisable energy per 100 g of food on a dry matter basis.
- Metabolisable energy is used to digest, absorb and utilise food (the heat increment) with the remainder being available for growth, lactation, reproduction, physical performance (the net energy for production) and repair, basic activity and thermoregulation (the net energy for maintenance).

Table 67 Estimated energy requirements in healthy cats in various physiological states

Physiological state	Cat (kcal/kg body weight)
<3 months (growth)	250
3–6 months (growth)	130
6–12 months	80–100
Inactive adult	70
Active	80
Gestation (<42 days)	88
Gestation (>42 days)	88–104
Peak lactation (3–6 weeks)	80 × (1 + [0.25 × number of kittens])

Resting energy requirement (RER)
- The basic energy expended by an animal at rest in a thermoneutral environment.
- RER (kcal) = 70 × (body weight in kg)$^{0.75}$.
- For cats over 2 kg, this approximates to 30 × (body weight in kg) + 70 (see Table 68).

Maintenance energy requirement (MER)
- The amount of energy that is used by an active animal in a thermoneutral environment.
- Does not include the energy required for growth, pregnancy or lactation.
- Various formulae used, MER (kcal/day) =
  - 1.4 × RER.
  - 110 × (body weight in kg)$^{0.75}$.
  - 1100 × body surface area (m^2).

Life stage nutrition
- Pre-weaning fed by queen if not then fostering is the best approach.
  - Large litters, queen with inadequate/ no milk, then a proprietary mild substitute is required; goat/cow milk has inadequate nutrient density and protein and excess carbohydrate.

Table 68 Resting and maintenance energy requirements of adult cats by weight

Weight (kg)	RER (kcal)	MER (kcal)
2.5	140	220
3	160	250
3.5	180	280
4	200	310
4.5	215	340
5	235	365
5.5	250	390
6	270	420

4.13.3 Dietary formulation

Types of diet

Complete
- Formulated to meet all the dietary needs for that group of animals.
- Some diets are complete for all life stages whilst others will only be complete for one life stage, e.g. maintenance.

Complementary
- Unsuitable as a single source of food as they lack one or more essential dietary component and are not necessarily balanced in terms of vitamins and minerals.
- Intended to be fed with another diet component to produce a complete diet.
- Used as a minor dietary component as a treat or to add textural variety.
- Clients often do not appreciate that foods are complimentary rather than complete which can lead to dietary deficiencies particularly if they are gourmet meat varieties.
  - Labelling on some cat foods can be poor/inadequate.

Moist foods
- High water content, usually 70–80%.
- Preserved by heat sterilisation, vacuum packing or freezing.

ORGAN SYSTEMS

- Tend to be highly digestible and palatable.
- Energy density is such that relatively large volume needs to be fed.

Semi-moist foods
- Rarely used.

Dry foods
- Low water content, around 10%.
- Preservation is achieved by drying; storage life can be relatively short.
- Nutrient density is high.
- Cats fed dry food tend to be at greater risk of obesity.
- Some dry diets may contribute to the development of FLUTD, depending on the formulation used.

4.13.4 Dietary deficiency and toxicity
- Dietary deficiencies and toxicities sufficient to cause clinically significant disease are generally rare.
  - Dietary recommendations for nutrients are based on an inclusion rate per 100 kcal ME. BUT this assumes an appropriate calorie intake, so severely anorexic cats may have dietary deficiencies even when fed a complete diet due to their low total intake.
- Dietary deficiencies are usually associated with neglect or with the owner feeding a home-prepared diet, particularly all lean meat or liver or attempting to feed a cat dog food.
- Dietary toxicity occur occasionally due to manufacturing errors (e.g. excess vitamin D), malicious (e.g. melamine poisoning), contamination (e.g. coccidiostats) or a lack of understanding of cats' nutritional requirements (e.g. inadequate potassium).
- Disease states, usually of the intestinal system, can lead to deficiencies in some or all of the dietary components especially vitamin B_{12}.
  - PU/PD can lead to low levels of water-soluble vitamins.

Common dietary problems in cats
Meat and poultry
- Lean meat which has excessive amounts of phosphorus relative to calcium and is deficient in sodium, iron, copper, iodine and vitamins.
- All meat diet can lead to severe and potential fatal skeletal abnormalities, classically nutritional secondary hyperparathyroidism and joint malformations.

Fish
- Raw fish can contain thiaminase leading to thiamine (B_1) deficiency.
- Can containing parasites, e.g. liver fluke.
- Excessive amounts of fish can cause a relative deficiency of vitamin E especially if packed in oil.
- Cheap fish can cause histamine release.

Liver
- Liver contains excessively high levels of vitamin A (see Section 4.10.4).

4.13.5 Nutrition of the hospitalised cat
When to feed?
- Cats should not starve for more than 3 days without addressing their nutritional needs.

Consequences of malnutrition
- Critical patients are catabolic despite starvation.
- Lack of enteral nutrition causes reduced epithelial cell turnover within the intestinal tract and increased bacterial translocation from the intestine into the systemic circulation.
- Poor nutritional status is associated with decreased immune function.
- Wound healing is delayed.
- The risk of sepsis is increased.
- Poor nutritional status may affect the prognosis.

What to feed?

- In general, hospitalised patients should be offered highly palatable, highly digestible nutrient dense foods in SMALL quantities.
- Frequent feeding (four to six times per day) is essential for critically ill or anorexic patients.
- There is probably nothing more unappetising for a hospitalised cat than to be presented with a large bowl of food which is left to go stale in the kennel and from which they cannot get away.
- Uneaten wet food should be removed 20–30 minutes after feeding.
- Dry food can be left longer especially if a cat is known to be a 'grazer'.
- Sometimes cats will only eat at night when the hospital is quiet.

How much to feed?

- Calculations should be based on the RER.
- On the first day between a third and a half of that calculated amount should be given and built up to the calculated amount over 2–3 days.
- In man, few additional health benefits have been demonstrated by feeding more than 50% RER, so this should be the minimum aim in conjunction with daily weighing of the patient.

How to feed?

Assisted feeding

- Many cats will eat voluntarily especially if given highly palatable, warmed, odorous food.
- Time should be taken to encourage a hospitalised cat to eat, by sitting with the patient and offering food by hand or from the end of a syringe.
- Sometimes inviting the owner to feed the animal can have positive benefits.

- Ensure the feeding environment is optimised, feeling safe and secure for the cat.
- Chemical appetite stimulants can be of value in the short term, but are only appropriate when the underlying problem causing the inappetence is resolved.

Recommended oral appetite stimulants for cats

- Mirtazapine – 3.75 mg/cat PO q48–72h:
  - Side effects – sedation can be profound, vocalization, increased affection in cats, hypotension and tachycardia. Rarely anticholinergic side effects, e.g. urinary retention, intestinal ileus.
  - Should not be used if monoamine oxidase inhibitors used in past 14 days, e.g. selegiline.
- Cyproheptadine – 1–2 mg/cat PO q12–24h:
  - Side effects – CNS depressant (sedation) and anticholinergic effects (dryness of mucous membranes, etc.). Cats can develop a paradoxical agitated state that resolves upon dose reduction or discontinuation. There have been reports of cyproheptadine-induced haemolytic anaemia in cats.
- Oxazepam – 1–2 mg/cat PO q24h:
  - Side effects – sedation and occasionally, ataxia. Paradoxical effects such as excitability, vocalization or aggression are possible. Rarely precipitates tonic–clonic seizures; use with caution in susceptible patients. Potentially, oxazepam could cause hepatic toxicity in cats, but this occurs very rarely.

Other methods

- Force-feeding is counter-productive as this only increases a cat's aversion to food and is stressful for the patient and staff.

ORGAN SYSTEMS

ORGAN SYSTEMS

- Some form of tube feeding is appropriate in most medium–long stay, anorexic, hospitalised cats that have not responded to assisted feeding.
- In extreme case parenteral nutrition may be required.

Other supplements
- The true value of augmenting the diet of hospitalised cats with rate-limiting or conditionally dependent nutrients is unclear but may be of value.

Glutamine
- Major substrate for gluconeogenesis.
- Principal amino acid in plasma and muscles.
- Important to the normal stress response of many tissues such as the kidney, white blood cells and fibroblasts.
- Additional glutamine supplementation may therefore be beneficial and improve recovery rates,

Branched chain amino acids
- Supplementation may be advantageous in septic animals or those with encephalopathy.

Arginine
- Supplementation may promote wound healing and immune function.
- Encephalopathy rapidly occurs in cats fed arginine-deficient diets (usually human enteral preparations).

Tube feeding (Table 69)
- Important in the management of hospitalised patient.
- It is better to fit a tube early and then not use it than have to fit a tube in a sicker, more cachexic patient several days later.
- Initially focus on frequent, small feeds:
  - If the tube diameter is narrow or the patient difficult to handle then drip

feeding the required calories over 18 hours/day using a syringe pump/driver may be appropriate.
- Type of tube fitted will depend on:
  - Length and time that supplementary nutrition is required.
  - Disease status:
    - Tube appropriate for that disease.
    - Effect of disease on risk/benefit of anaesthetising the patient.
  - Equipment availability.
  - Other procedures being performed, e.g. if the patient is having a laparotomy and tube feeding may be necessary then an oesophagostomy or gastrostomy tube can be placed at that time.
- *Specialist techniques.*

Jejunostomy tubes
- J-tubes are indicated in patients with intractable vomiting or pancreatitis. They can be used for medium-term support but are difficult to place and seem to fall out relatively easily. There is a lack of availability of suitable monomeric diets for use; using other liquid diets designed to pre-digest in the stomach and requiring pancreatic enzymes for further breakdown will often lead to chronic diarrhoea. Leakage around the insertion site will cause peritonitis.
- Endoscopic placement is possible.

Parenteral nutrition
- Partial parenteral nutrition may be suitable for some cats to increase calorie intake in the short term. Feeding can be delivered via a peripheral line but most will fail after 48–72 hours due to the hypertonic nature of the solution.
- Total parenteral nutrition requires a jugular catheter as the solutions are very hyperosmolar. It is a complex technique and suitable feeding solutions are not available, so need to be made

Table 69 Indications, contraindications and technique for placing feeding tubes in cats

Method	Equipment	Technique for placement	Indications	Contraindications and complications
Naso-oesophageal	Topical anaesthetic PVC/silicone feeding tube (3.5–5 Fr) Lubricating jelly Suture/adhesive Sterile water/saline Elizabethan collar	Generally this technique can be performed in the conscious or lightly sedated patient. Tube measured to 9th rib in cats. Nostril desensitised and the tube advanced in a ventral and medial direction with the neck flexed to the pre-measured point. Tube position can be checked with sterile water/saline or by radiography. Tube can be secured by butterfly tapes sutured to the nose and top of the head. Super glue can be used but is associated with thermal burns	Short-term feeding (5–7 days)	Vomiting, megaoesophagus, oesophagitis obstruction of the nares or pharynx, semi-conscious or comatose patients. Long-term nutrition Rhinitis, aspiration of the tube
Oesophagostomy	10–14 Fr feeding tube or Foley catheter Long curved haemostats Scalpel and suture Tape and collar	A small incision is made in the oesophagus under light general anaesthesia and the tube fed 9th rib in cats. Rapid and relatively risk-free procedure with few complications	Short-/medium-term feeding	Vomiting, megaoesophagus, oesophagitis, obstruction of the nares or pharynx, semi-conscious or comatose patients Wound infection, oesophageal stricture
Percutaneous endoscopic gastrostomy (PEG tube)	General anaesthetic Endoscope or percutaneous (van Noort) kit 20 Fr mushroom-tipped or flanged gastrostomy tube 16 g catheter	The cat is lightly anaesthetised in right lateral recumbency and an area caudal to the last rib clipped and prepared. The endoscope is guided into the stomach which is inflated and the indentation made by a fingertip placed on the	Long-term feeding (months to years)	Vomiting, unacceptable anaesthetic risk Leakage around the tube and peritonitis, necrosis of the stomach wall (tube pulled too tight), splenic laceration, interference with gastric emptying

(Continued)

Table 69 Indications, contraindications and technique for placing feeding tubes in cats (Continued)

Method	Equipment	Technique for placement	Indications	Contraindications and complications
	Monofilament nylon Scalpel blade Adapters Stockinet bandage	appropriate skin site located. An over-the-needle catheter is then pushed into the stomach and nylon threaded through. The nylon is grasped by the biopsy forceps and withdrawn with the endoscope out of the mouth. The tube is tied to the nylon which is drawn back taking the feeding tube via the oesophagus into the stomach. A small skin incision allows the tube to be drawn out through the stomach and body wall where it is secured. The end of the tube is then attached to a suitable connector to which a syringe can be fitted	Long-term feeding (months to years)	Vomiting, unacceptable anaesthetic risk Leakage around the tube and peritonitis, necrosis of the stomach wall (tube pulled too tight), splenic laceration, interference with gastric emptying
Blind gastrostomy	General anaesthetic Lubricated vinyl/metal tube as for PEG	Essentially similar to a PEG tube except that the locating tube is inserted into the stomach blindly and manipulated until it can be seen distorting the body wall in the correct place. A catheter is then placed into the lumen of the tube and stiff wire attached to suture material drawn through to the mouth. The tube is attached and drawn through as for the PEG tube	As PEG	As PEG – greater risk of obstruction and iatrogenic damage due to the blind technique. Difficult in obese patients. Lower equipment costs
Surgical gastrostomy	Laparotomy pack Feeding tube Stockinet	Right lateral incision, gastrostomy, placement of tube, secured by purse-string sutures. Standard closure	As PEG	As PEG. Anaesthetic longer – most suitable when a laparotomy is already being performed

with the associated concerns over sterility. Poorly formulated total parenteral nutrition (TPN) solutions can cause severe acid–base and metabolic issues.

4.13.6 Nutritional management of organ-related disease
- Nutritional requirements for specific disease conditions are addressed in the relevant organ-specific sections.

Food intolerance and food hypersensitivity (allergy)

Non-immunological adverse reactions to food – food intolerance
Where a non-immunological cause of the intestinal signs is implicated prior exposure to the diet is not required and signs generally resolve rapidly on withdrawal of the offending product.

Causes
- Foods may contain pharmacologically active micronutrients such as caffeine or theophylline (in chocolate) that can cause GI disturbances.
- Food preservatives, additives and dyes have also been implicated in adverse reactions.
- Toxic contamination from bacteria or chemicals can be associated with acute onset GI signs.
- Some canned fish, e.g. tuna, have high concentrations of histamine present resulting in significant intestinal signs.
- Dietary indiscretion is a less common cause of GI signs in cats.
- Lactose intolerance is perhaps the best known non-immunological dietary intolerance in cats. Due to their unique physiology, cats are, in general, poorly able to tolerate large amounts of carbohydrates in their diet (due to a lack of pancreatic amylase).
- Novel diet – as with any individual, if cats are subjected to a sudden, radical,

change in diet type GI signs are likely to ensue.

Dietary hypersensitivity
- Usually associated with food that has been fed for some time and not recent introduction of new diets.
- Non-seasonal, wide age range, no breed or sex predilection, often occurs suddenly, not associated with an apparent dietary change.
- Food types – beef, fish, dairy products, gluten.
- Dry foods may be more likely to cause problems than wet foods.
- Clinical signs – dermatological (pruritus particularly head and neck in cats) or GIT.
- GIT signs – usually causes weight loss, vomiting and diarrhoea. Vomiting is probably the most consistent feature. Some cats, however, present without obvious GI signs showing weight loss in the face of a normal to increased appetite.
- Other possible associations – anorexia, rhinitis, conjunctivitis, bronchoconstriction, seizures, lethargy, FLUTD, urinary incontinence, glomerulonephritis.
- If an immunologically based adverse reaction to food is suspected then this should be investigated using an elimination diet.
- Ideally, the new diet should contain a novel protein and carbohydrate source or, if this is not possible, then a source that the patient has not seen for 6 months.
- Strict adherence to the trial is essential which may be necessary for up to 10 weeks, although most cases will be showing a response in 1–2 weeks.
- If signs resolve, then the patient should be re-challenged with the original diet to show that the symptoms recur. Understandably many owners are reluctant to pursue the second phase!

ORGAN SYSTEMS

Hypoallergenic diets
- Chicken or fish is not innately less aller-genic than beef, it is the novelty of the protein source that is important.
- Hydrolysed diets – proteins in the diet have been digested into smaller frag-ments that are thought to be less immu-nogenic and therefore these diets are classified as 'hypoallergenic'.
  - Efficacy in the diagnosis and manage-ment of allergic GIT disease has yet to be validated in large scale, field, trials.
  - Most contain protein fragments of around 100 amino acids. A truly hypoallergenic diet would need to digest these peptides further to <9–10 amino acids.
  - Which proteins in the diet are hydro-lysed varies – meat proteins vs. all proteins.
  - Some highly hydrolysed diets have peptide fragments that are genu-inely too small to excite and immune response.
  - May be acting as a very novel protein diet.
  - Which proteins within the diet have been hydrolysed varies between diets

GIT disease
- Acute self-limiting diarrhoea is usually non-immunologically based.
- Food allergy is often *unassociated* with a recent change in diet.
- Single-source protein or hydrolysed diets are appropriate as part of the man-agement of most GI diseases.
- Value of low-fat diets in the manage-ment of intestinal disease is unproven.
- Most home-prepared diets are nutri-tionally inadequate and are not recom-mended for long-term (months) main-tenance.
- High-fibre diets are only appropriate in the management of constipation and some motility disorders.

Aims of diets suitable for treating cats with CKD
- Reduced phosphorus.
- Moderate protein restriction (usually required to achieve low phosphorus).
- Increased omega-3:omega-6 ratio.
- Energy provided from fats.
- Increased potassium levels.
- Value and risks of salt restriction is unclear.
- Supplementation of water-soluble vita-mins, especially B group.

Aims in the treatment of lower urinary tract disease
- Wet foods are generally preferred as they increase urine output.
- Crystalluria does NOT necessitate die-tary manipulation, unless associated with urolithiasis.
- Urolith analysis is vital to the appropri-ate management of urolithiasis.
- Oxalate uroliths should be managed by
  - Avoiding high salt levels.
  - Avoiding low or high phosphorus diets.
  - Ensuring adequate magnesium levels.
  - Encouraging alkaline urine pH.
  - Avoiding high protein/high calcium diets.
  - It is not possible to dissolve existing calcium oxalate uroliths with diet.
- Struvite uroliths should be managed with
  - Reduced magnesium and phosphate diets.
  - Moderate calorie density.
  - Increased salt.
  - Encouraging an acid urine pH.

Aims in the treatment of hepatic insufficiency causing encephalopathy
- Control ammonia production by mod-erate protein restriction.
- Moderately reduce fat levels.
- Provide significant calories as carbo-hydrate.

- Increase vitamin levels.
- Supplement with vitamin E.
- Restrict copper.
- Supplement with zinc.

Cats with non-encephalopathic reduction in liver function; normal function but raised liver enzymes

- Protein restriction in these cases is of no value and may affect liver repair.
- Improved antioxidant capacity is likely to be valuable.

4.13.7 Management of obesity

- Cats that are more than 20% above their ideal weight are defined as obese.
- Obesity affects 10–20% of cats.
- Some endocrinopathies are associated with weight gain due to an increased appetite, organomegaly or hypometabolism but are rare in cats.
- Hyperadrenocorticism.
- Acromegaly.
- Hypothalamic disorders.
- Insulinoma.
- Hypothyroidism.
- Hypopituitarism.
- In the vast majority of cases weight gain is associated with over-nutrition due to increased caloric intake or reduced requirement (e.g. less exercise).

Diseases associated with obesity

- Respiratory difficulties – Pickwickian syndrome.
- Skin disease.
- Decreased cardiac reserve.
- Insulin resistance.
- Poorer response to infectious diseases.
- Fatty infiltration of the liver.
- Increased surgical risk – anaesthesia, fat necrosis, slower wound healing, technical difficulty of procedure.
- FLUTD.
- Increased joint stress and exacerbation of osteoarthritis.
- Dystocia.

Weight reduction

- Reduce caloric intake.
- Increase exercise.
- Behavioural modification of owner and pet.

Causes of overfeeding

- Generally cats regulate their caloric intake better than dogs.
  - Major issue is highly palatable energy-dense diets fed *ad libitum*
- Failure to adjust feeding to individual needs.
- Additional energy from snacks or treats ignored.
- Encouraging eating as a sign of good health.
- Indulging begging behaviour.
- Providing food when the pet is left alone.
- Associated with owner attempts to diet.

Reducing caloric intake

- Cut out high- calorie snacks and treats and replace with low- calorie ones, e.g. proprietary low- calorie treats.
- Reduce the amount of normal food:
  - Change from ad *libitum* to portion feeding.
  - Prevent obese cat from eating food for other cats in household.
- Maintain current volume of food, but reduce caloric density of food:
  - Increase water content of diet.
  - Increase fibre content of diet – preferably non-fermentable fibre.
  - Increase calories provided by carbohydrates.

Other diet features

- It is essential that the diet has
  - Adequate protein levels to minimise tissue protein loss.
  - Essential components such as EFAs, vitamins and minerals should be included at sufficient levels, i.e. weight loss is not an excuse for a poor quality diet!

ORGAN SYSTEMS

Calculation of caloric requirement
- Initially the target should be a 15% reduction in body weight.
- Feed 55–60% of the calculated energy requirements at that target weight.
- Most cats require a calorie intake of 40–45 kcal/kg for effective weight reduction.

Rate of weight loss
- Safe weight loss is considered to be 1–1.5% per week.
- May be as little as 50 g/week for a 5 kg cat.

Failure to lose weight
- Majority of cases are due to poor owner compliance and support is therefore important.
- If the caloric intake is reduced a cat's BMR falls reducing their caloric requirement.
- The reduction in BMR can be partially prevented by increasing exercise.

Check
- Owner compliance with diet particularly scraps and type of fluids being given.
- For alternate feed sources particularly when dieting cats (hunting, being fed next door).
- If sufficient time has been given to show a change within the accuracy of the practice scales.
- Re-calculate requirement and recommendations to client.
- Reconsider the possibility of an endocrinopathy.
- If the client appears to be following the diet adequately then the caloric intake should be reduced by 15%.

Risks and complications of weight loss
- In general, controlled weight loss in healthy adult animals is a safe procedure.

Hepatic lipidosis
- Potentially fatal disease that can be associated with a sudden fall in caloric intake.
- Usually associated with the cat refusing to eat the new diet and not being offered an alternative.
- See hepatobiliary disease section 4.4.7.

4.14 INTOXICATION

4.14.1 Introduction
- Intoxication is generally uncommon in cats and it is most commonly associated with
  - Contamination of food being fed to the cat.
  - Contamination of the coat with the intoxicant subsequently being ingested during grooming.
    - These are usually solvent-based compounds, e.g. petroleum products.
  - Drug toxicity associated with dog products being used in cats, e.g. permethrins or paracetamol.
  - Cats that chew and ingest plant material often those containing saponins, particularly
    - Spider/ribbon plant.
    - Cordyline and Dracaena.
    - Cyclamen.
    - Poinsettia.
    - Lilies (NB genus *Lilium* and *Hemerocallis*).
    - Catnip/catmint/catrup.
    - Peace lily/white sails.
- All pharmaceutical drugs, herbal products and nutraceuticals are potentially poisonous.
  - Some cats will show an idiosyncratic reaction to a licensed pharmaceutical given at an appropriate dose.
- Poisoning cases can present with a variety of clinical signs and therefore are included in many differential lists. Generally the presentation is acute with many having a clear history of known or likely exposure.

- Specific diagnostic tests are available for some poisons; results are slow and therefore confirmatory rather than therapeutically useful.
- Routine haematology, coagulation profiles and biochemistry are helpful in establishing which and how significantly affected the patient is.

4.14.2 Approach to suspected intoxication

Decontaminate skin

- If immediate decontamination not possible fit an Elizabethan collar to prevent further absorption.
- Isolate from other pets/children.
- Clip hair especially long-haired cats.
- Wash skin with copious tepid-warm water and mild detergent.
  - Stronger degreasing detergents required for oily substances – wash out well.
  - Check that this will not increase rate of absorption.
  - Ensure washer adequately protected.
  - Be careful when washing not to cause hypothermia.

DO NOT

- Use solvents, e.g. alcohol.
- Neutralise acids with alkalis/bases or vice versa.

Decontaminate GIT

- Induce vomiting if recent ingestion (within last 2–3 hours).

DO NOT USE APOMORPHINE
DO NOT INDUCE VOMITING IF

- The substance is a hydrocarbon (petroleum-based), caustic or volatile.
- Patient may not be able to defend airway, e.g. CNS depression when vomits.
- Ingested poison may cause seizures.
  - Reduce absorption, may be better given by naso-oesophageal or orogastric tube.

- Activated charcoal preferably as slurry at 1–4 g/kg q4–6h for 24–48 hours:
  - Continued use important if enterohepatic circulation, e.g. salicylates, methylxanthine.
  - Consider effect absorption of drugs used for treatment.
  - Cathartics increase elimination of activated charcoal.
- Other options include kaolin, chalk or barium.

Induction of emesis

- Washing soda crystal at back of tongue.
- Xylazine (3 mg/kg) or medetomidine (10 µg/kg) or dexmedetomidine (5 µg/kg) – more effective if stomach full/ small meal fed prior to administration.
- Will cause sedation and hypotension that may be undesirable.
- Other options may be used in an emergency.
- Syrup of ipecacuanha 1:1 with water – 2–5 ml.
- Salt (2 tsp) or mustard in cup warm water.
- 3% hydrogen peroxide – 2 ml/kg PO.

Gastric lavage

- Appropriate if not safe to induce emesis/emesis induction been ineffective.
- Lightly anaesthetised and intubated.
- Stomach tube – large bore, end hole.
- Instil 10–20 ml warm water, agitate and drain with gravity.
- Repeat 10–20×.
- Instil activated charcoal, kaolin, chalk or barium at end.

Further treatment

Use appropriate symptomatic and supportive care dependent on the intoxicant and clinical presentation.

Patient suspected of contacting/ ingesting potential toxin

- Ensure patent airway and adequate ventilation.

ORGAN SYSTEMS

- Support CO.
- Monitor heart rate and rhythm and BP.
- Check PCV, renal and hepatic parameters, electrolytes and acid–base status.
- Manage hydration – IVFT with crystalloids (Hartman's usually appropriate) and colloids if BP low.
- Treat CNS signs.
- Manage seizures with benzodiazepines or barbiturates.
- Excitation as for seizures or sedation (medetomidine, ACP/opioid).
- Maintain body temperature within normal range.
- Once stable establish diagnosis and treat appropriately.

4.14.3 Specific intoxications

Common pharmaceutical intoxications in cats

- Benzodiazepines – idiopathic hepatic necrosis, ataxia, incoordination, drowsiness.
- Dichlorophen – vomiting, hypersalivation, tachycardia, pyrexia, neurologic signs, collapse.
- Fluoroquinolones – GIT signs, hypersalivation, neurologic signs including convulsions. Central blindness with enrofloxacin.
- Imidaclopramide – GIT signs commonly, rarely neurologic signs, tongue inflammation and ulceration.
- Milbemycin – rarely lethargy, ataxia and twitching.
- Nitenpyram – increased scratching, hypersalivation, vomiting, diarrhoea, hyperactivity and panting. Rarely tachypnoea and tachycardia.
- Nitroscanate – ataxia and incoordination usually; rarely depression agitation, pupil changes.

- NSAIDs – GIT signs, abdominal tenderness, ataxia, PU/PD. Rarely tremor, weakness, drowsiness, convulsions, AKI.
- Paracetamol – signs due to methaemoglobinaemia; brown mucosa, GI and respiratory signs, facial and paw oedema, hypothermia.
- Permethrins – GIT and neurologic signs of hyperstimulation, respiratory distress, urinary retention.
- Piperazine – GIT signs; weakness, ataxia, incoordination, tremor, convulsions.
- Praziquantel – GI signs, hypersalivation, depression.
- Tramadol – CNS depression, GI signs, foaming at mouth, dilated pupils. Rarely respiratory depression, CNS stimulation, hyperthermia.

Common non-pharmaceutical intoxications (Table 70)

- As many of these compounds are ingesta following skin contamination, careful inspection of the skin and coat is important. Some compounds cause local inflammation, irritation blistering.

Key to management options
1. Emesis
2. Supportive
3. Activated charcoal and/or demulcent
4. Specific therapy
5. Removal surgically, endoscopically or by lavage
6. Laxative
7. Clean skin
8. Lipid infusions

Table 70 Common non-pharmaceutical poisonings in cats

Signs dependent on type of battery, location and whether leaking

	Abdominal pain	Anaemia/bruising	Blindness	Coma/collapse	Constipation	Convulsions	Depression/lethargy	Diarrhoea	Dilated/constricted pupils	Dyspnoea	Excitement	Fever	Haematuria	Inappetence	Incoordination/ataxia	Jaundice	Muscle tremor	Olig/anuria	Paralysis	Salivation	Sudden death	Thirst	Vomiting	Management
Acids/alkalis	X							X						X						X			X	2, 3
Adder bites		X		X				X				X											X	2, 4
Alcohol				X			X				X				X									2
Alphachloralose						X			X		X				X		X							1, 2, diazepam
Ant powders, etc.				X		X		X	X	X					X									2
Anticoagulant rodenticides								X	X	X			X		X		X						X	2, 4
Cannabis						X	X		X		X				X		X							1, 2, 3, 5
Carbamate						X		X				X			X		X			X				1, 2, 3, 5, atropine
Carbon monoxide					X					X					X					X				2
Chocolate						X		X			X										X		X	2, 3
Christmas trees								X													X		X	2
Ethylene glycol			X			X	X								X		X				X			2, 4
Washing products								X						X						X			X	2, 7
Lilium							X							X				X					X	1, 2, 3, 5, 7
Luminous necklaces	X						X													X			X	2, 3
Organophosphate				X		X		X	X			X			X		X			X				1, 2, 3, 4, 7
Petroleum products	X							X						X						X			X	2, 7
Saponins	X						X		X	X					X					X			X	1, 2, 3, 5
Slug pellets				X		X			X	X		X	X		X		X		X					2, 5
Toad toxicity				X			X		X	X					X		X			X		X		Flush mouth, 2
Xylitol (diet sugar)				X		X									X				X				X	2, 4

SECTION 5

INFECTIOUS DISEASE

INFECTIOUS DISEASE

Notes on Feline Internal Medicine, Second Edition. Edited by Kit Sturgess. ©2013 John Wiley & Sons, Ltd.
Published 2013 by Blackwell Publishing Ltd.

SECTION 5

INFECTIOUS DISEASE

Huntington's Disease, Second Edition... Edited by... Published 2013 by Blackwell Publishing Ltd.

5.1 BORDETELLOSIS

Other sections

5.1.1 Introduction

- Aerobic, Gram-negative coccobacillus.
- Precise role and importance of *Bordetella bronchiseptica* in feline respiratory disease is unknown.
- Can cause respiratory disease as a sole agent experimentally.
- Originally associated with bronchopneumonia in kittens in laboratory colonies.
  - Clinical cases occur sporadically in adults.
- Also isolated in association with respiratory viruses in cases of respiratory disease in pedigree and household cats.

5.1.2 Epidemiology

- Antibodies are very prevalent within the cat population (25–80%).
- Isolation rates of up to 50%.
- Active shedding in 10% of cats especially in multicat households and rescue facilities.
  - Association with respiratory disease found in rescue catteries.
- May be a carrier state.
- More common in households that also have dogs.
  - Clinical infection from symptomatic dogs reported.

Route of infection

- Presumed to be oronasal transmission.
- Short-term contamination of the environment may be involved.

5.1.3 Pathogenesis

- Attaches to the cilia causing ciliostasis and destruction of the cilia.
- Able to overcome mucociliary clearance and colonise respiratory tract.
- Releases toxins that cause local and systemic inflammation.
- Presumed to cause tracheobronchitis, but coughing is not a major clinical sign.
  - Will also target the lower respiratory tract.

5.1.4 Clinical findings

Upper respiratory tract
- Pyrexia.
- Sneezing.
- Oculonasal discharge.
- Submandibular lymphadenopathy.
- Signs resolve after around 10 days.

Lower respiratory tract
- Bronchopneumonia in kittens; rarely in adults.
- Dyspnoea.
- Cyanosis.
- Coughing.
- Mortality can be relatively high in young kittens.

5.1.5 Diagnosis

- Culture or PCR from oropharyngeal or nasal swab, but can be cultured from healthy cats:
  - Requires charcoal Amies transport medium and selective culture medium.
  - Both culture and PCR lack sensitivity.
- Cytology and culture of bronchoalveolar lavage.
- Serology is of limited value as up to 80% of cats have antibodies.

INFECTIOUS DISEASE

5.1.6 Therapy and control

Therapy

Upper respiratory tract

- Antibacterial – tetracyclines, e.g. doxy-cycline, trimethoprim-sulphonamides, fluoroquinolones.
- May not eliminate infection.

Lower respiratory tract

- Antibacterials as above.
- Intensive care may be required including
  - Bronchodilators.
  - Supplementary oxygen.
  - Gentle coupage.

Control

Management

- Reduce stress levels – stable groups.
- Reduce density of cats.
- Kitten in isolation.
- Quarantine new arrivals.
- Regular cleaning and dedicated food bowls/litter trays.

Vaccination

- Inactivated intranasal fimbrial vaccine licensed for use in the UK and other countries.
  - Vaccine efficacy against challenge is good and duration of immunity is at least 12 months.
- Use of the canine intranasal vaccine in outbreaks appears to be safe and may be efficacious.

5.2 VIRAL UPPER RESPIRATORY TRACT DISEASE

Other sections

2.12 Chronic Coughing
2.15 Dyspnoea
2.29 Ocular changes caused by systemic disease
2.34 Ptyalism
2.38 Sneezing and nasal discharge

5.2.1 Introduction

- Variety of causes of feline URTD.
- Viral infections account for more than 80% of cases.
- Two viruses are responsible for 'cat flu'; they may be seen separately or in combination.

Causal agent

- FHV-1 (Feline viral rhinotracheitis – FVR) – an alpha herpes DNA virus.
- FCV – an RNA virus.

5.2.2 Epidemiology

Route of infection

- Inhalation following direct or close contact.
- Particularly aerosol infection over 1–2 m.
- Indirect spread and environmental contamination are minor problems, except where cats are very densely housed.

Survival in the environment

- FHV-1 <24 hours.
- FCV 8–10 days.

Incubation period

- 2–10 days.
- Dependent on
  - Strain.
  - Infectious dose.
  - Host immunity.
  - Intercurrent disease.

5.2.3 Pathogenesis

- Rare FCV isolates appear to cause severe systemic disease.
- See Figure 31.

5.2.4 Clinical findings

Systemic FCV

- Uncommon variant strains.
- High fever, facial and paw oedema.

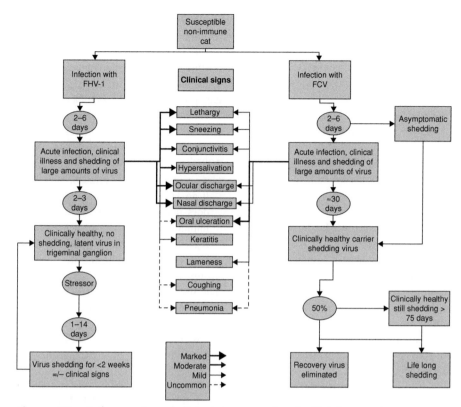

Figure 31 Pathogenesis and clinical signs associated with feline respiratory virus infection

INFECTIOUS DISEASE

- Oculonasal discharge, ulcerative stomatitis.
- Haemorrhage from GIT and nose.
- Jaundice, pneumonia, pleural and peritoneal effusion, pancreatitis reported.
- Mortality 30–50%.

Sequelae
- Both viruses are associated with chronic disease even where the virus has apparently been eliminated.
- Chronic FHV-1-associated keratitis.
- FCV-associated gingivitis and stomatitis.
- Chronic rhinitis.

5.2.5 Diagnosis
- Clinical signs.
- VI or PCR from oropharyngeal swabs.
- Rising antibody titres.

Differential diagnosis
- *Mycoplasma* infection.
- *Bordetella bronchiseptica*.
- Irritant chemicals.
- Allergic disease.
- Cowpox virus.

5.2.6 Therapy and control
Treatment
- Symptomatic and supportive.
- Rehydration, naso-oesophageal or oesophagostomy tube feeding.
- antibacterials to control secondary bacterial infection for 2–3 weeks.
- Steaming.
- Mucolytics such as bromhexidine hydrochloride (Bisolvon).

- Vitamins.
- General nursing:
  - Grooming.
  - Cleaning discharge from eyes and nose.
  - Tempting to eat and drink.

Antiviral drugs
- Acyclovir is of little use against FHV.
- Ophthalmic antiviral drugs for herpes keratitis are more effective:
  - Trifluorothymidine.
  - Idoxuridine.
  - Vidarabine.
- Interferon has been used with some success in FCV infection.
- Oral lysine has been recommended for treating FHV-1 infection; clinical trials to date have not shown clear benefit.

Control
- Decrease population density.
- Introduce sneeze barriers or cage separation (1–2 m).
- Hygiene – fomites (particularly hands).
- Rear kittens away from adults.
- Early wean kittens from queen at 3–4 weeks.
- Regular vaccination.
- Decrease stress.
- Quarantine new cats on arrival.

Isolation
- Important especially in a colony situation as the condition is highly contagious.
- Viruses are labile; they survive poorly in the environment and are susceptible to most commonly used disinfectants.

Carriers
- FCV carriers shed continuously (at varying levels); most clear the infection within 3–6 months.
- All cats infected with FHV-1 are assumed to become carriers, shedding is intermittent associated with stressors.

Vaccination
- Modified live and dead vaccines are available.
- Neither virus is particularly immunogenic.
- Only one serotype of FHV-1; the vaccine protects around 85–90% of cats.
- FCV shows significant strain variation; dual strain vaccines available; breadth of cover still significantly less than 100% (traditional vaccine strains protect against ≈65% of isolates).
  - If an FCV strain enters a colony that does not cross react with the vaccine immunity then disease will spread regardless of the group's vaccinal status.
- Six-monthly vaccination of 'at-risk' groups has been suggested.
- The need for yearly boosters has been questioned by the American Association of Feline Practitioners.
- Transient limping syndrome has been reported following FCV vaccination.

5.3 AVIAN INFLUENZA

Other sections
2.5 Ataxia
2.15 Dyspnoea
2.27 Jaundice
2.35 Pyrexia (fever) of unknown origin

5.3.1 Introduction
- H5N1 avian influenza virus.

5.3.2 Epidemiology
- Infected via contact with infected birds or cat–cat contact.
- Moderate amount of virus required.
- Incubation 2 days experimentally.
- Virus shed in nasal secretion and faeces from days 3–7.

Route of infection
- Respiratory and oral (from feeding on infected chickens).

5.3.3 Pathogenesis
- Virus replicates at site of infection (respiratory tract or gut).
- Virus-associated inflammation and necrosis of lungs, heart, brain, kidneys, liver and adrenals.

5.3.4 Clinical findings
- Fever.
- Lethargy/depression.
- Dyspnoea.
- Conjunctivitis.
- Less commonly jaundice and neurologic signs (circling and ataxia).
- Usually fatal within 1 week.

5.3.5 Diagnosis
- VI or PCR from oropharyngeal, nasal or rectal swab.
- PM samples from lungs, GIT, mediastinal lymph node for immunohistochemistry.

5.3.6 Therapy and control
Therapy
- None described.

Control
- Isolate infected cases.
- Virus sensitive to all standard disinfectants.
- Avoid contact with infected chickens or chicken carcases.
- Owners should seek medical advice.
- Veterinary authorities should be notified.

5.4 CHLAMYDOPHILA FELIS

Other sections
2.15 Dyspnoea
2.29 Ocular changes caused by systemic disease
2.38 Sneezing and nasal discharge

5.4.1 Introduction
- *Chlamydia psittaci* var. *felis* has been renamed *Chlamydophila felis*.

- Obligate intracellular bacterium.
- Originally thought to be involved with URTD (feline pneumonitis).
- Primarily a conjunctival pathogen.
- Respiratory signs are rare and usually indicate a co-infection with a respiratory virus.

5.4.2 Epidemiology
- Serological studies have shown that 5–10% of cats have had recent exposure.
- Most commonly isolated pathogen from conjunctival swabs taken from cats (around 30%).
- 50% of cases are in cats <6 months old.
- Antibodies do not appear to be protective.
- Recurrent infections in adult cats occur.
- Cats can continue to excrete *Chlamydophila* for 8 months, and occasionally longer, following infection.
- Main sources of infection are apparently healthy cats excreting infectious elementary bodies and clinical cases.
- Maternally derived antibodies appear to protect kittens against infection until 5–8 weeks of age.
- Existence and role of carriers is unknown.

Route of infection
- Direct cat-to-cat contact is required.
- Bacteria in conjunctival secretions need to contact conjunctiva of susceptible individuals.
- *Chlamydophila* may also be spread over limited distance as it is present in nasal discharges.
- Poor survival outside the cat (<24 hours), so indirect spread unlikely.
- Susceptible to most disinfectants.

Incubation period
- 4–14 days.

5.4.3 Pathogenesis
- Conjunctival epithelium main target.
- Replication in the conjunctival cells causing destruction and inflammation.
- Cell-mediated response is crucial to recovery.

5.4.4 Clinical findings
- Begins unilaterally.
- Typically serous or mucopurulent ocular discharge.
- Blepharospasm and chemosis (very marked in acute cases).
- Mild pyrexia and inappetence initially in some cases.
- Chronically hyperaemia and folliculitis of the conjunctiva may develop.
- Secondary damage to the eye, such as corneal ulceration.
- Most cases are self-limiting and will eventually improve without treatment.

NB – *Sticky eyes seen in kittens of around 10 days of age is more commonly FHV related, but can occasionally be a non-specific bacterial problem which resolves with symptomatic therapy.*

Other clinical syndromes
- Role in infertility in cats:
  - Reproductive failure.
  - Abortion.
- Also has been isolated from the gastro-intestinal tract, though its role, if any, is unknown.

5.4.5 Diagnosis

Differential diagnosis of conjunctivitis (Box 13)

Laboratory confirmation

Isolation and culture
- Provides a definitive diagnosis of *Chlamydophila* involvement.
- Correct swabbing technique is vital.

Box 13 Differential diagnosis of conjunctivitis

Infectious causes	Secondary bacteria
Environmental	Trauma
	Foreign body
	Irritants
Anatomic	Eyelid problems – distichiasis, etc.
Tear ducts	Inflammation
	Foreign body
Immune-mediated	Allergic
	Autoimmune – pemphigus
	'Dry eye'
Other	Neoplasia
	Periorbital disease

- Use a small ENT swab.
- BE FIRM – epithelial cells must be dislodged.
- Topical anaesthetic can be used if the eye is painful.
- Place swab immediately into VCTM.
- Needs to be at the laboratory within 24 hours.

  Limited value
- In chronic cases (>6 weeks).
- Where topical or systemic treatment is being used.
- May miss low numbers of infectious agent.

Polymerase chain reaction
- *Chlamydophila* does not have to be viable.
- Swabbing technique as for culture.
- Slightly more sensitive than culture; stays positive for longer (5 vs. 1 day) in treated cases.

Serology
- Demonstrates infection has occurred.

Interpretation of Chlamydia serology
- 1:1024 – recent or current exposure, but high titres can persist for up to 12 months.
- 1:128 – may indicate infection; take a second sample 2–4 weeks later to demonstrate a rising titre.
- <1:128 – equivocal.

Conjunctival smears
- Stain with immunofluorescence (IF) antibodies valuable in detecting acute (first few weeks) infection.

ELISA techniques
- Test sensitivity very variable depending on kit used.
- False positives and negatives do occur.
- Viability is not important.

5.4.6 Therapy and control
- Systemic antibacterials are vital to successful treatment of chlamydiosis.
- Topical ointments (tetracycline) are of some value; need to be given q2h.
- Minimum treatment 4 weeks or 2 weeks after all clinical signs have been resolved.

Systemic
- All cats in the group should be treated:
  - Oxytetracycline at 20 mg/kg q8h.
  - Doxycycline at 10 mg/kg q24h.
  - Clavulanic acid potentiated amoxicillin at 25 mg/kg q12h.
  - Azithromycin at 5 mg/kg q24–48h is less effective as recrudescence is common.

Contraindications
- Use of tetracyclines in pregnancy and young kittens due to the risk of causing staining of the tooth enamel in the kittens.
- Doxycycline binds less readily to calcium than oxytetracycline; hence the risk of tooth discoloration is probably reduced but is associated with oesophageal stricture in some countries.

Treatment of a colony outbreak of Chlamydophila
- All cats in the colony should be treated.
- Continue treatment for 2 weeks longer than clinical signs are present.
- When all cats are healthy vaccination *may* reduce the likelihood of recrudescence of clinical signs.
- Once endemic in a colony, *Chlamydophila* can prove difficult to eradicate.

Management changes
- Routine hygiene should be employed, such as washing hands and using disinfectants.
- Clinical cases should be isolated from the others.
- Non-affected cats should always be handled first when performing daily tasks and medication.
- Queens should kitten in isolation.
- Kittens can be early weaned at 4 weeks of age and isolated.
- In colonies without a problem, only seronegative cats should be introduced.

Vaccination
- Will reduce but may not prevent infection, shedding or development of carrier status.
- Care during vaccine reconstitution of modified live products is important; aerosolised droplets can cause clinical disease if they come into contact with the conjunctiva.
- Vaccination as a sole method of management in endemic infection is unlikely to be successful.
- Generally not considered a 'core' vaccine.

Zoonotic potential
- No confirmed cases in people.
  - No increase in conjunctivitis in people with cats with chlamydiosis.

INFECTIOUS DISEASE

- Zoonotic potential not been completely excluded, so advise sensible hygiene precautions especially in young, old or immunosuppressed people.

5.5 FELINE INFECTIOUS ANAEMIA

Other sections
2.9 Collapse/syncope and weakness
2.15 Dyspnoea
2.27 Jaundice
2.30 Pallor
2.35 Pyrexia (fever) of unknown origin
2.43 Weight loss
3.1 Low haematocrit

5.5.1 Introduction
- Many cats are probably infected with low levels of haemoplasma.
- Vast majority of cats successfully control the parasite and never show disease or a circulating parasitaemia.
- Studies suggest a prevalence of 20% in the sick cat population.

5.5.2 Epidemiology
Causal agent
- Epicellular red cell parasite.
- Reclassification from *Rickettsia* to *Mycoplasma*:
  - Previously *Haemobartonella felis*, large and small forms.
  - Now *Mycoplasma haemofelis* and *Mycoplasma haemominutum*.
- Recently a third haemoplasma, *Mycoplasma turicensis* has been identified; its significance as a cause of anaemia in cats is unknown.

Route of infection
- Unknown.
- Queen to kittens (in the absence of arthropod vector) possibilities include

- *In utero*.
- At parturition.
- During nursing.
- Blood-sucking parasites, primarily fleas.
- Increased incidence in cats known to fight.
- Iatrogenic-blood transfusion/operating instruments.

Incubation (preparasitaemic) period
- 1–3 weeks following experimental IV inoculation.
- Many cats are asymptomatic carriers with clinical signs occurring after periods of stress.

5.5.3 Pathogenesis
- *M. haemominutum* is associated with minimal clinical signs – no significant differences in parameters in anaemic cats with or without *M. haemominutum* infection.
- *M. haemofelis* is uncommon in the UK; generally it is associated with more severe disease.
- Precise role of haemoplasma as a primary pathogen is unclear.

Acute phase
- Time from first to last major parasitaemia – can last months.
- Some cats will die (30% if left untreated) at this stage due to a massive drop in red cell count.
- Parasites appear in blood in a cyclical manner peaking 1–5 days into each cycle.
  - Can be cleared from the blood within hours.
- Associated with rapid changes in PCV, presumably associated with splenic sequestration.
- Parasite adheres to feline red cells damaging the cell surface and leading to removal of erythrocytes from circulation by the liver and spleen.
- Minimal intravascular haemolysis occurs.

- A very high percentage of red cells can be parasitised.
- Significant immune-mediated component to the disease.

Recovery phase
- From last major parasitaemia to return of PCV to normal.

Carrier phase
- Lasts months or years; may be lifelong.
- Balanced state between replication of parasite and removal.
- Repeat acute episodes can occur following a period of stress or intercurrent disease; most closely associated with cat bites.
- Low numbers of parasites intermittently identified in blood.

Prognosis
- Generally good unless
  - Underlying cause.
  - Very young kittens.
  - Severe anaemia at presentation.

5.5.4 Clinical findings
- Very variable:
  - Health status and intercurrent disease.
  - Age of cat.
- Nil → mild → severe anaemia – usually regenerative.
- Lethargy, anorexia.
- Weight loss, depression.
- Intermittent pyrexia.
- Splenomegaly.
- Dyspnoea and pleural effusion.
- Jaundice.
- Lymphadenopathy, GIT and skin signs may be seen if there is coincident FeLV infection.

5.5.5 Diagnosis
Haematological changes
- Regenerative anaemia.
- Average PCV 15–18%.

- Anisocytosis, polychromasia, macrocytosis.
- Reticulocytosis.
- Non-regenerative anaemia is reported:
  - Very early in a parasitaemic episode.
  - Intercurrent disease, e.g. FeLV.

Blood smears
- Romanowsky-type stains.
- Smear from fresh, non-anticoagulated blood.
- Differentiate from other feline erythrocyte inclusions and artefacts:
  - Stain precipitate – variable position and size, often larger – filter stains before use.
  - Howell–Jolly bodies – round and densely staining, within erythrocyte.
  - Heinz bodies – round or irregular with a clear appearance, within erythrocyte but may protrude if at periphery.
  - Refractile artefact – irregular borders and colourless.
- Detects only 40% of infections.

Polymerase chain reaction
- More sensitive, diagnostic of choice.
- Can distinguish between strains.
- Quantitative PCR to measure degree of parasitaemia.

5.5.6 Therapy and control
- Supportive – fluids, nutrition.
- Antibacterials decrease but do not entirely eliminate parasite:
  - Doxycycline at 10 mg/kg q24h for 14–21 days – recrudescence will occur in some cats.
  - Enrofloxacin at 10 mg/kg q24h may also be effective – recrudescence will occur in some cats.
  - Azithromycin is ineffective.
- Blood transfusion may be necessary.
- As there appears to be an immune-mediated component of the disease,

INFECTIOUS DISEASE

glucocorticoids may be of value in the acute haemolytic phase at 2 mg/kg q24h tapering over 3 weeks.

- Intractable disease usually indicates some underlying cause, e.g. FeLV, and carries a poor prognosis.
- Control of ectoparasites.
- Recrudescence may occur during periods of stress.

5.6 FELINE INFECTIOUS PERITONITIS

Other sections
2.1 Abdominal enlargement
2.13 Diarrhoea
2.15 Dyspnoea
2.27 Jaundice
2.29 Ocular changes caused by systemic disease
2.35 Pyrexia (fever) of unknown origin
2.43 Weight loss

5.6.1 Introduction

- Major viral infectious disease of cats.
- Almost invariably fatal.
- Part of a group of closely related viruses including canine coronavirus (CCV) and porcine transmissible gastroenteritis virus (TGEV).
- Infection with FCoV is very common in cats, but few cats develop FIP.
- Different strains of FCoV have markedly different infectivity and virulence.

NB – *Despite its name once FIP develops it does not seem to be easily transmissible to other cats.*

5.6.2 Epidemiology

- Up to 40% of the general cat population have serological evidence of prior coronavirus exposure.
- In catteries and multicat households, this figure commonly approaches 90% of the cats in the group.

- Some groups are coronavirus negative.
- Incidence of disease is low, at less than 1% (some studies suggest about 0.02%) in the general cat population.
- Sporadic disease occurs more commonly in larger multicat households.
- More common in pedigree than non-pedigree cats, due to
  ○ Pedigree cats tending to live in groups.
  ○ Genetic factors.
- In catteries where FIP is endemic
  ○ Cases tend to occur irregularly.
  ○ Mortality rate rarely exceeds 5%.
  ○ It is often kittens that are affected.
  ○ Not uncommonly, several kittens from the same litter may develop FIP over a period of weeks or months.
- Estimated that up to 50% of the risk of developing FIP following coronavirus infection is due to genetic factors.
- FCoV is a relatively labile virus; most strains do not survive longer than a few days in the environment.
  ○ Some strains may survive several weeks under the right conditions.
- Faeces from infected cats are the main source of virus; some cats appear to shed at higher levels than others.
  ○ Many cats shed for >10 months following FCoV infection.
- Other reservoirs of FCoV may exist.
- 75% of cases of FIP occur in cats <1 year old.
- Second peak occurs in old cats >12 years.

Route of infection
- Oronasal infection is likely to be the most common route.
- Saliva from grooming.
- Litter trays and shared food bowls may be a significant source of infection.
- Transplacental transmission can occur, but is probably uncommon.
- Most cats are infected at a young age when the major source of infection to kittens is the queen.

Incubation period

- In experimental challenge models in which a single, large dose of virus is administered, the incubation period is usually around 5–10 days.
- In field situations, it is much harder to determine as a cat may have harboured a low virulence FCoV for many months or years before it happens to mutate to virulence.
- Clinical disease often follows a stressful event that acts as a trigger, rather than a source of infection.
  - Common stress triggers are rehoming, vaccination, neutering, changes in the household.
  - Stressors are cumulative – multiple stressors occurring concurrently, increasing the risk.
- Incubation period is generally shorter in wet FIP compared with the dry form.

5.6.3 Pathogenesis

- Initial replication taking place in the mucosa of the pharynx and small intestine.
- There is rapid spread to regional lymphoid tissue where infection of macrophages/monocytes occurs, within which the virus replicates.
- Infection of macrophages leads to dissemination of infection throughout the body (a cell-associated viraemia).
- Whether a cat resists challenge with FCoV depends on many factors, the most important of which are
  - Virulence of the particular strain of virus.
  - Genetic background of the cat.
  - Cat's immune status and immune response.
  - Concurrent disease or stress.
- FIP is an immune-mediated condition in which the antibodies are important in the production of the disease (ADE).
- Cell-mediated responses are a crucial factor that determines whether FIP develops.

- The fidelity of copying of the viral RNA is poor, with the virus making around three errors per replication cycle resulting in
  - Each cat having unique swarms of similar viruses (quasispecies).
  - The potential for low pathogenicity FCoV mutating to cause disease months or years after infection.
- Consistent mutation points conferring virulence have not been found.

5.6.4 Clinical findings

- FIP can mimic almost any disease process and therefore should be high on the differential diagnosis list of all sick, especially young cats, until another diagnosis is reached.
- Onset of FIP is usually marked by a number of vague clinical signs including fluctuating pyrexia, inappetence, weight loss and lethargy.
- Signs often develop following a period of stress.
- More specific signs develop after a variable period of time, sometimes several weeks.
- The disease is usually divided into one of the two types – effusive or non-effusive disease.
  - In reality, many cats develop disease with a mixture of both types, although often one form will predominate.
- Once clinical signs develop, FIP is almost invariably fatal.

Effusive (wet) FIP

- Accounts for around 60–70% of FIP cases.
- Protein-rich exudate accumulates in a variety of body cavities.
- Most common site for this is the abdominal cavity, but the fluid may also accumulate in the thoracic cavity (and/ or pericardial sac).

INFECTIOUS DISEASE

- Around 10% of wet FIP cases show pleural fluid alone.

Common clinical signs
- Dull and anorexic (some cats remain bright and appetent).
- Weight loss.
- Dyspnoea.
- Jaundice.
- Abdominal swelling with a fluid thrill.

Non-effusive (dry) FIP
- Little or no exudation into body cavities.
- Granulomatous inflammatory lesions develop in a variety of different sites throughout the body.
- Clinical signs will depend on which organs are affected and the extent to which they have been damaged.
- 50% of cases show ocular signs:
  - Uveitis.
  - Chorioretinitis.
  - Hyphaema.
- CNS signs are also common – 13% of cases:
  - Neurological deficits.
  - Paresis.
  - Ataxia.
  - Seizures.
  - Hyperaesthesia.
  - Hydrocephalus occurs in 75% of neurologic cases.
- Abdominal involvement is very common with signs relating to renal, hepatic or gastrointestinal disease.

Intestinal FIP
- GIT is the only organ affected.
- Ileocolic or colonic pyogranulomatous lesions.
- Thickened intestines on palpation.
- Typical clinical signs:
  - Chronic diarrhoea.
  - Weight loss.
  - Vomiting.
  - Constipation.

5.6.5 Diagnosis

Presentation, biochemical and haematologic changes
- Cats <2 or >10 years old, pedigree cats, multicat households.
- Recent episode of stress – rehoming, vaccination, neutering.
- Ascites (75% of cases).
- Dyspnoea (pleural fluid 25% of effusive cases).
- Ocular or CNS disease.
- Unexplained, poorly responsive fever.
- More rarely, intestinal and renal forms of FIP occur with primary signs relating to the organ involved.
- Haematology – non-regenerative anaemia (40%), lymphopenia (75%), neutrophilia (50%).
- Biochemistry – hyperglobulinaemia (50%), hyperbilirubinaemia (25%).
- Serum protein electrophoresis – raised α_1- & γ-globulins.
- Normal α_1-glycoprotein levels have shown good discrimination for cases that do not have FIP with high levels (>1.5 g/l) being supportive of FIP.

FIP fluid
- Straw coloured and proteinaceous (tacky feel) and may clot.
- Total protein of ascitic fluid >35 g/l with at least 50% globulin:
  - Ascitic fluid where albumin > globulin is a good rule out for FIP.
- Cellular content is very variable but usually low numbers of mixed inflammatory cells.

Rivalta test
- Assesses protein content of fluid:
  - Some published reports suggest high accuracy, but test seems very operator dependent; apart from time factors, it offers no advantage over standard biochemical analysis of effusions.

CSF
- Increased protein and pleocytosis are common in neurological cases of FIP.
- Dry taps are not uncommon in FIP cases.
- Risk of herniation associated with hydrocephalus secondary to obstruction of CSF flow.

Coronavirus serology
- Considerable variation in reliability and consistency between diagnostic laboratories has been shown with the same sample having significantly different titres at different laboratories.
- A POSITIVE TITRE ONLY INDICATES EXPOSURE TO CORONAVIRUS.
- In healthy cats, coronavirus titres do not predict the likelihood of a particular individual subsequently developing FIP.

Coronavirus titres for diagnosis of FIP
Coronavirus serology can be used as an aid to diagnosis but
- Confirmed cases can have titres of zero particularly cats with effusive FIP.
- Non-effusive FIP cases are rarely seronegative.
- General association between higher titres and having FIP.
  - Actual titres of limited value in an individual case.
- Positive CSF titres are suggestive of neurologic FIP; titre should be higher than in the blood.

Coronavirus titres in cattery screening
- Serial coronavirus testing to try and establish whether virus has been cleared from a group of cats is complicated by cats whose titre falls to zero and then rises again.
- In general cats with higher coronavirus titres are more likely to be shedding the virus.
- A group of cats is only likely to become seronegative if
  - Number of cats is small.
  - No new cats are introduced to the group.
  - Cats within the group do not have contact with cats outside the group.

Coronavirus testing to try and establish coronavirus-free group
- Controversial as
  - Coronavirus is highly infectious, so a single failure likely to infect whole group.
  - Very reliant on the laboratory to which the sample has been sent.
- Test all cats and divide into serologically positive and negative groups.
- Continue testing and separating until all cats have become negative or persistent positive cats have been identified and moved out of the group.

Screening prior to mating
- Some breeders with seronegative cats will request testing prior to mating to ensure that their negative status is maintained.

PCR testing
- Reverse transcriptase PCR can be used to identify presence of coronavirus.
- To date unique DNA sequences associated with virulence have not been identified.
- Reverse transcriptase PCR (RT-PCR) is most useful in confirming the presence of coronavirus in antibody negative cats and for detecting shedding.

Histopathology
- FIP causes pyogranulomatous change with evidence of vasculitis, perivascular mononuclear cell infiltration and central necrosis.
- Recent studies have suggested standard histopathology is not definitive for a diagnosis of FIP in all cases; immunohistochemistry is required.

INFECTIOUS DISEASE

Immunohistochemistry

- Viral detection in tissue biopsies, cytologic specimens or macrophages in effusive FIP.
- Can help to establish a diagnosis of FIP where histologic changes are not typical.
- Virus has to be associated with lesions identified.

5.6.6 Therapy and control

Therapy

- At present there is no effective treatment available for FIP.
- Symptomatic/supportive treatment using immunosuppressive drugs may be effective for some time, particularly in cases where there is only ocular involvement.
  - Antiviral drugs have been investigated; the use of low-dose, oral, human, recombinant, interferon-alpha (0.5–5 iU/kg/day for 7 days on alternate weeks) or feline omega-interferon may increase mean survival time in non-effusive FIP.

Polyprenyl®

- Polyprenyl is a mixture of polyphosphorylated, linear polyisoprenols. It has reportedly low toxicity and is orally absorbed.
- Recent work using a dose rate of 3 mg/kg twice weekly given to three cats with dry FIP improved survival time over that expected with two cats being alive, 24 months after diagnosis.
- A larger trial is currently being conducted with reported response rates of dry FIP cases of around 20%.

Control

General recommendations

- Minimise stress in young kittens – avoid multiple procedures close together; rehoming, vaccination, neutering.
- Reduce overcrowding and fighting in rescue facilities.
- Maintain stable groups of cats.

Management of endemic colonies

- Any cats developing clinical signs of FIP should be kept in isolation until a diagnosis is achieved.
- Review hygiene procedures particularly regarding disposal of cat litter, cleaning of litter trays and feeding bowls/utensils.
- Ensure sufficient litter trays are available.
- Review breeding records to
  - Identify queens whose kittens have had FIP, as they are likely to be shedding the virus.
  - Identify lines with increased susceptibility to FIP.

Options to reduce recurrence

- No new cats should be allowed into the household for a period of 6 months.
- Stop any breeding activity and, where possible, do not recommence for a period of 6 months from the last case of FIP.
- Do not continue to breed from queens who have had previous litters of kittens with FIP.
- If breeding is continued, queens should be kittened in isolation and the kittens remain isolated until sold.
- Early weaning of the kittens at 3–4 weeks of age into an isolated environment can further reduce the risks of FIP in the kittens, but can have adverse consequences on their socialisation.
- Establish a coronavirus negative colony (see above).

Vaccination

- Temperature-sensitive modified live intranasal vaccine is available in the USA and in parts of Europe.
- Based on a serotype II isolate, but serotype I is more prevalent.
- Concerns remain over its efficacy and the risks of ADE should a cat develop FIP following vaccination.
- Field studies have not indicated there is a risk of ADE.

- Most studies have shown a reduced incidence of disease in vaccinated cats.
- Limited value in endemic colonies where most individuals are coronavirus positive.
- Less effective in cats that are already coronavirus seropositive, as some are incubating disease.
- Preventable fraction reported to be 50–75%.

5.7 FELINE SPONGIFORM ENCEPHALOPATHY

Other sections
2.5 Ataxia
2.6 Behavioural changes
2.32 Polyphagia
2.33 Polyuria/polydipsia

5.7.1 Introduction
Feline spongiform encephalopathy is one of a group of prion-related, transmissible, neurodegenerative diseases.

5.7.2 Epidemiology
Route of infection
- Unknown, probably food.
- Non-domesticated cats can be affected.
- Prion proteins are very stable in the environment, but it is very unlikely that cat-to-cat transfer occurs.

Incubation period
- Prolonged.
- Not seen in cats <2 years of age.
  o No age, sex or breed predisposition.
- Average age at clinical presentation is 7 years.

5.7.3 Pathogenesis
- Causes a modified prion protein to be produced that is misfolded and resistant to enzyme degradation.
- Induces additional copies of itself acting like an infectious agent accumulating in the CNS causing degenerative changes

with vacuolation of the neutrophil and nerve cells.
- Strain experiments support FSE being derived from bovine spongiform encephalopathy (BSE).

5.7.4 Clinical findings
- Chronic progressive locomotor disturbances.
- Abnormal behaviour.
- Aggression.
- Hyperaesthesia.
- Changes in grooming behaviour.
- Ataxia.
- Polyphagia/polydipsia.
- Once clinical signs occur, they are rapidly progressive.
- Most cats euthanised within 2–3 months of presentation.

5.7.5 Diagnosis
- Suggestive clinical signs.
- Characteristic spongiform changes in the brain at post-mortem.
  o NOTIFIABLE POST-MORTEM DIAGNOSIS IN THE UK
- Fibrils in CNS tissue on EM.
- Positive for prion protein on immunostaining.

5.7.6 Therapy and control
- None available.
- Symptomatic and supportive.
- BUT clinical signs are progressive.

Control
- Prion proteins resistant to inactivation with heat, formalin, glutaraldehyde, alcohol and radiation.
- Avoid exposure.

Public health
- Zoonotic risk unknown.
- Likely to be extremely low for the general public.
- Major risk is during handling of brain, spinal cord or CSF.

INFECTIOUS DISEASE

- Care should be taken when performing a CSF tap or myelogram in cats with suspected FSE – surgical masks and gloves should be worn.

5.8 MYCOBACTERIAL INFECTIONS

Other sections
2.12 Chronic coughing
2.13 Diarrhoea
2.15 Dyspnoea
2.28 Lymphadenopathy
2.35 Pyrexia (fever) of unknown origin
2.43 Weight loss

TUBERCULOUS MYCOBACTERIUM

5.8.1 Introduction
- Highly resistant, intracellular, non-spore-forming bacteria.
- *M. tuberculosis* – rare in cats in the UK, tends to cause respiratory infection; reverse zoonosis from man.
- *M. bovis* – more common in cats than dogs, primarily alimentary infection via milk, often seen in farm cats.
- *M. lepraemurium* – young cats exposed to infected rodent prey, winter months.
- Fast and slow growing opportunistic mycobacteria.
- *M. tuberculosis – M. bovis* variant – predominantly in rural hunting cats, source of infection may be prey. Relationship with *M. microti* is uncertain.

5.8.2 Epidemiology
- Cat exposure associated with infection of other species in its environment.
- Cat → cat infection likely to be very rare.
- Siamese cats are over-represented.

5.8.3 Pathogenesis
- Entry via respiratory, alimentary tract or skin.

- Local replication to form granuloma at site of infection is uncommon in cats.
- Dissemination to draining lymph node and localisation is more common.
- Immune response often limits further replication.
- Persistent or disseminated disease occurs when the cell-mediated response is poor.
- Infection localised and viable in granuloma – may break out later if the cat is immunosuppressed.

5.8.4 Clinical findings
- Signs relate to the organ infected (see Table 71).

Disseminated disease
- Anorexia, fever, weight loss.
- Dermal nodules and non-healing, draining ulcers.
- Disseminated disease can involve any organ and may occur without initial localising signs.
- Granulomatous uveitis and CNS signs have been reported.
- Abdominal organomegaly.

Table 71 Clinical signs associated with different mycobacterial infections

M. tuberculosis	Respiratory signs; can disseminate
M. bovis	GIT signs and weight loss may spread to involve respiratory, cutaneous or lymphatic system. Mesenteric lymph nodes enlarged and sometimes calcified
M. tuberculosis – *M. bovis variant*	Nodular draining cutaneous lesions, peripheral lymphadenopathy, local myositis, arthritis and osteomyelitis; can disseminate

5.8.5 Diagnosis

- Likely exposure.
- Dermal nodules and non-healing, draining ulcers.
- Calcification of abdominal lymph nodes.
- Moderate leucocytosis.
- Non-regenerative anaemia.
- Hyperglobulinaemia.
- Identification of acid-fast bacillus on biopsy, in leucocytes, bone marrow smears or urine.
- Nodular to diffuse interstitial pneumonia.
- Pleural/peritoneal fluid.
- Intradermal skin testing produces inconsistent results – a positive test is supportive of infection.
- Serology is also unreliable.

Bacterial isolation

- Takes 4–6 weeks to establish visible colonies.
- Rapid culture techniques have been developed that deliver results in 2 weeks.

PCR

- Can be used on tissue specimens or fluid; can detect non-culturable forms.
- Shortens time to definitive identification.

5.8.6 Therapy and control

Treatment (see Table 72)

- Instituted on the basis of histological/cytological diagnosis.
- Multi-agent as resistance will develop to single-agent therapy.
- Complex and expensive.
- Continue for a minimum of 6–9 months.
- Side effects are not uncommon.
- Public health risks need to be considered.

Public health

- Actual risk is unknown.
- *M. tuberculosis–bovis* variant risk is lower as it is not known to infect people.
- Families with non-immune competent individuals should not keep *Mycobacterium*-infected cats.

OTHER MYCOBACTERIA

5.8.7 Feline leprosy syndrome

- *M. lepraemurium* + other mycobacterial organisms.
- Unculturable – obligate intracellular agents.
- FeLV or FIV may be involved in pathogenesis.

Clinical signs

- Multiple cutaneous and subcutaneous, non-painful nodules in skin.
- Young cats.
- Face, forelimbs and trunk.
- Cat systemically well.
- Regional spread.
- Regional lymphadenopathy.

Table 72 Treatment of *M. tuberculosis–bovis* variant[a]

Rifampin	10–20 mg/kg	q24h	Hepatotoxicity, pinnal erythema
Enrofloxacin[b]	5–10 mg/kg	q12–24h	Vomiting, retinal degeneration, blindness
Marbofloxacin	2 mg/kg	q24h	Retinal toxicity low
Azithromycin	7–15 mg/kg	q24h	Rarely causes side effects
Clarithromycin	62.5 mg	q12h	Pinnal erythema

[a]Rifampin + fluoroquinolone + either azithromycin or clarithromycin for 2 months then fluoroquinolone + one other for a further 4–6 months (possibly lifelong).
[b]Use with care as can be retinotoxic in cats.

INFECTIOUS DISEASE

INFECTIOUS DISEASE

- Tends to cause ulcers, abscesses and fistulae.
- Second group of older cats (>9 years) also identified.

Diagnosis
- Clinical findings.
- Acid-fast bacillus on histopathology.
- PCR.

Treatment
- Complete surgical excision.
- Where surgery is not feasible, response to clofazimine at 8–10 mg/kg once daily for 8 weeks or longer is reported.
  - Combination therapy with rifampin, clarithromycin and other drugs may be more effective.

5.8.8 Opportunistic, non-tuberculous mycobacterial infections
- Saprophytic.
- Slow growing forms rarely cause disease.
- Acquired following trauma to skin or soft tissue.
- *M. avium* – innate resistance, infection rare but can cause dermal granulomas.

Clinical signs
- Cutaneous and subcutaneous granuloma.
- Especially inguinal.
- Draining ulcers and fistulae.
- Regional spread.
- Cats are generally systemically well.

Diagnosis
- Acid-fast bacillus in tissue biopsies (may be in very low numbers).
- Bacterial culture of deep tissues.
- PCR.

Therapy
- Treatment based on susceptibility data for at least 6 weeks with fluoroquinolones, sulphonamides, doxycycline, gentamicin, ciprofloxacin or clarithromycin can be effective.
- Surgical debulking, but risk of dehiscence at wound edge.

Prognosis
- Guarded.
- Lifelong therapy may be required.
- Long-term dissemination to internal organs.

5.9 RABIES VIRUS

Other sections
2.6 Behavioural changes
2.9 Collapse/syncope and weakness
2.14 Dysphagia
2.31 Paresis and paralysis
2.32 Polyphagia
2.34 Ptyalism

5.9.1 Introduction
Rabies is a viral disease affecting the CNS of dogs, cats, foxes, man and, potentially, all warm-blooded animals. Dogs, cats and foxes are important vectors for the virus. Worldwide, dogs constitute a greater risk to man than cats, being responsible for 99% of cases transmitted to man but this pattern is changing in some countries e.g. USA.
- An enveloped RNA virus.
- Member of the Rhabdovirus family.
- Genus *Lyssavirus*.

5.9.2 Epidemiology
In Europe for 2010, 5801 cases of rabies were reported, 45% in domestic animals and 55% in wildlife. Twelve cases of human rabies occurred. The number of infections in domestic animals in Europe has fallen by 35% over the past 10 years. Cases mainly occurred in Eastern Europe. In the USA for 2007, 6940 cases in animals were recorded with only 7% in domestic pets. Of these 274 were in cats, a rate of infection three times higher than in dogs.

Route of infection

- Infected saliva from bite wounds accounts for nearly all cases.
- Rarely other routes of infection have been reported in man.
- Exhaled excreted virus from cave-dwelling bats.
- Ingestion of infected tissue/secretions.
- Transplacental.
- Fomites.
- Corneal transplants.
- Cases of latent rabies with prolonged periods of salivary excretion without neurologic signs are reported; their importance as a route of infection is unknown.

Incubation period

- 10 days–4 months.
- Depends on
  - Site of the infection (distance from the spinal cord).
  - Severity of the bite.
  - Degree of innervation of the bite site.
  - Dose of virus inoculated.
  - Host immunity – previous exposure/vaccination.
- Average 4–6 weeks in cats.

NB – *Cases exceeding 6 months have been reported in dogs.*

5.9.3 Pathogenesis

- The virus multiplies in the muscle fibres and connective tissue cells at the site of infection and may remain there for some time (days to months).
- Enters nearby nerves and spreads by intra-axonal flow towards the CNS.
- Initially enters the spinal cord on the ipsilateral side but rapidly spreads to contralateral side and ascends to the forebrain.
- Damage to the motor neurones causes a LMN-type disease – flaccid paralysis.
- Direct damage to CNS is compounded by programmed cell death (apoptosis) and accentuated by the immune response causing inflammation and necrosis.
- Further replication occurs within the CNS and the virus moves outwardly along the nerves to other parts of the body including and especially the salivary glands (this results in hypersalivation).
- The presence of virus in the saliva means CNS infection has already occurred and death follows.
- Cats shed virus from 1–2 days before to 3 days after the onset of clinical signs.
- Rarely the course can be chronic and subclinical, with recovery possible, probably occurring secondary to pre-existing antibodies.

5.9.4 Clinical findings

- Prodromal phase lasting 2–3 days associated with a change in temperament and pyrexia.
- Constant licking of the site of infection.
- Classically described as furious and dumb forms, presentation can be very variable and atypical signs are commonly seen.

Furious form

- Most common form in cats.
- Gradual marked hyperexcitability; affected animals are restless and irritable due to forebrain involvement.
- May be associated with a depraved appetite.
- Avoid people and hide in dark and quiet places.
- Cats are described as having an anxious, staring, wild, spooky or blank look in their eyes.
- Become very vicious if confined.
- Some cats will run until they die of exhaustion.
- Gradually generalised signs develop.
- Weakness.
- Difficulty in swallowing.

- Drooping of the jaw and eyelids.
- Disorientation.
- Muscular incoordination.
- Death follows and may take the form of convulsive seizures or paralytic coma.

Dumb form
- Less common in cats.
- Signs include
  ○ Congestion of the conjunctivae.
  ○ Sagging of the lower jaw and drooling saliva.
  ○ Change in meow.
  ○ Can appear to be choking.
  ○ General progressive muscle paralysis.
- Death occurs due to respiratory failure.
- This form usually follows the furious form at around 5 days after the onset of clinical signs in cats.

5.9.5 Diagnosis
No pre-mortem tests are considered reliable enough for rabies diagnosis and should not be attempted in suspected case.

Post-mortem
- In the UK, diagnosis is made post-mortem on the brain, which has to be removed with extreme care at specialised facilities.
- Diagnosis is established by direct fluorescent antibody testing of tissue which is both rapid and sensitive.
- Diagnosis is confirmed by intracerebral inoculation of mice.
- PCR techniques have also been developed.

5.9.6 Therapy and control

Treatment
- No attempt should be made to treat suspected cases.
  ○ A suspected case should be securely confined and the relevant authority notified.

Control

Disinfection
- Rabies virus is labile and is inactivated by UV light, heat, detergents and disinfectants.

Suspected exposure of people
- Immediate thorough washing of wounds have been shown to significantly reduce the risk of infection.
- Local treatment with >40% ethanol or irrigation with a 1–4% solution of a quaternary ammonium compound under pressure.
- Deep wounds should be irrigated with saline alone to avoid further tissue damage.
- Seek immediate medical advice and follow appropriate post-exposure protocols.

Procedure for suspected cases
- Notifiable disease in the UK.
- All cats with unexplained and compatible nervous signs should be considered and particularly those with a history of having travelled abroad.
- These animals should be securely confined and the Department for the Environment, Food and Rural Affairs informed.
- There is obvious danger in handling suspect animals and it should be avoided at all costs.
- Any attempts to cage a suspected case should be undertaken with great care using remote devices – e.g. trap cage, cat catcher.
- Thick gloves should be worn when carrying the cage.

Vaccination
- A variety of vaccine types are available, although modified live virus vaccines are undoubtedly effective and cause fewer reactions, there remains a risk of vaccine-induced rabies and for this

reason such vaccines are not licensed in most areas of the world.

- Inactivated cell culture, recombinant and nucleic acid vaccines are available.
  - In the UK, inactivated and recombinant vaccines have licenses for use in cats.

Vaccine recommendations (UK vaccines)
- Primary course from 4 weeks of age; but usually from 12 weeks of age.
- Booster every 3 years (some vaccines recommend a first booster after 1 year and then 3 yearly).

NB1 – *With the wider use of rabies vaccines in the UK, the likelihood of maternally derived antibody (MDA) becoming a significant factor is greater.*
NB2 – *It is important to check that the national recommendations for vaccination frequency rather than the manufacturer recommendations are used in cats that are to travel abroad.*

Post-exposure vaccination recommendations (not UK)
- Previously unvaccinated – destroy or quarantine – vaccinate 1 month before release.
- Vaccine not current – assess likelihood of protective immunity remaining.
- Vaccinated – re-vaccinate immediately and keep under owner's control for 45 days.

Post-vaccinal complications
- Fever.
- Anaphylaxis.
- Local soreness, lameness and local lymphadenomegaly (if injected into a limb).
- Focal cutaneous vasculitis and granulomas occurring 3–6 months post inoculation – well-circumscribed inflammatory reactions involving the dermis.

- Polyradiculoneuritis with inactivated suckling mouse brain-derived vaccines.
- Vaccine-induced sarcomas.

PETS travel scheme (UK)
The author strongly advises that up to date information is sought from the relevant authorities well in advance of likely travel to ensure that sufficient time is available to comply with the regulations current at the time.

The travel scheme has recently been revised; at the time of writing (2012) the current regulations for the UK are

Cats resident in the UK
The cat MUST be
- Microchipped.
  - Manufacturers do not guarantee the chip unless it has been shown to have remained in place on a subsequent visit.
- Vaccinated against rabies using a licensed vaccine.
- Issued with an official health certificate recording the animal's details, its chip number and vaccination.

Cats entering the UK
- Cats entering from the EU and listed countries MUST be
  - Vaccinated against rabies, microchipped, have a valid passport and travel with an approved transport company on an authorised route.
- Cats entering from non-listed countries MUST be
  - Vaccinated against rabies and blood sampled to show an adequate antibody titres, microchipped, have a valid passport and travel with an approved transport company on an authorised route.

Zoonosis
- In man, the disease is considered fatal after the onset of clinical signs.

INFECTIOUS DISEASE

5.10 TOXOPLASMOSIS

Other sections

2.5 Ataxia

2.13 Diarrhoea

2.15 Dyspnoea

2.29 Ocular changes caused by systemic disease

2.35 Pyrexia (fever) of unknown origin

2.37 Seizures

2.42 Vomiting

3.13 Muscle enzymes

5.10.1 Introduction

- *Toxoplasma gondii*
- Obligate intracellular coccidian parasite

5.10.2 Epidemiology

Life cycle

- Definitive host – cats and other felidae.
- Intermediate hosts – all non felidae, therefore *zoonotic*.
- Cats generally become infected by ingesting tissue cysts in intermediate hosts.
- Both cats and other hosts can be infected by ingestion of oocysts that have been passed in cat's faeces.
- Transplacental spread can also occur.
- Level of antibodies to *T. gondii* in cats increases with age and varies with lifestyle.
  - Highest prevalence in cats fed raw meat or are outdoors, shelter or homeless.

5.10.3 Pathogenesis

Life cycle (see Figure 32)

- Incubation period for clinical toxoplasmosis in cats is very variable.

5.10.4 Clinical findings

Asymptomatic infections

- By far the most common.
- Cats shed oocysts for 10–14 days during which time they develop immunity and rid themselves of the organism.

- Surveys have shown oocysts in only 1% of faecal samples analysed.

Transplacental infections

- Seen as stillborn kittens or neonatal deaths.
- Liver, lungs and CNS are typically affected in kittens.
- Ascites.
- Kittens with *Toxoplasma* encephalitis are very sleepy or cry a lot.

Acute infection

- Lasts 2 weeks.
- Rare and most frequently seen in young kittens.
- Typical signs are pyrexia, anorexia, dyspnoea and pneumonia.
- Occasionally diarrhoea, vomiting, myositis, myocarditis, jaundice and enlarged lymph nodes occur.

Chronic infection

- More commonly seen in older cats.
- Time course of several months.
- Clinical signs are very non-specific, toxoplasmosis is said to mimic almost any disease.
- Signs most commonly reported are
  - Intermittent pyrexia.
  - Vomiting and diarrhoea.
  - Dyspnoea and pneumonia.
  - Neurological signs – ataxia, convulsions and blindness.
  - Ocular lesions.

5.10.5 Diagnosis

- On clinical signs.
- Looking for oocysts in faeces.
- Organisms can be found in ascitic or pleural fluid in acute infections.
- Biopsies showing Toxoplasma cysts.

Serology

- At least a fourfold antibody (IgG) rise on paired samples taken 2–3 weeks apart.

- IgG levels remain high for prolonged periods following infection, of little value in chronic disease.
- IgG levels may not begin to rise until several weeks following infection.
- IgM titres rise earlier and then fall again relatively rapidly; a single high titre is indicative of recent infection.
- Not all serological test methods measure feline anti-Toxoplasma IgM accurately.

5.10.6 Therapy and control

Treatment
- Antimicrobial therapy.
- Clindamycin is the drug of choice at 12.5 mg/kg q12h for 2–4 weeks.
  ○ GIT side effects can be a problem.
- Potentiated sulphonamides and sulphonamide/pyrimethamine combination are also used, but can be bone marrow suppressive.
- Doxycycline may be effective.
- Treatment will not eliminate latent infection.
- Penetration of antimicrobials into the CNS and eye can be poor.

Prevention
- Oocysts are highly infective for other animals and man therefore
  ○ Cats shedding oocysts should be confined to a cage until faeces are negative for three consecutive days.
  ○ Litter trays should be emptied daily and disinfected (faeces should be burned).
  ○ Children and pregnant women should avoid soil contaminated with cat faeces and handling litter trays. Gloves should be worn whilst gardening.
  ○ Cats should be fed only cooked meat and discouraged from hunting.
- Oocysts can remain infective for at least 18 months.
- Earthworms have been shown to contain oocysts.

Vaccination
- A vaccine is marketed in the USA.
- Not available at present in the UK.

Zoonosis (see Figure 32)
- Infection is much more likely from
  ○ Handling/eating raw or undercooked meat.
  ○ Soil contamination of hands.

INFECTIOUS DISEASE

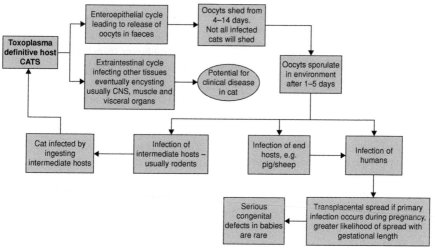

Figure 32 Life cycle of *Toxoplasma gondii*

5.11 FELINE LEUKAEMIA VIRUS

Other sections

2.13 Diarrhoea

2.28 Lymphadenopathy

2.30 Pallor

2.42 Vomiting

3.1 Low haematocrit

3.3 Platelet abnormalities and clotting system

3.4 White blood cells changes

5.11.1 Introduction

- FeLV is a retrovirus.
  - Retroviruses contain their genetic material as RNA so they also have to produce reverse transcriptase that makes a DNA copy of the viral RNA (the provirus) which is then inserted into the host DNA where it initiates new virus production or can lie dormant (latent infection).
- FeLV is a member of the oncornavirus family which are tumour forming.
- Major infectious disease of cats.
- Accurate current estimates of persistent infection in the UK are lacking and there are distinct, often very localised variations in incidence.
  - Prevalence of infection fallen since introduction of vaccination:
    - 0.5–1% of healthy cats (50–100 000 individuals).
    - 5–10% of sick cats.

Viral structure

- Surface envelope glycoprotein spikes responsible for viral subgroup.
  - Neutralising antibodies confer immunity.
- p27 is the major core protein – detection of p27 is the basis of ELISA and IC tests as it is produced in excess by the virus.

Subgroup A

- Present in almost all positive cats – major transmitted form and the basis for other subgroups.
- Both subgroups B and C may arise in infected cats but are defective requiring the presence of subgroup A for effective replication.

Subgroup B

- Present in 50% of cases. It occurs by genetic recombination between subgroup A and endogenous FeLV sequences that exist within the normal feline genome.
- Important in tumour generation. Infection with A and B may be more pathogenic than with A alone.

Subgroup C

- Rare 1–2% cats arising through mutation.
- Particularly associated with severe anaemia due to bone marrow suppression.

5.11.2 Epidemiology

Route of infection

- Prolonged close direct contact is necessary for effective transmission.
- The major source of virus is saliva.
  - Transfer can result from biting and grooming, also in high concentration in respiratory secretions.
- Urine and faeces from litter trays.
- Milk from mothers to kittens.
- Blood from transfusions or contaminated surgical instruments.
- Congenital (vertical) transmission can occur *in utero*.
- Kittens less than 12 weeks are generally more susceptible than adults.

Incubation period

- 2–4 weeks following infection there is a pyrexia, dullness and lymphadenopathy (that often goes unnoticed).

- Only around 30% of cats infected by FeLV become persistently viraemic.
- Another 30% may become latent carriers of the virus.

FeLV-related disease

- 2–52 months (average 23 months) in persistently viraemic cats before clinical evidence of immunosuppressive or neoplastic disease is evident.
- Period depends on strain of FeLV, recombination in the host, infectious dose and age at initial infection.

5.11.3 Pathogenesis

- Oronasal infection of a susceptible cat.
- Local viral replication in the oropharyngeal epithelium and in the lymphocytes and monocytes of the tonsils and associated local lymph nodes.
- Infected leucocytes then migrate away from the local lymph nodes and are able to infect systemic lymphoid tissue and the bone marrow.
- Persistent viraemia, of bone marrow origin, then develops (at 2–12 weeks post-exposure) – primarily within neutrophils and thrombocytes, along with the release of free virus and core viral antigens, including p27.
- Finally, dissemination of replication sites occurs, to include mucosal and glandular tissue (salivary glands, GIT, pharynx and bladder).
- Shedding of virus is primarily in the saliva, but smaller amounts may be present in other body secretions.

Resistance to persistent infection (Figure 33)

- FeLV infection can be eliminated by an effective immune response at any stage, but this occurs in most infected cats before viraemia (productive bone marrow infection) is established.

- Around 30% of all cats that become viraemic have a transient (1–12 weeks) viraemia before overcoming the infection.
- Macrophage function is an important part of the immunity to FeLV and can be significantly reduced by pharmacological doses of corticosteroids.
- Of the recovered cats some appear to eliminate the infection completely. The majority appear to harbour a latent infection, primarily in the bone marrow, but in some cases in other tissues also (focal infections).
- The latently infected bone marrow cells appear to be gradually eliminated with time, so only 10% are still latently infected 2 years after exposure.
- Latent and focally infected cats are not important epidemiologically, but are associated with development of FeLV-related disease.

FOCMA

- Expressed on the surface of FeLV transformed cell.
- Thought to originate from expression of endogenous retrovirus sequences present in normal feline DNA.
- FOCMA expression does not occur exclusively in cells that have been infected with FeLV.
- Anti-FOCMA antibodies confer protection against tumorigenesis.

Outcome of infection

- Persistent viraemia.
- Transient viraemia and complete elimination.
- Transient viraemia and latent or focal infection.
- Resists viraemia.

5.11.4 Clinical findings

- 80% of persistently FeLV-positive, viraemic cats die within 3 years of diagnosis.

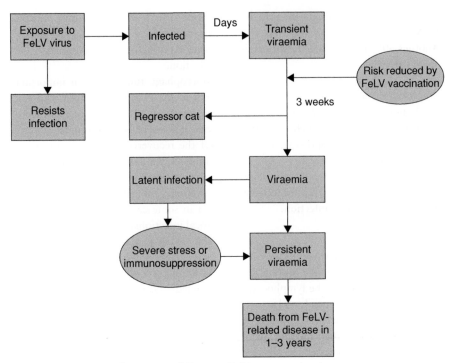

Figure 33 Potential outcomes following FeLV exposure

- No specific FeLV-related clinical signs
- Most cats encountering the virus will develop immunity to it and eliminate the infection (70%).

Neoplastic disease

Myeloid or lymphoid leukaemia
- Rare – anorexia, depression, lethargy, pallor and pyrexia.

Lymphoma
- Solid organ lymphoid neoplasias.
- Specific signs depend on the site of the tumour.

Mediastinal – thymic lymphoma
- Primarily respiratory signs.
- Mainly young cats.
- Pleural fluid frequently present with decreased thoracic compliance.
- Diagnosis on radiography, cytology of pleural fluid or mass.

- Percentage of FeLV-positive cases of mediastinal lymphoma is declining.

GIT
- Tend to be diffuse rather than focal masses.
- Vomiting, diarrhoea.
- Weight loss.
- Mesenteric lymphadenopathy.
- Jaundice.
- Older cats with abdominal masses.
- <30% FeLV positive.

Multicentric
- Peripheral lymphadenopathy.
- Non-specific signs of illness.
- Young to middle-aged cats.
- <60% FeLV positive.

Solid organ
- Non-specific signs include anorexia, depression, weight loss and intermittent pyrexia.

- Signs will depend on the site; most common sites
  - Renal.
  - CNS/spinal.
  - Ocular.

Non-neoplastic disease

- Immunosuppression resulting in a susceptibility to other diseases – the most common presenting complaint.
- Fading kittens.
- Vomiting and diarrhoea in older cats associated with co-infection.
- Infertility, abortion and endometritis in breeding queens.
- Autoimmune disease.
- Immune complex glomerulonephritis.
- Polyarthritis.
- Immune-mediated haemolytic anaemia or thrombocytopenia.
- Bone marrow suppression – anaemia is one of the most frequent disorders seen especially with FeLV infection. Anaemia tends to be non-regenerative and macrocytic. Can be a primary FeLV effect, or secondary to chronic disease or feline infectious anaemia.
- Uveitis and spastic pupil syndrome.
- FPV-like gastroenteritis.
- Osteochondroma.
- Osteopetrosis (excessive bone formation).
- Cartilaginous exostoses.
- Incontinence.
- Non-neoplastic CNS disease – ataxia, behavioural change.
- Stomatitis.

5.11.5 Diagnosis

- A variety of tests are available, all have their strengths and weaknesses and will identify different types of infected cats
- Ideally multiple techniques and repeated tests should be used to confirm persistent viraemia particularly in a healthy cat.
  - ELISA.
  - IC.

  - VI.
  - IF.
  - PCR.

Reasons to consider testing for FeLV

- The cat is sick and FeLV is a potential diagnosis.
  - At-risk group – cats housed or living in social groups.
  - Common clinical signs – tumours primarily lymphoma, anaemia, panleukopenia, immunosuppression with increased prevalence of infectious disease or recrudescence from carrier status.
  - Other syndromes – FeLV-associated enteritis, reproductive disorders, fading kitten syndrome, neuropathy and hepatopathy.
- A new cat of unknown status is being introduced into a multicat household – particularly a breeding unit.
- A feral cat that has been rescued or a cat of unknown viral status that has been relinquished to an owner.
- In-contact cats in a household with a known positive FeLV cat – test at least 28 days after exposure.
- Newly acquired kitten/cat or part of general health screening.

FeLV antigen by ELISA or immunochromatographic methods

- Antibody-based capture systems that are used to identify the presence of p27.
- ELISA and rapid immunomigration (RIM) tests are the most widely marketed for in-practice use.
- Most commercial laboratories will use a plate ELISA system.
  - In-house tests are robust and easy to use although relatively expensive compared with laboratory-based systems.
- False-positive results do occur for a variety of reasons, most commonly
  - Sample mix-up or contamination.
  - Recent routine vaccination.

INFECTIOUS DISEASE

○ Anti-mouse antibodies.
○ Inadequate washing.

Immunofluorescent antibody testing (IFA)

- Detects cell-associated p27 antigen primarily in circulating platelets and granulocytes.
- A positive result reflects viral replication within the bone marrow.
- Leucopoenia can reduce the chance of detecting genuinely positive cat.
- Occasional false-positive results due to uptake of fluorescent conjugates by normal eosinophils.
- ELISA tests will become positive before IFA tests.
- A group of IFA-positive, ELISA-negative cats has been reported; the cause for this is unclear.

PCR

- Very sensitive technique and will detect very low levels of FeLV infection.
- Quality of the test is very dependent on methodology used particularly primer sequences and the way that the DNA is prepared.
  ○ Environmental contamination; this will lead to false-positive results.

Two types of PCR are available.

1. Identifies and magnifies FeLV RNA that is first reverse transcribed into DNA.
   - Demonstrate active infection with ongoing viral replication.
2. Identifies and magnifies FeLV proviral DNA that is incorporated into host tissues (bone marrow).
   - Will identify latently infected cats.
   - Real-time PCR (qPCR) is a relatively recent quantitative methodology. The fewer number of cycles to positivity the higher the number of FeLV RNA or proviral DNA copies present in the sample.

FeLV antibody testing

- Support response to previous FeLV challenge but antibody levels do not correlate well with degree of protection.
- This test is not generally advised as a diagnostic tool for an investigation of FeLV infection.

VI

- Not used for routine diagnosis as technically demanding and expensive – only test that would demonstrate viable virus to be present.

Performing the test

- The way that in-house tests are performed can significantly affect the results.
- The testing protocol should be closely followed in particular appropriate warming of reagents and accurate timing to read the results.
- Anticoagulated blood samples should be used:
  ○ Serum/plasma less likely to give false-positive results than whole blood.
  ○ Saliva or tear testing is significantly less accurate.

What does a positive result mean?

- Interpretation will depend on the test method used (Table 73).
- When performing an ELISA/RIM 'test and removal' policy in a cattery with endemic FeLV, all negative cats should be retested after 12 weeks as viraemia may take this length of time to develop in a recently exposed cat.
- >90% of IFA-positive cats will remain persistently viraemic.
- Persistently viraemic cat – retest in 12 weeks will remain positive.
- Transiently viraemic cat – retest in 12 weeks will become negative.
- Single test is generally reliable in sick cats.

- Single-test ELISA/RIM tests are unreliable in healthy cats; may be as high as 60% false positives in this group.
- No healthy cat should be euthanised on the basis of a single positive test result:
  - Positive results in healthy cats should be confirmed by another method and then the cat should be retested in 12 weeks.

Interpreting a negative result
- Generally reliable in an unexposed cat.
- Recovered transiently infected cat.
- Latent/focally infected cat (see Table 73).
- Early infection – retest in 12 weeks if the cat has been recently exposed to FeLV.

Table 73 Types of FeLV infection detected by different test methodologies

	ELISA	IFA	PCR	Antibody
Persistent infection	✓	✓	✓	✓
Latent infection	✗	✗	✓[a]	✓[b]
Focal infection	✗	✗	✓[a]	✓[b]
Previous exposure	✗	✗	✗	✓[b]
Vaccinated cats	✗	✗	✗	✓[b]

[a]With appropriate tissue sampling.
[b]Depending on time from viraemia.

Discordant results
- Discordant results – on a single individual sometimes one test gives a positive and another a negative result.
  - Majority of discordant results become concordant with time.
  - A small percentage of cats remain persistently suggesting –

- Latent/focal infection.
- Test methodology problems.
- Anti-mouse antibodies.

5.11.6 Therapy and control
Treatment
- Secondary problems associated with infection can be treated symptomatically as they arise.
- Glucocorticoids should be avoided as they may reactivate infection.
- FeLV-positive lymphoma can be treated surgically or with standard chemotherapy protocols (Section 4.12).
  - Prognosis is not markedly worse than for FeLV-negative cats.
- Immune stimulants are of unproven value.
- Antiviral agents do not appear to be effective.
- Maintain vaccination protection against other infectious disease.
- Ensure good health care programme – diet, worming, flea treatment.

Vaccination
- Provides significant, but not 100% protection.
- Variety of vaccine types are available.
- All cats that are likely to face exposure should be vaccinated (i.e. cats that are free to roam outside).
- Direct comparisons have not generally been made.
- Vaccine-associated sarcomas are reported in about 1 in 10 000 cats that are vaccinated. NOT solely a FeLV vaccine problem.
- Vaccination does not replace testing in large colonies.
- FeLV should still be considered as a cause of disease in vaccinated cats.

Pre-vaccination testing
- Controversial.
- Problems of interpreting a positive result in healthy cats are significant.

INFECTIOUS DISEASE

- May be of value to test kittens/cats that originate from areas where the prevalence of infection is high, BUT all positive cases should be retested as above.

Management

FeLV-positive, healthy, single cat
- Where possible, the cat should be encouraged to live indoors particularly at night to reduce the risks of spreading disease to other cats and of the infected cat picking up secondary infections.
- New cats should not be introduced to the household.
- Aggressive treatment of infections is necessary.

FeLV-positive, healthy, colony cat
- Ideally such a cat should be isolated or rehomed to a single-cat household.
- If this is not possible then other cats in the group should be tested and vaccinated.
- Positive cats should be housed in small, stable groups.

FeLV-positive sick cat
- Decision to treat a FeLV-positive sick cat has to be based on

- ○ The type of illness from which the cat is suffering.
- ○ Whether the FeLV infection is an intimate part of the disease process or an incidental finding.
- ○ Sick cats tend to excrete more virus and therefore are a considerable risk in a colony situation.
- ○ The prognosis for a sick cat with FeLV-related disease is poor.

Isolation
- Not essential to control the disease in the short term as prolonged contact is required for transmission of the virus.
- FeLV-positive cats are a source of virus for others in the household/group.
- Survival of virus: only 24–48 hours in the environment, so of minor concern in veterinary hospitals.

Public health risk
- No person has been found to be viraemic with FeLV.

5.11.7 Other retroviruses
See Table 74

Table 74 Other retroviruses

Name	Feline sarcoma virus	Feline foamy virus (syncytium-forming)	RD114
Importance	Multicentric fibrosarcoma in young cats Cutaneous or subcutaneous nodules Locally invasive, rare metastasis to lungs Wide surgical excision and radiation	Associated with polyarthritis	May play a role in fetal development
Relationship to FeLV	Requires co-infection to cause disease	Potentiated by FeLV	None

INFECTIOUS DISEASE

5.12 FELINE IMMUNODEFICIENCY VIRUS

Other sections

2.5 Ataxia

2.13 Diarrhoea

2.28 Lymphadenopathy

2.29 Ocular changes caused by systemic disease

2.30 Pallor

2.35 Pyrexia

2.37 Seizures

3.1 Low haematocrit

3.4 White blood cells changes

5.12.1 Introduction

- RNA virus that contains reverse transcriptase and an enzyme that makes a DNA copy of the viral RNA (the provirus) which is then inserted into the host DNA where it initiates new virus production.
- FIV is a member of the *lentivirus* (slow virus) family due to the length of time between infection and the development of disease.
- FIV is not directly oncogenic.
- Surveys suggested that up to 19% of sick cats and 6% of healthy cats in the UK are FIV positive, but this is likely to be a significant overestimation in most areas.
- Nationwide the prevalence of FIV in healthy cats is likely to be around 1–2%.
- In some parts of the UK, FIV is becoming more prevalent than FeLV, e.g. Southeast.
- In other areas of the world, the prevalence of FIV is very high, e.g. in Australia 30–40% of cats are FIV positive.

Viral structure

- Surface envelope glycoprotein spike (gp120) associated with a transmembrane protein (gp41).

- Internally a variety of proteins including p24, the capsid protein.
- ELISA and IC tests look for antibodies generated against either p24 or gp41.

Genetic variation

- Considerable variation in the gene sequences from isolates from the USA, Europe and Japan.
- Changes in the genome also occur once the virus has entered the host; most variation occurs in the envelope region of the gene.
- Genetic variation is important as different isolates are known to have different *in vivo* and *in vitro* properties, both in infectivity and pathogenicity, e.g. FIV in Australia has not been associated with severe disease.

FIV in exotic cats

- FIV antibodies have been detected in captive cats (lion, white tiger, snow leopard, jaguar) and indigenous species (Florida panther, bobcat).
- FIV-like virus has been isolated from an indigenous Russian cat.
- FIV-like virus is endemic in many groups of African lions.
- Relationship between the virus and disease in large cats is unclear.
- FIV testing should be considered when dealing with a sick exotic cat.

5.12.2 Epidemiology

Route of infection

- Principal route of transmission is by biting (inoculation of saliva, which contains FIV, into tissues).
  - A single bite can result in successful transmission.
- FIV infection is significantly more common in
  - Cats allowed outdoors vs. cats kept entirely indoors.

INFECTIOUS DISEASE

- Cats known to fight vs. cats never known to fight.
- Cats with a history of abscesses vs. cats with no history of abscesses.
- From an infected queen to her kittens – occurs infrequently (because few breeding queens are infected with FIV), but it can be important.
  - About one-third of kittens born to an infected queen are likely to become viraemic.
  - Current indications are that transmission occurs via the milk or close queen to kitten contact rather than transplacentally.
- Other routes of transmission occur rarely.
  - Cats with oral lesions sharing feeding bowls.
  - Fomites.
  - Contaminated surgical instruments.
- There is no evidence to suggest that sexual transmission occurs though FIV in cat semen and vaginal transmission has been demonstrated experimentally.
- Transmission through prolonged close contact with infected cats is extremely inefficient, but may occur (around 1–2% risk – about one-tenth of the risk for FeLV).
- If a cat is allowed outdoors, the risk of it becoming infected from a cat *outside* the household is very much greater than the risk of it becoming infected through contact with an FIV-infected cat in the same household.
- Role of blood-sucking parasites is unknown.

5.12.3 Pathogenesis

Incubation period
See Figure 34.

Pathogenesis
- Progressive decline in immune function.
- Ability to respond to new infection is lost before amnestic responses.
- The virus targets the CD4 lymphocytes.

5.12.4 Clinical findings

Clinical signs
- Cause or effect?
- A diseased cat is likely to be more susceptible to the effects of FIV, and an FIV-infected cat is likely to be more susceptible to the effects of disease/other infections.

Three phases (see Figure 34)
- Acute – pyrexia, lymphadenopathy.
- Latent – asymptomatic.
- Chronic – AIDS-like stage as a result of immunosuppression; secondary infection from commensal organisms occurs.

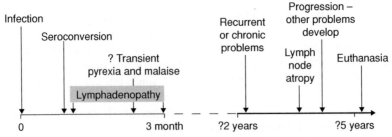

Figure 34 Incubation period and development of clinical signs following FIV infection

Primary FIV effects
- Lymphadenopathy in around 50% of cases, can last for months.
- Lymphoid depletion and node atrophy in later stages.
- Non-regenerative anaemia, neutropenia, lymphopenia and thrombocytopenia.
- Chronic gingivostomatitis
- Pyrexia.
- Diarrhoea.
- Uveitis, chorioretinitis.
- CNS disease – dementia, aggression, seizures, ataxia.
- Glomerulonephritis.
- Renal failure.
- Neoplasia (presumed to be as a result of decreased immune surveillance).

Clinical syndromes associated with immunosuppression
- Chronic upper respiratory tract infections.
- Conjunctivitis, keratitis, uveitis, chorioretinitis.
- Chronic diarrhoea.
- Wasting and pyrexia.
- Anaemia secondary to haemoplasma.
- Meningitis, encephalitis.
- Pyothorax and pneumonia.
- Skin infections.
- Otitis.
- Cystitis.
- Glomerulonephritis, pyelonephritis, renal failure.

5.12.5 Diagnosis

Haematological and biochemical changes
- More frequently associated with FIV-positive sick cats (rather than FIV-negative sick cats):
  - Lymphopenia.
  - Hypoalbuminaemia.
  - Hypergammaglobulinaemia.
  - Raised BUN and creatinine.
- Statistical link between FIV and gingivitis, pyrexia, anaemia and neoplasia (lymphoma, myeloproliferative disorders and others).

Staging of infection
- Generally there is an acute phase, an asymptomatic phase and a phase of immunological decline with the appearance of chronic, recurrent and poorly responsive disease which has been termed FAIDS.
- FAIDS does not appear to be directly analogous to AIDS in people, lacking specific disease associations, e.g. Kaposi's sarcoma, *Pneumocystis carinii*.
- Parameters used to stage HIV infection such as CD4 cell counts, neopterin levels have proved to be of limited value in cats.
- Quantitative PCR measuring viral load may be of value.

Reasons to consider testing for FIV
At-risk group
- See above.

Cats showing compatible clinical signs
- A wide variety of non-specific clinical signs have been associated with the acute and chronic phases of FIV infection.
- Fever and malaise.
- Diseases associated with chronic infection (see above).

Cats in a multicat household
- A new cat of unknown status – particularly a breeding unit.
- A feral/relinquished cat of unknown viral status.
- In-contact cats in a household with a known positive FIV cat.
- Newly acquired kitten/cat or part of general health screening – not recommended if not from an at-risk group.

Available tests
FIV antibody by ELISA or IC methods
- As very few, if any, cats will clear the virus once infected, it is assumed that the presence of antibodies reflects persistent infection.

- False-positive results do occur similar to FeLV.
- False positive associated with FIV vaccination where available.
- Weak or equivocal results are more of an issue with FIV testing than for FeLV.
- Negative results are less reliable than for FeLV testing as around 10–15% of FIV-infected cats are antibody negative:
  - Not yet seroconverted – can take 3–6 months.
  - Do not produce anti-FIV antibodies.

PCR for proviral DNA
- Detects DNA from FIV provirus:
  - FIV proviral DNA is not produced as a result of vaccination with inactivated vaccinal strains.
  - Low viral loads in the subclinical phase of infection means that high cycle numbers or nested PCR is sometimes required, increasing the risk of false positive.
- FIV exists as a number of clades throughout the world with significant genetic differences between strains:
  - Universal primers that will detect all strains of FIV are lacking.
  - Geographic clustering of isolate subtypes; hence primers specific for the clades seen in the area of origin of the cat should be used to reduce the likelihood of false-negative results.
- PCR can be used in kittens born to FIV-positive queens to distinguish passive maternal antibodies from active infection.
- Real-time PCR can be used to estimate viral load and therefore the likelihood in a sick FIV-positive cat that the signs being shown are related to their FIV infection or not.

Western blot analysis
- Rarely used on a clinical basis.

Virus isolation
- Rarely used on a clinical basis – technically demanding and time-consuming.

Problems in FIV diagnosis
Interpreting a positive ELISA/RIM result
- Infected cat – positive results are generally reliable in sick cats.
- Kitten born to infected queen – retest when kitten is 6 months old.
- False positive – common in healthy cats – retest in 6 weeks or use another method, preferably PCR.

Interpreting a negative ELISA/RIM result
- Not infected with FIV.
- Infected but antibody negative:
  - Around 10–15% of infected cats are antibody negative.
  - Recent infection not yet seroconverted.
- PCR will reliably distinguish between uninfected and infected antibody non-producing cats; it may not detect very recent infection.

Equivocal results
- In some cases, the ELISA result is at or near the positive threshold, or there is an equivocal colour change in a RIM test:
  - Report as low positive by some laboratories – this is meaningless.
- Higher proportion of these are false positives than of the clear positive results.
- Retest in 4–8 weeks or use an alternative method (PCR).

5.12.6 Therapy and control
Antiviral drugs
AZT and PMEA
- Azidothymidine (3′-azido-3′deoxythymidine) and another nucleoside analogue phosphonomethoxyethyl adenine have some success with cats showing

improvement in clinical signs (gingivitis) and immune parameters:

○ Potentially severe side effects (anaemia).
○ Close monitoring is required.
○ Relatively expensive.
○ Of no value in preventing infection becoming established, e.g. if a cat is bitten by another known FIV-positive cat.
○ Does not prevent eventual deterioration in the immune system.
○ Dose:
  ▪ AZT – 10 mg/kg daily.
  ▪ PMEA – 5 mg/kg daily.

Immunomodulators

- A wide variety of immunomodulators have been trialled in FIV-infected cats.
- There is limited evidence of efficacy:
  ○ Omega-interferon may be of value.
  ○ Lactoferrin reduces gingivitis/stomatitis signs.

Essential fatty acids

- Definite benefits with EFAs have been reported.
- Increases in weight, improved coat quality and well-being.
- Cats in the earlier stages of infection benefited more than those in the later stages.
- Immunological parameters were not improved in the long term.
- Dose:
  ○ Evening primrose oil at 550 mg once daily.

Non-specific therapy

- Vaccination should be kept updated – non-live vaccines should be used.
- Regular worming, ectoparasite control.
- Good diet.
- Aggressive management of infection.
- Immunosuppressive agents should be used with care.

Vaccination

- Not currently available in the UK.
- Is licensed in the USA – efficacy is unproven.

Management of FIV-positive cats

- FIV survives poorly in the environment (hours to 1–2 days) and is susceptible to most disinfectants.
- Keep cat in at night – reduces the risk of spread and the likelihood of the positive cat developing intercurrent infection.
- In multicat households, minimise fighting and stress.
- Feed cats from separate food bowls.
- Regularly disinfect litter trays.
- Do not breed from FIV-positive queens:
  ○ Kittens born to infected queens should be hand-reared.

Public health risk

- No person has been found to be viraemic with FIV.

5.13 FELINE VIRAL ENTERITIS

Other sections
2.5 Ataxia
2.13 Diarrhoea
2.20 Haematochezia and melaena
2.35 Pyrexia (fever) of unknown origin
2.42 Vomiting

5.13.1 Introduction

A number of viruses have been shown to cause vomiting and diarrhoea in cats.

Causes of viral enteritis in cats

- FPV (feline infectious enteritis, feline panleukopenia virus):
  ○ Widespread in nature causing serious and potentially fatal disease in cats.
  ○ Targets cells that are rapidly dividing, causing distinctly differing disease syndromes depending upon the age at which the animal is infected.
  ○ FPV (unlike canine parvovirus) has long been associated with cats; only one serotype of FPV exists.
- Feline rotavirus – mild diarrhoea in kittens as a single infection.

- Feline reovirus – experimentally causes mild diarrhoea in kittens.
- Feline leukaemia virus – a severe, often fatal parvovirus-like disease has been reported.
- Feline astrovirus – green, watery diarrhoea, sometimes vomiting, pyrexia and depression.
- Feline torovirus – linked to diarrhoea/ nictitating membrane protrusion syndrome in cats.
- Feline coronavirus – Some low pathogenicity coronaviruses will cause diarrhoea in cats and have been named feline enteric coronavirus:
  ○ Does establish a systemic viraemia and therefore seroconversion occurs.
    ▪ Differentiation from FIP is problematic.
  ○ Has been associated with mild leucopenia in some cases.

5.13.2 Epidemiology of FPV

Route of infection
The success of the parvovirus is due to the hardiness of the virus allowing it to survive for long periods (possibly years) in the environment. Infected animals shed virus for up to 6 weeks after infection, contaminating the environment and remaining potentially infectious even though they appear to have recovered themselves.

- Principal route of infection is by a faecal-oral route.
- Indirect spread occurs due to environmental contamination or via fomites (e.g. food bowls, grooming equipment, toys). This can be a particular problem in some situations such as rescue, boarding or breeding catteries.
- Fleas may act as mechanical vectors.
- Transplacental spread is now relatively rare.

Incubation period
- Usually around 5–6 days, but will depend on infectious dose, age of animal and intercurrent disease.

5.13.3 Pathogenesis of FPV
See Figure 35.

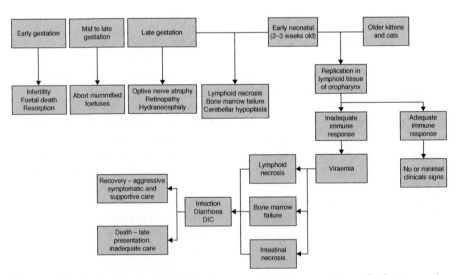

Figure 35 Pathogenesis of FPV infection according to age at time of infection and immune response

5.13.4 Clinical findings in FPV infection

In utero/perinatal infection

- This is now extremely rare and is most likely to be caused by the inadvertent vaccination of pregnant animals with a modified live vaccine or seen in kittens that have not received adequate colostrum (see Figure 35).

Older kittens and adult cats

Enteritis

- Fever, depression and anorexia progressing to vomiting and then foetid diarrhoea ± jaundice.
- Typical posture crouched with head between front paws.
- Some cats may die *before* diarrhoea develops probably due to dehydration, electrolyte imbalance, septicaemia/endotoxaemia and DIC.
- Vomiting is frequently bile tinged.
- Diarrhoea usually contains blood and pieces of intestinal mucosa giving the typical 'parvovirus smell'.
- Subacute FPV – depression, fever and diarrhoea lasting a few days.

Subclinical infection and carriers

- Subclinical – common in adult cats, mild fever and fall in white count. May be significant in the epidemiology of infection.
- Carrier status has not been demonstrated, but some epidemiological evidence suggests that carriers may exist.

Differential diagnosis of foetid enteritis

- Foreign bodies – especially linear foreign bodies.
- Intussusception – especially in kittens.
- *Salmonella, Campylobacter, Leptospira, C. perfringens, Tritrichomonas, Giardia*.
- Irritant chemicals/poisons.
- Liver disease.
- Neoplasia.

- Immune-mediated diseases.
- Bleeding disorders.
- Gastric or duodenal ulceration.
- Hypoadrenocorticism.

NB – *Any case of foetid gastroenteritis should be treated as potentially contagious and cases isolated until proven otherwise.*

5.13.5 Diagnosis of FPV

- Typical clinical signs
- Haematology – leucopenia, the magnitude of which is usually related to the severity of the disease and is both a neutropenia and lymphopenia. The white cell count is usually around $0.05–3.00 \times 10^9/l$.
- Mild anaemia may be present.
- Biochemistry – changes are usually non-specific, frequently BUN levels are raised primarily due to dehydration. Liver parameters (AST, ALKP, ALT and bilirubin) are sometimes elevated in cats. Hypoglycaemia and hypokalaemia are common.
- Radiology/ultrasound – gas-filled static intestinal loops.

NB – *Differential diagnoses include FB and intussusception.*

Virus detection

- Faecal sample (not a swab) submitted, as removal of viable virus from the fibres of a swab is unreliable. This can lead to a false-negative result particularly if viral numbers are low:
  - Direct visualisation – negative staining EM.
  - VI – cell culture from faeces.
  - Haemagglutination of pig red blood cells – the virus causes red blood cells to 'stick' together preventing the formation of a pellet in the test well.
  - ELISA test – a commercially antigen ELISA test is available for the diagnosis of CPV-2; its reliability in detecting FPV seems variable.

Problems with using virus detection for diagnosis

- The number of parvoviruses in the faeces falls rapidly once enteric infection is established. Numbers can be further reduced by the dilution effect of the diarrhoea; this can lead to false-negative results for virus detection.
- FPV is quite frequently identified in normal cat faeces.

Serology

- Strong antibody response to FPV occurs within about 7 days. Antibody levels are measured using a haemagglutination inhibition test.
- A titre could be due to vaccination, maternally derived antibodies, previous infection, current infection, use of hyperimmune serum.
- In order to establish that the titre is due to a current infection a second (convalescent) sample showing a rising titre in an animal that has not been recently vaccinated needs to be taken. Serology is therefore slow and of limited value. It is most commonly used to check response to vaccination.

Post-mortem

Usually intestinal congestion that may be mild or severe. Typically, the intestines feel thickened or inelastic and the serosal surface has a roughened, granular appearance. The mucosa may appear ragged with a catarrhal (mucoid) or even diphtheritic (grey, membranous) exudate and the contents may be fluid containing floccules of mucosal debris, blood tinged or even frankly dysenteric. The lymph nodes may be swollen and oedematous or congested. In kittens there is frequently thymic atrophy.

5.13.6 Therapy and control

Disinfection and hygiene

Strict attention to hygiene is essential and any areas where the cat has been should be disinfected, and as many procedures as possible carried out in isolation. Parvoviruses are resistant to many commonly used disinfectants. Effective compounds include

- Hypochlorite-based disinfectants (bleach).
- Formaldehyde/glutaraldehyde, care must be taken when using aldehyde-based disinfectants, particularly with the concentrate.
- Peroxygen compounds.

NB1 – *It is important that disinfectants are used at the correct concentration and that gross organic matter is removed prior to disinfection. Formalin, whilst very effective, is only of value if the premises can be emptied, cleaned, sealed and fumigated.*

NB2 – *Separate over-garments should be worn when handling infected cats, if at all possible. Many cases, however, will be small kittens that have recently been weaned and sometimes rehomed as well. In order to maintain good hygiene there is a tendency to abandon them in a bleak, sterile, isolation area. Tender loving care (TLC) is very important in helping these animals cope with and fight a very debilitating disease, so efforts should be made to spend time with them.*

Therapy

No specific treatment is available. Supportive care is vital with the majority of animals dying of dehydration and secondary infections.

- Fluids – intravenous or intraosseous wherever possible, lactated Ringer's (Hartman's solution) with a potassium supplement, due to the acidosis and potassium loss caused by vomiting. In severely dysenteric animals in circulatory collapse, whole blood, plasma or colloids can be beneficial.
- 2.5% glucose may be required to treat hypoglycaemia.

- Good i/v catheter management is important as cases may need to be on fluid therapy for up to 7–10 days and are immunosuppressed – a central line should be considered.
- Broad-spectrum antibacterials – potentiated amoxicillin, cephalosporins, potentiated sulphonamides, metronidazole, gentamicin can be used with care in severely neutropenic animals.
- Anti-emetics – maropitant, metoclopramide (either as bolus or by continuous infusion), chlorpromazine or prochlorpromazine can also be useful.
- Vitamin supplements – may be helpful as part of supportive care, especially B group vitamins.
- Hyperimmune serum – has not been shown to be of value in established cases, but may be helpful for non-immune in-contacts, e.g. colostrum-deprived littermates.
- Nutrition – once vomiting has ceased a suitable convalescent diet should be used. If anorexia is persistent and non-responsive to appetite stimulants a oesophagostomy tube should be considered.

Drugs of doubtful value
- Intestinal protectant, e.g. kaolin pro or prebiotics, vitamin K.

Contraindicated drugs
- Motility modifiers, e.g. anticholinergics or opiates. Such drugs act to reduce gut motility; this can lead to increased absorption of bacterial toxins and increased bacterial/viral penetration of the bowel wall. Fluid is still sequestered into the lumen of the gut leading to abdominal distension/discomfort and further dehydration. The apparent absence of diarrhoea can lead to premature cessation of fluid therapy.
- Glucocorticoids are immunosuppressive and may well promote viral replication;

there is no evidence that they are beneficial.

Control

In the veterinary surgery
- Isolation of suspected cases and disinfection of any contaminated areas.

Vaccination
- In the general population, parvoviruses are highly immunogenic and show little antigenic variation, hence vaccination is very effective. Yearly boosters are probably unnecessary as immunity lasts for 2–3 years.
- FPV vaccination – modified live and killed vaccines. All manufacturers recommend two injections in kittens under 12 weeks and a single injection for kittens over 12 weeks.
  - Booster frequency is generally driven by combination with respiratory viruses in the same vaccine.
- Modified live vaccines are contraindicated in pregnancy and cats known to be FIV or FeLV positive.
- Some modified live vaccines have caused problems in Burmese, Siamese or similar breed kittens; this may reflect a decreased resistance to FPV infection in this group.

Endemic catteries
- Vaccination alone is unlikely to be effective in controlling parvoviruses on such premises. Several problem areas exist:
  - No vaccine will provide absolute protection, if the weight of challenge is sufficiently heavy particularly if other intercurrent diseases are present or if only one vaccination in a course has been given.
  - In all cats, there tends to be an immunity gap where maternally derived antibodies have declined to the point where they are no longer protective, but are still too high to allow

INFECTIOUS DISEASE

vaccination. On endemic premises many animals become infected at this time (i.e. around 6–10 weeks old).

o In a large group of kittens it is impossible to predict when a particular individual will become susceptible to infection or suitable for vaccination.

o In poorly managed establishments little attention is often given to adequate colostral intake. Such kittens can then become susceptible to infection at a much younger age.

Prognosis

- Clinical parvovirus infection is now rare in many rural and semi-rural areas; the temptation is to stop vaccination. This should be strongly discouraged as a susceptible population will gradually build up with no vaccinal or acquired immunity resulting in the risk of a parvovirus epidemic.
- With prompt, aggressive, intensive care the outlook for adult animals is good.
- In kittens presenting with acute FPV, mortality ranges from 25% to 90% depending on their state at presentation; if presented early the outlook is fair to good.
- Fluid therapy in tiny kittens can be difficult, intraosseous fluids may be more easily maintained than intravenous.

Note – Fluid requirements for neonates are significantly higher than adults (80–120 ml/kg/day) but fluid volumes may be low (2–3 ml/hour).

5.14 OTHER INFECTIOUS DISEASE

5.14.1 Viral infections

Non-suppurative meningoencephalitis ('staggering disease')

- Bornavirus suspected as the causal agent because

- Borna disease virus (BDV) titres are high in clinical cases.
- Virus has been isolated from some clinical cases.
- Similar clinical signs in rats after passage.
- Described in several European countries, North America, Australia and Japan.
- Causes a non-suppurative meningoencephalitis affecting the cortex, brainstem and cord grey matter.
- Bornavirus causes encephalopathy in sheep and horses, psychiatric disorders in man.

Signalment

- Peak age 2–3 years (mean 3.8).
- Neutered male predominant.
- Outdoor cats.
- A number of households had other cats with clinical signs.

Clinical signs

- Usually slow and gradual decline.
- Loss of appetite.
- Fever.
- Neurologic signs.
- Hind limb ataxia – gradually progressive.
- Increased attention seeking.
- Aggression.
- Inability to retract claws.
- Sacral pain.
- Ptyalism.
- Urinary incontinence.
- Constipation.
- Dysphagia.
- Pruritus.
- Seizures.

Diagnosis

- Difficult.
- Haematology/biochemistry normal.
- Histopathology.
- MRI or CSF not described, but may be helpful.

Treatment
- Symptomatic and supportive.

Cowpox

Cause
- Orthopox group, family Poxviridae.

Epidemiology
- Wide host range in Eurasia.
- Cats are the most commonly recognised host in the UK – responsible for about 50% of human cases.
- Most cases in cats and man occur in autumn.
- Most common in adult, rural living cats.
- Also occurs in large felidae.
- Route of infection in cats.
  - Primary route is from small mammals whilst hunting.
  - Cat-to-cat transmission can occur, but is of minor importance tending to cause asymptomatic infection in the recipient.

Clinical signs
- Widespread skin lesions usually originating from a single lesion on the head, neck or forelimb.
- Spreading occurs around 10 days after initial wound.
- Not pruritic unless secondarily infected.
- Scabs dry and separate in 2–3 weeks.
- Healed by 6–8 weeks.
- Mild systemic – oculonasal or GIT involvement occurs in 20% of cats.
- Severity increased by secondary bacterial infection, intercurrent disease (especially FeLV/FIV) or the use of immunosuppressive drugs, e.g. corticosteroids.
- Cats with severe secondary signs particularly pneumonia have a poor prognosis.

Diagnosis
- Clinical signs.
- Fixed biopsy material.
- Eosinophilic intracytoplasmic inclusion bodies.
- Virus seen on electron microscopy.
- VI on unfixed scabs.
- Serology.

Treatment and prevention
- No specific treatment.
- Antimicrobials for secondary infection.
- Avoid corticosteroids.
- Prevent self-trauma.
- Virus is very hardy.
- Remains infectious in scab material for years in cool conditions.
- Susceptible to most disinfectants, particularly hypochlorite.

Zoonosis
- Source of 50% of human infections.
- Often a single lesion in man.
- Widespread and severe disease in immunocompromised individuals.
- Careful handling and labelling of potential infectious material.
- Advise owner about careful handling of the cat.

Hantavirus
- Member of bunyavirus group.
- Single-stranded RNA virus.
- Transmitted by urine and saliva from reservoir rodent hosts.
- Causes variable disease in man.
- Human haemorrhagic fever and renal syndrome (Asia).
- Pulmonary disease with high mortality (North America).
- Generally mild and subclinical (Europe).
- Antibodies detected in ≈10% of cats in the UK, levels variable across Europe.
- Virus isolated from a cat in China.
- Clinical significance of infection to the cat is unknown.
- In man, epidemiological association with outdoor lifestyle and contact with rodents.
- Cats unlikely to be significant source of infection to man.

INFECTIOUS DISEASE

Other viral disease
- Paramyxovirus.
- Arthropod-borne viruses.
- Feline herpes type 2 infection.
- Parapoxvirus (Orf).
- Aujeszky's disease (pseudorabies).
- Feline adenovirus.
- Feline viral papillomatosis.

5.14.2 Bacterial infections

Cat scratch disease

Bartonella henselae and B. clarridgeiae
- Fastidious, arthropod-transmitted, Gram-negative bacteria.
- Vector thought to be fleas or ticks.
- Variable rates of seropositivity from <10–60%, dependent on region.
- Estimated 6000–20,000 cases a year in the USA.
- Also linked to hepatic peliosis and bacillary angiomatosis.

Disease in cats
- Does not appear to cause clinically apparent disease in cats.
- Cats appear to be chronically infected.
- Due to the high percentage of cats infected, establishing a cause and effect relationship is difficult.
- May become significant in association with other diseases.

Disease in man
- Usually associated with self-limiting disease.
- Febrile.
- Most commonly in children.
- Possibility of flea transmission has not been excluded.

Primary skin lesion
- At site of scratch.
- Non-pruritic, erythematous papule.
- Develops to vesicle then papule.
- Ruptures, scabs over and heals.

Regional lymphadenitis
- Develops weeks to months after skin lesion.
- Can be recurrent.

Atypical symptoms
- Bacillary angiomatosis – proliferative disease of the skin, multiple, blood-filled cystic tumours.
- Bacillary peliosis.
- Relapsing fever with bacteraemia.
- Endocarditis.
- Granulomatous hepatosplenic syndrome.
- Retinitis and swelling of the optic nerve.
- Parinaud syndrome.
- Arthritis.
- Osteolytic lesions.
- Possible role in development of encephalopathy in AIDS patients.

Diagnosis

Cats
- Serology.
- PCR.

Man
- Lymph node biopsy.
- Histopathology.
- Identification of bacteria on silver staining.
- PCR.

Treatment

Cats
- Doxycycline (10–20 mg/kg q12h) or fluoroquinolone has eliminated the infection.

Man
- Doxycycline, enrofloxacin and rifampin are recommended.
- Should be considered following significant cat bites/scratches.
- Other antimicrobials have also been effective.

Borreliosis (Lyme disease)

- Tick-borne disease.
- Seropositivity has been demonstrated in cats (around 4% in the UK).
- Distinct disease association has not been made.
- Experimentally it has been associated with arthritis and meningitis.

Cat bite abscess

- Associated with multiple infectious agents.
- Anaerobes and facultative anaerobes most common.
- Fungal elements sometimes found – relevance is unclear.
- More common in entire, male, free-roaming cats.

Diagnosis

- Usually follows cat fights.
- Bite wounds can sometimes be very hard to find and require thorough clipping and cleaning of area.
- Differential diagnosis of puncture wounds should be considered.
- Grass seeds.
- Air gun pellets.

Clinical signs

- Variable.
- Anorexia, lethargy, pyrexia.
- Usually painful (unless ruptured) causing altered gait, apparent tail paralysis, altered behaviour.
- Local lymphadenopathy.
- Palpable, soft, fluctuant swelling.
- Foetid discharge.
- Most common head, legs, back and base of tail.
- May lead to systemic disease, e.g. pyothorax, endocarditis, osteomyelitis.

Treatment

- Local drainage wherever possible.
- Warm water compress.
- Lavage of abscess cavity with very dilute hydrogen peroxide or antiseptic.
- NSAID as appropriate.

Antibacterials

- *Only* indicated where there is evidence of systemic infection or where the cat is at high risk of becoming septic, e.g. FIV positive.
- Antibacterial levels within the abscess cavity will be too low to be effective.
- Pencillins or cephalosporins usually effective.

Failure to respond to treatment

- Reconsider diagnosis, e.g. associated with foreign body.
- Retrovirus serology.
- Characterise infectious agent, e.g. *Mycobacterium*, *Cryptococcus*.

Feline leptospirosis

- Clinically rare.
- Antibodies in 7% of cats in the UK with various serovars detected.
- Experimental infection rarely produces clinical signs.
- Excretion of leptospira in the urine can continue for up to 3 months.

Salmonellosis

- Infection rates are significantly higher than clinical disease.
- Cats seem very resistant to developing salmonellosis.
- Occasional outbreaks in kittens occur.
- Transmission to man is possible.

Tetanus

- Cats seem very resistant to disease.
- Often develop localised signs.
- Diagnosis is based on clinical signs – spastic paralysis.
- Treatment is symptomatic and supportive.
- Wound should be debrided and cleaned.
- Antitoxin is of limited value in established disease.

INFECTIOUS DISEASE

INFECTIOUS DISEASE

Other bacterial disease

- Botulism – cats are very resistant and disease is rare.
- *Actinomyces* and *Nocardia* – commonly found in pyothorax.
- *Streptococcus* – septicaemia in kittens.
- Tyzzer's disease.
- Colibacillosis.
- *Yersinia*.
- Plague.
- Tularaemia – hepatosplenomegaly.

5.14.3 Rickettsial infections

Ehrlichiosis and anaplasmosis

- Rare.
- Older cats.
- Non-specific signs – fever, lethargy, anorexia and weight loss.
- Splenomegaly, lymphadenopathy, joint pain.
- Diagnosis – serology and demonstration of morulae in leucocytes.
- Treatment – doxycycline at 10 mg/kg PO q12h for 3 weeks.
- Potential zoonosis.

5.14.4 Fungal infections

Aspergillosis

- Rare in cats.
- Chronic nasal disease.
- Systemic infection causing pyogranulomatous pneumonia or infiltrative intestinal lesions.
- Treatment is usually ineffective.

Cryptococcus neoformans *var.* gattii

- Most common systemic mycosis in cats.

Common clinical signs

- Sneezing, snuffling and nasal discharge.
- Skin lesions.
- Nasal mass.
- Anterior uveitis, chorioretinitis.
- CNS disease.
- Siamese cats may be over-represented.

Diagnosis

- Cytology on nasal discharge.
- Serology – latex agglutination or ELISA.
- Tissue biopsy.
- Fungal isolation.

Treatment

- Surgical debulking of large masses.
- Imidazoles – fluconazole is the drug of choice at 5–15 mg/kg once or twice daily for at least 6 months.

Prognosis

- Variable.
- Better outcome associated with a tenfold decline in antibody titre within 2 months.
- FIV-positive cats are likely to require lifelong maintenance therapy.

Sporotrichosis

- Infection following traumatic inoculation.
- Nodular ulcerating lesions on limbs, head and tail.
- Diagnosis – cytology/histology, culture, IFA testing.
- Treatment – antifungals but toxicity often an issue.
- Potential zoonotic risk.

Other fungal and algal disease

Marked geographical variations occur in the prevalence of fungal disease with fungi being common causes of disseminated infections in some parts of the world. The following should be considered although in general cats appear much more resistant to fungal infection than dogs.

- Blastomycosis.
- Histoplasmosis.
- Coccidiomycosis.
- Candida.
- Trichosporonosis.
- Prototheocosis.
- There are case reports of a wide range of other fungal and algal diseases.

5.14.5 Protozoal infections

Cryptosporidia

- Mild diarrhoea in kittens.
- Zoonotic risk.
- Infection probably from contaminated water.
- Diagnosis of oocysts on sugar flotation.
- Clinical signs usually self-limiting.
- Tylosin, azithromycin or clindamycin may be helpful.

Cystoisospora (Isospora)

- Direct faecal-oral infection or via rodent intermediate host.
- Diarrhoea major clinical signs.
- Clinical signs usually seen in kittens.
- Diagnosis on demonstration of oocysts on faecal flotation.
- Treatment-potentiated sulphonamides and supportive care.

Other protozoal disease

Protozoal diseases can be regionally dependent and are relatively rare in cats; consider

- Leishmania.
- Hepatozoonosis.
- Cytauxzoonosis.
- Babesiosis.

5.15 FELINE ZOONOSES

5.15.1 Introduction

- Reliable incidence figures for feline zoonoses are not available.
- There are little data that suggest cat ownership is associated with specific health issues other than allergy to cats:
  - Immunocompetent individuals appear to be at very low risk of contracting zoonotic disease from cats.
  - Children are at slightly higher risk because of increased likelihood of putting items such as fleas into their mouth and they are less likely to wash their hands before eating.
- As cats tend to bury their faeces, the risk of surface environmental contamination is less.
- The evidence that feral cats present a greater zoonotic risk is equivocal.

5.15.2 At-risk groups

- Age – fetuses, new-born, infants and the elderly.
- Concurrent illness – diabetes, renal or liver failure, burns, malnutrition.
- Immunodeficient disease – AIDS, congenital immunodeficiency, splenectomy.
- Immunosuppression – chemotherapy, organ transplantation, drug use.
- Implants – catheters, indwelling tubes, synthetic implants.

Guidelines for reducing the zoonotic risk for people with reduced immune function

- Wash hands after handling the cat and before eating.
- Choose a cat over 1 year of age as kittens are more likely to scratch/bite and contract infectious diseases.
- Seek early veterinary intervention if the cat becomes sick.
- Regular vaccination, worming and ectoparasite control.
- Feed a commercial ration and discourage hunting.
- Avoid games that are likely to lead to scratching/biting.
- Avoid being licked by the cat especially if the person has open wounds.
- Wear gloves when handling and giving medication – especially oral medication or removing ticks.
- Any bites or scratches should be washed thoroughly and prompt, aggressive medical management sought as appropriate.
- Gloves should always be worn for cleaning litter trays – use scalding water, bleach or ammonia.
- Always wear gloves for gardening.

INFECTIOUS DISEASE

5.15.3 Methods of disease spread
- Major routes of spread of zoonotic disease:
  - Bite wounds and saliva.
  - Scratches or close physical contact to skin/mucosal surfaces.
  - Faecal-oral.
  - Urogenital.
  - Vector-borne.

5.15.4 Potential zoonoses and estimate of risk (Table 75)

Table 75   Potential zoonotic diseases and their estimated risk

Minor risk	Minimal risk	Unknown risk	Regionally variable	Probably not zoonotic
Toxoplasma	Giardia	*Pneumocystis carinii*	Tularaemia	Helicobacter
Bartonella spp.	Cryptosporidia	Listeriosis	Nipah virus	Lyme disease
Cat scratch disease	Cryptococcosis	Feline parapox	Histoplasmosis	*Clostridium difficile*
Bacillary angiomatosis	Aspergilla	Borna virus	Blastomycosis	
Coxiella burnetii (Q-fever)	Anthrax	Hantavirus	Flaviviruses, e.g. yellow fever	**Not zoonotic but public concern**
Group A *streptococci*	Salmonella	Feline spongiform encephalopathy	Togaviruses – Venezuelan equine encephalitis	
Tuberculosis	Influenza – including H5N1			FeLV
Dermatophytosis	Leptospirosis	*Chlamydophila*	*Rickettsia felis*	FIV
Toxocara/Toxascaris	*Campylobacter*	*Echinococcus*	Sporotrichosis	
Fleas	*Sarcoptes*	*Dermatophilus congolensis*		
Cowpox	*Diphylidium*	*Dirofilaria*		
Cat bite – pasteurellosis	*Notoedres*	Enterocytozoonosis		
Anaerobiospirillum	Cheyletiella			
Opistharchiasis	*Clostridium perfringens*			
Rabies	*Bordetella*			
Plague – *Yersinia pestis*	Cutaneous larva migrans – *Ancylostoma braziliense* *Ancylostoma tubaeformae* *Uncinaria stenocephala*			

Nelson, R.W. & Couto, C.G. (2008) *Small Animal Internal Medicine*, (4th Edn), Mosby.
Useful lists of differential diagnosis of presenting clinical signs although not cat specific.
Ettinger, S.J. & Feldman, E.C. (2010) *Textbook of Veterinary Internal Medicine*, (7th Edn), W.B. Saunders.
Comprehensive text although general bias is towards canine internal medicine.
Sherding, R.G. (ed.) (1994) *Cat Diseases and Clinical Management*, W.B. Saunders.
Text covers all aspect of feline medicine although getting increasingly out of date.

Specific texts

Feldman, E.C. & Nelson, R.W. (2004) *Canine and Feline Endocrinology and Reproduction*, (3rd Edn), W.B. Saunders.
Comprehensive coverage of all aspects of endocrine disease.
Ware, W.A. (2011) *Cardiovascular Disease in Small Animal Medicine*, Manson Publishing.
Covers all aspects of feline heart disease, well written and readable.
Greene, C.E. (ed.) (2012) *Infectious Diseases of the Dog and Cat*, (4th Edn), Elsevier Saunders
Comprehensive review of infectious disease diagnosis and treatment.
Guilford, W.G., Center, S.A., Strombeck, D.R., Williams, D.A. & Meyer, D.J. (1996) *Strombeck's Small Animal Gastroenterology*, (3rd Edn), W.B. Saunders.
Excellent and comprehensive coverage of gastrointestinal and hepatobiliary disease although getting dated in places.
Hand, M.S., Thatcher, C.D., Remillard, R.L. & Roudebush, P. (2000) *Small Animal Clinical Nutrition*, (4th Edn), Walsworth Publishing.
Major work, lots of detail useful for specific problems.
Horwitz, D.F. & Mills, D.S. (2009) *BSAVA Manual of Canine and Feline Behavioural Medicine*, BSAVA
Covers feline behavioural medicine not dealt with in this text.
England, G.C.W. & von Heimendahl, A. (2010) *BSAVA Manual of Small Animal Reproduction and Neonatology*, (2nd Edn), BSAVA.
Covers reproduction and some paediatric medicine.
Stades, C., Wyman, M., Boevé, M.H. & Neumann, W. (2007) *Ophthalmology for the Veterinary Practitioner*, (2nd Edn), Manson Publishing
Good general text for approaching ophthalmic disease
Fitzmaurice, S. (2010) *Saunders Solutions in Veterinary Practice – Small Animal Neurology*, Saunders/Elsevier.
Easy access material on approach and management of neurology cases
Withrow, S.J., Vail, D.M. & Page, R.L. (2013) *Small Animal Oncology*, (5th Edn), Saunders/Elsevier.
Excellent text covering all aspects of oncology although there is a general canine bias.

FURTHER READING

Notes on Feline Internal Medicine, Second Edition. Edited by Kit Sturgess. ©2013 John Wiley & Sons, Ltd.
Published 2013 by Blackwell Publishing Ltd.

Jackson, H.A. & Marsella, R. (2011) *BSAVA Manual of Canine and Feline Dermatology,* (3rd Edn), BSAVA.
Good comprehensive guide to dermatological disease
Bonagura, J.D. (ed.) (2000) *Kirk's Current Veterinary Therapy XIII,* W.B. Saunders.
Bonagura, J.D. & Twedt, D.C. (ed.) (2008) *Kirk's Current Veterinary Therapy XIV,* W.B. Saunders.
Excellent sections covering new developments and reviews in a wide range of areas. Useful list of laboratory values and drug dose rates in appendices.
August, J.R. (2009) *Consultations in Feline Internal Medicine,* Volume 5, Saunders
August, J.R. (2005) *Consultations in Feline Internal Medicine,* Volume 6, Saunders
Covers current topics in feline medicine and reviews system-based areas of feline medicine, doesn't have an index that includes references to previous volumes
Imaging – *no single text covers both radiology and ultrasound, in general BSAVA manuals are comprehensive reviews of anatomic regions.* Penninck, D. & d'Anjou, M-A. (2008) *Atlas of Small Animal Ultrasonography,* (2nd Edn), Blackwells *provides beautiful ultrasound images of ultrasound structures*
Journal of Feline Medicine and Surgery – W.B. Saunders, ISSN: 1098-612X.
Bimonthly Journal providing research articles, editorials.

FURTHER READING

Note – key references are in bold.

For common terms where there are multiple citations these are aimed to help the reader find relevant references within a known section e.g. lymphoma within GIT disease section.

Notes on Feline Internal Medicine, Second Edition. Edited by Kit Sturgess. ©2013 John Wiley & Sons, Ltd.
Published 2013 by Blackwell Publishing Ltd.

INDEX

INDEX

INDEX

INDEX

Printed and bound by CPI Group (UK) Ltd, Croydon, CR0 4YY

09/10/2024

14571432-0001